The

POWER
and the GRACE

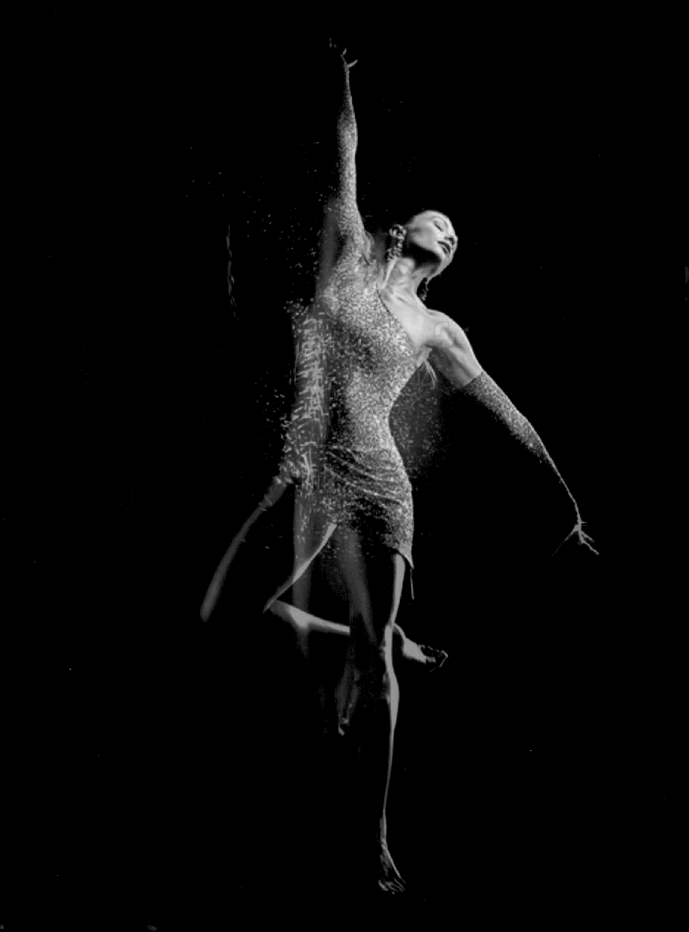

The
POWER
and the
GRACE

A Professional's Guide to Ease and
Efficiency in Functional Movement

Joanne Elphinston

Forewords **Thomas W Myers**
Elizabeth Larkam

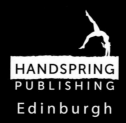

HANDSPRING
PUBLISHING
Edinburgh

HANDSPRING PUBLISHING LIMITED
The Old Manse, Fountainhall,
Pencaitland, East Lothian
EH34 5EY, Scotland
Tel: +44 1875 341 859
Website: www.handspringpublishing.com

First published 2019 in the United Kingdom by Handspring Publishing
Reprinted 2020

Copyright ©Handspring Publishing 2019

ISBN 978-1-912085-38-5
ISBN (Kindle e-Book) 978-1-912085-39-2

British Library Cataloguing in Publication Data
A catalogue record for this book is available from the British Library

Library of Congress Cataloguing in Publication Data
A catalog record for this book is available from the Library of Congress

Notice
Neither the Publisher nor the Authors assume any responsibility for any loss or injury and/or damage to persons or property arising out of or relating to any use of the material contained in this book. It is the responsibility of the treating practitioner, relying on independent expertise and knowledge of the patient, to determine the best treatment and method of application for the patient. The material within this book is designed to be used by healthy individuals with normal levels of fitness under the supervision of a healthcare professional. The author is not liable for misuse or misunderstanding of the material herein, nor any injury which may be incurred while performing the exercises provided.

All reasonable efforts have been made to obtain copyright clearance for illustrations in the book for which the authors or publishers do not own the rights. If you believe that one of your illustrations has been used without such clearance please contact the publishers and we will ensure that appropriate credit is given in the next reprint.

Commissioning Editor Mary Law
Project Manager Morven Dean
Photographer Ian Llewelyn
Designer Bruce Hogarth
Indexer Aptara, India
Typesetter DSM Soft, India
Printer Finidr, Czech Republic

The
Publisher's
policy is to use
paper manufactured
from sustainable forests

CONTENTS

FOREWORD *by Thomas W. Myers*

Joanne Elphinston has accomplished – and you now hold – a comprehensive but accessible new book for all contemporary teachers of movement. Books on human movement abound these days, many with the word "functional" attached – surely we do not need another one? Yes, we do, because so many of these contemporary books focus not on "movement" but on "training" – strength, conditioning, skill building, endurance, or the proper specifics of a system like Pilates or yoga.

Of course, all these explorations are very useful to athletic endeavor, but this book is aimed at something much more universal: we have a crisis in non-performative, everyday movement – walking, standing, sitting, relating, and transferring from place to place. Joanne's book addresses the everyday incorporation of healthy movement with a zest, verve, and loads of immediately practical advice that is refreshingly free of any particular method's axe to grind. In this way, the book is unique and belongs on your shelf, or better – open on your desk.

No matter what your modality, you will be able to fit these insights into your work. This book is for the student, certainly, but primarily for the professional who wants to make a real difference – not just on the gym floor or the yoga mat, but in our everyday relationship to our body in motion.

It is easy to imagine a life without sight or hearing – as essential as these windows on the world can be people make wonderful lives while blind or deaf. It is more difficult to imagine a life without a sense of the body's movement, without kinesthesia. Even though much of our body's coordination happens below the conscious level, our assembly of ourselves, so wrapped into our proprioceptive and interoceptive sensations, contributes so much to our emotions, our outlook, and our sense of where we are that life without it is, in Moshe Feldenkrais' term, "unthinkable."

How do I tackle common problems like head-forward posture in practical terms with my everyday clients? Joanne's varied experience is conveyed in a light manner that belies the depth of understanding that went into constructing the exercises and approaches. She does not skirt the issues of biomechanics and proper hygiene in our "acture" (another Feldenkrais term for "posture in action"); you will find exercises to tackle such common problems directly. So much of our movement, however, is modulated unconsciously, and thus our ability to "conquer" our movement through conscious replacement of habits with "better" ones is so often an exercise in frustration (or worse, yet another self-esteem abasement project like trying to diet and change our sleep habits).

Joanne instead incorporates the unconscious elements in habitual movement, so that her explorations work *with* the unconscious mind to improve movement *naturally*, rather than trying to beat the "below the conscious" parts of movement to death with our conscious "hammer" of good ideas we got from whichever "coach." Conscious retraining of movement often hammers at the wrong nail, and then we are surprised when the client's improvement subsequently "falls apart." Good movement is never imposed, it simply needs to be exposed within you – here is *how*, and here is the explanation – as far as we know, for there is much yet to be discovered about movement – for *why*.

Rely on this book with confidence. It covers the underlying patterns that contribute to the modern collapse of posture and impoverishment of movement. It does not tell you how to move, it shows you how to uncover your own inner mover. It is written by someone who has been there. Joanne's programme is cleverly designed to remove the blocks imposed on your movement by accident, injury, imitation, or attitude to leave you moving as you were intended – uniquely you, fitting inside your skin, as she says, like your favorite old sweater. That surely beats moving as if in a suit of armor imposed by "good" or "correct" movement. The best movement is your movement. Use this book to get there.

Thomas W. Myers LMT, BDSI
Director, Anatomy Trains
Walpole, ME
August 2019

FOREWORD *by Elizabeth Larkam*

Joanne Elphinston has created a magnificent resource that informs the future of movement education. Therapists, athletic trainers, coaches, personal trainers, and educators from every discipline will find inspiration, clarity, and valuable guidance in *The Power and the Grace: A Professional's Guide to Ease and Efficiency in Functional Movement*. The premise of this unique book is that you do not have to choose between being science-based or heart-centered. It is not a choice to work holistically, but an imperative. Each chapter encourages the development of the qualities of proprioception (where am I?) and interoception (how am I?) that are essential for the experience of embodiment. Practitioners of Anatomy Trains®, Continuum®, dance, fascia fitness, Feldenkrais®, 5Rhythms®, Gyrotonic®, Gyrokinesis®, martial arts, Pilates, qi kung, t'ai chi and yoga will find that every chapter enhances their personal practice and their work with clients.

Joanne Elphinston is a courageous, critical thinker. She exposes myths that impede progress in best practices of teaching functional movement, explaining: "It is a position of integrity and strength when a discipline can look at itself objectively to see what is outdated, misunderstood, or limiting."

The Power and the Grace is designed to lead the reader into kinesthetic experience, demonstrating the value of integrating learning through the sensing brain with learning from the thinking, analytical brain. Ample "Movement explorations" engage the reader with embodied experience, converting theory into grounded practice of proprioception and interoception. Every chapter includes "Real life studies" – descriptions of client transformation that result from movement practice. Each chapter closes with "Power points" that summarize key concepts and explain their ability to facilitate powerful, graceful movement.

The Power and the Grace is an essential reference for every movement educator and therapist throughout the career arc. Joanne Elphinston observes: "Movement is usually considered to be an activity of the body, but could more accurately be seen as the brain visibly expressing itself." Movement professionals mature in their appreciation of this profound statement through the enriching experience of every client interaction.

Movement educators in training and those who have recently completed their coursework will welcome the clarity with which sophisticated concepts of movement complexity are distilled into exercises accessible to every client. These ingenious movement practices have a profound effect in that they focus power in order to liberate a state of graceful flow.

Practitioners early in their careers will turn to *The Power and the Grace* as a reliable mentor, guiding their observations of and experiences with clients, modeling how to integrate the art and science of movement education in order to inspire new movement possibilities.

Seasoned movement professionals will turn to *The Power and the Grace* for inspiration to refresh their skills and for compassionate encouragement to critically examine the efficacy of their familiar teaching strategies that have become habitual. Joanne Elphinston explains how to evaluate the benefits and limitations of training methods that interfere with the graceful power of natural movement then demonstrates how to elegantly connect each training system with natural movement.

The message of *The Power and the Grace* is essential for health in our times. Every chapter includes practices that enhance movement comfort, ease, and efficiency. The World Health Organization ranks physical inactivity – sitting too much – as the fourth biggest preventable killer globally, causing an estimated 3.2 million deaths annually.[1] Dr. James Levine, professor of endocrinology at the Mayo Clinic, Phoenix, Arizona, writes, "Sitting is more dangerous than smoking, kills more people than HIV and is more treacherous than parachuting."[2]

People of all ages spend increasing amounts of time absorbing information from screens of all sizes – handheld devices, desktop devices, and large screen media devices. Focusing one's gaze on screens for an extended period of time may compromise whole-body movement with dysfunction concentrated in the head, neck, thorax, shoulder girdle, arms, and hands.

All movement educators may be assured that they can easily access the wisdom generously offered in *The Power and the Grace* while respecting scope of practice guidelines. In her pioneering book Joanne Elphinston brings to life a masterful guide to powerful concepts and tools that inspire the art and the heart of teaching functional movement. Freedom to move with graceful power enriches embodied experience and suffuses life with grace.

Elizabeth Larkam
Author, *Fascia in Motion: Fascia-focused movement for Pilates* (Handspring Publishing, 2017)
Mill Valley, California, USA
September 2019

1. World Health Organization. Physical Inactivity: a global public health problem. [Accessed September 6, 2019] Available: www.who.int/ncds/prevention/physical-activity/inactivity-global-health-problem/en/.

2. Levine JA. Get Up! Why Your Chair Is Killing You and What You Can Do About It. New York: St. Martin's Press; 2014, pp. 70–71.

ABOUT THE AUTHOR

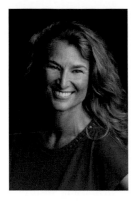

International movement expert Joanne Elphinston is a high performance consultant for professional dancers, musicians, and elite athletes at Olympic level; a consultant physical therapist specializing in chronic and persistent neuromusculoskeletal conditions; a former coach and fitness instructor; and the author of several popular books in the field of movement.

Joanne has been developing and teaching her unique JEMS® approach for over 20 years, training rehabilitation, health and fitness professionals around the world to explore, inspire, and optimize movement in people of all ages and walks of life. Her work is the subject of current research into the management of hypermobility-related pain, falls prevention, stroke rehabilitation and sports performance, and her programs are used in such diverse fields as child development, chronic pain management, and athletic training.

Joanne has a passion for communicating complex concepts in simple, elegant ways that enable practitioners to work holistically yet functionally, supported by science, and balancing knowledge with skill and humanity.

PREFACE

This is a book that I have wanted to write for some time. I am now able to bring more of my whole self than ever before to my work, because there is a growing tribe of wonderful movement and rehabilitation professionals who can reach beyond the mechanics and grasp the essence of movement as one of our most authentic forms of self-expression. They are a gift beyond price to me.

When I look back, I see the profound influences that have shaped my development over the past thirty years, and understand how fortunate I have been to have discovered very early in my career the illuminating writings of Moshe Feldenkrais, Thomas Hanna and F. M. Alexander; the concepts of such movement theory pioneers as Rudolf von Laban, Irmgard Bartenieff and Shirley Sahrmann; and the early 3D anatomy writings of Thomas Myers, which married form and function so brilliantly. I am profoundly grateful for their wisdom and creativity, the keenness of their intellects, and humanity of their vision. Their example showed me how to pursue a life of professional exploration and independence of thought, and their philosophies are woven into the fabric of my work.

We are fortunate to live in a time now where our practice can be informed by an ever-expanding contemporary research base to explore, deepen, and modify our understanding of what influences our movement, our physical health, and our psyche. However, there is an art to applying the science in a meaningful way when it comes to movement. This sparked the genesis of the *JEMS*®G approach many years ago, as I wanted to help movement and rehabilitation professionals to confidently integrate and apply this growing body of knowledge with sensitivity, skill, and insight. From managing the emotional dynamic in the room, to the language that we use, to the informed use of hand, body, and voice to cue and facilitate change, skill is the sword through which we wield knowledge. Through skill we can begin to practice the art of working with movement.

However, it's no longer enough to talk about the art and the science of working with movement. It is the heart that makes movement work transformative.

Our movement is more deeply emotional than we are usually prepared to admit. Our relationship with our deepest selves can be reflected in how we carry ourselves, our posture and movement choices signaling our self-image and even our sense of identity. It is our armor, our costume, and our vulnerability. Helping someone to experience movement as something to be revealed, explored, and experimented with, as something that is uniquely theirs, and as something that can feel satisfying, even joyful, is a privilege that I treasure every week as a practitioner.

To make this experience of self-expression and self-discovery possible, we must have ways to bring seemingly complex concepts to life. It is absolutely possible, indeed essential, to transform the potential complexity involved into concepts and language that are accessible and readily understandable. Do not mistake simplicity for being simplistic – to achieve simplicity, you must have true understanding. It is worth the effort, as through simplicity the magic happens.

That's what I want to achieve with this book, written for the diverse array of movement professionals who inspire me and give me hope. To help to build connections between you, I have where possible used everyday language to describe poses and exercises that you might use in your chosen discipline, to enable everyone to benefit from the examples. I want to share simple ways to deploy and communicate the rich science available to us, a way to resolve some of the apparent conceptual conflicts that sit between different movement disciplines, and some of the keys to unlocking the magic.

This book is written for those who want to work holistically, intelligently, and in a scientifically informed manner while embracing the idea of movement as a deeply sensory and emotional experience.

I have been waiting for the opportunity to write about the deliciousness of movement, the feeling of it, and how we feel about it. I hope you find something to dive into and roll about in.

Joanne Elphinston
Cardiff, United Kingdom
May 2019

ACKNOWLEDGMENTS

I am exceptionally fortunate to have received incredible generosity and support throughout the development of this book from a number of special people, and I am so grateful for their encouragement, their enthusiasm, and their help.

At inception, Mary Law's gentle but persistent persuasion transformed an idea that I had toyed with into a reality, and between Mary's enthusiasm and Andrew Stevenson's steady and reassuring hand, this project was guided onto the tracks at Handspring Publishing.

Through the writing of the text, I have been lucky enough to have had a team of trusted readers from different professional backgrounds who have shared with me their impressions, ideas, concerns, and insights. Each one represented a different lens, creating a three-dimensional view of incomparable value.

Andrew Nice's deep knowledge as an experienced Pilates teacher, movement coach, and JEMS® Certified Rehabilitation Practitioner has been utterly priceless. Andy's extensive understanding of Pilates culture and methodology has been essential to the integrity of this book, and his absolute conviction regarding the value of the content carried it through some of its most vulnerable times. Andy has been one of my most constant supporters over more years than I can remember, and his belief in me has been a blessing that I have counted time and again.

Claire-Louise Carter would be very surprised to be described as a muse, but, as she so beautifully represents the intended reader for the book, she was a constant source of inspiration as I was shaping its language and approach. She read each developing chapter with joy in her heart, and integrated the work immediately into her Pilates classes, reporting the responses of class participants with glee, and sharing her own discoveries as she went. Through Claire, I have experienced the exuberance of a passionately evolving and very talented teacher, through whom the JEMS approach has landed beautifully with the varied population it is intended to be used with.

Lesley Dike, physiotherapist, yoga teacher, and trainer of yoga teachers, responded to the task of reading preliminary chapters with an uncompromising rigor, robust honesty, and humor that still makes me smile. Lesley is one of the most genuine people I know and, with a triple-barreled background as a clinician, an educator, and a lifelong student of yoga, she was able to challenge me in all the best ways. The book is much the better for her contribution!

Experienced soft tissue therapist, Polestar Pilates teacher, and JEMS® Certified Rehabilitation Practitioner Laura Kavanagh embraced the reading with an infectious delight, applying her favorite gems immediately and positively with her clients to bridge the gap between rehabilitation and performance. A skilled practitioner both in a clinical setting as well as in her movement teaching, Laura buoyed me up in the latter stages of the process with her enthusiastic emails and immediate connection with the finer details that she uncovered.

The entire Handspring team has been incredible. Morven Dean has patiently guided the project with immense skill, drawing together the various threads involved in preparing a book for production with an impressive delicacy of touch and consummate diplomacy. I had said that I wanted to create a beautiful book, not just in its text but in its physical form, and Bruce Hogarth exceeded all my expectations with his design, as well as his marvellous interpretation of my illustration wish list. Ceinwen Sinclair has single-handedly reversed my adverse previous editorial experiences and, where I had dreaded that part of the process, I found myself thoroughly enjoying our collaboration. Proofreaders Laura Booth and Sally Davies have been truly awesome – I am beyond grateful for their sharp eyes and clear thinking.

I am so grateful to photographer Ian Llewelyn for his exceptional patience, expertise and sensitivity to what I was trying to communicate through the photographs. His images are a huge contribution to the beauty and effectiveness of the book, and his ability to draw the best out of us on long demanding shoots was magnificent.

That the brilliant Tom Myers and Elizabeth Larkam, both such well-respected and extraordinarily busy leaders in their fields, were willing to take the time to contribute forewords for the book is more than I could possibly have wished for, and I thank them for their kindness, generosity, and insights.

My family stands with me in everything I do with an absolutely unwavering belief which I have never taken for granted. My parents, Christopher and Suzanne Elphinston, cheered and encouraged throughout the writing phase and then waded through the initial drafts – I have a particularly wonderful photo of my father, aged 79, in a full squat in front of his laptop as he tested the cues for himself. Dad subsequently proofread the entire text not once, but twice, picking up what I missed myself. It was an amazing effort of detailed concentration, and an incredible gift for which I am overwhelmingly grateful.

And then, most profoundly, there is my husband, Kent Fyrth. Every step of the way, Kent has, as always, delivered unflagging belief, support and encouragement, and quite beyond this has on countless occasions arrived home after a long day's work to be asked to take up a position on the floor to test whatever crazy thing I had been creating that day. He has lived with this book daily just as I have, has borne my obsession with grace, and has patiently gone off downstairs to bake restorative muffins to keep the wheels of industry turning when the going got tough.

Finally, this book would not be what it is, and indeed, may have foundered in difficult times had I not been the beneficiary of the heartfelt, exuberant enthusiasm of my JEMS crew and the extended JEMS tribe. You have always been the inspiration for what I do. I really hope this book supports the wonderful work you do.

HOW TO USE THIS BOOK

A gem icon will appear throughout the book to guide you through an active experience of the content. When appearing in a purple box, it invites you to sense something personally for yourself. When appearing in a pink box, it indicates an activity for the movement professional to explore with a client or patient. A yellow box indicates a relevant point for the movement professional. A blue box emphasizes a key concept to reflect upon.

Words appearing in the Glossary are marked at first instance with a ^G next to the word.

INTRODUCTION

Human beings are a complex and wondrous blend of unique characteristics, habits, and histories. Every day we express ourselves through our movement strategies, beliefs, and emotions; every day we create and control *forces*^{G} with varying strategies, some more effective than others.

Even with no formal training, we innately recognize those who express their human potential through movement so effectively that it makes our hearts sing. We see people who unleash power as effortlessly as a lightning strike, and others whose grace makes us forget to breathe, but often perceive these two qualities to be somehow different, even polarized. However, it is the intimate control, impeccable timing, and coordinated dance of muscle tension and relaxation that connects power and grace such that one cannot exist without the other. This is what enables a ballet dancer to be powerful and demands that a discus thrower be graceful.

For the everyday person, this is just as significant. Movement forges an ongoing positive relationship between our minds, our bodies, and our lives. We may use specific exercises to strengthen ourselves, stretch ourselves, or stabilize ourselves, but these achievements are not necessarily meaningful to our brain without integrating them into movement. It is akin to learning a new language: acquiring new words doesn't make us fluent; it merely increases our potential. With movement it is the same – we may strengthen or stretch a muscle, but without making it meaningful through movement, the brain does not necessarily know what to do with this new potential. Despite dedicated effort, the expected improvement in health or performance may not emerge.

We are in fact rather good at training for potential. Gyms, clinics, and studios are filled with people developing physical potential. They pursue a course of training, whether it be yoga, Pilates, personal training, or rehabilitation – and may achieve wonderful improvements within these pursuits – but sometimes they are disappointed to find that they are not benefitting as expected in terms of their everyday lives, sports, or activities. This is frequently because although they have been building potential, often very effectively, they have not yet discovered how to make it meaningful to their brain. The great gap is usually in transference of this potential into more effective movement.

This is in fact great news! It means that most people already have a lot of what they need to move more effectively right now; they just need a bit of help to access it.

Many people carry an assumption that is quite the reverse, believing that they are fundamentally lacking in some way. I certainly used to think that through my assessments I was discovering a specific deficit in a patient or client, and I would set about filling that lack with therapeutic exercise in the belief that this would turn into better movement. With time and experience, I realized that this wasn't the case at all – if they could walk out the door after their first session moving better, they clearly had the potential there already. I just needed to help them to access it.

It's hard to believe sometimes, but most of us are capable of much more than we realize once we learn to get out of our own way. When we create a bridge between the science of physics, function, and structure, and the art of integrating the mind, the body, and even the heart, we connect with ourselves, our environment, and our aspirations. When applied with passion, positivity, and confidence, we touch our potential for the power and the grace.

At this point, perhaps you might be thinking: but surely people still need to work on *strength*^{G}, mobility, and control? You are absolutely correct, but remember we are talking about potential-building activities – they will give you the building blocks to use but won't automatically make you move any better.

I meet a lot of very strong people who move poorly, and even more who are bewildered to find that their movement performance has eroded as their strength has increased. I meet people who, although they have the *flexibility*^{G} to put their limbs into positions that defy the imagination, or can command perfect control when supported on a piece of equipment, find it impossible to recover from a trip or stumble, or move in harmony and dynamism over the ground. Each in their way has developed an aspect of potential. This is wonderful. Each has the further possibility for rich, adaptable, satisfying movement, and the opportunity to experience the power and the grace that moving beautifully offers. To achieve it, however, we must convert potential into meaning for the brain.

To do this, we must understand the intimate relationships that underpin our movement, and how we organize ourselves to meet the functional challenges of our daily lives. In this book we consider the major players: our musculoskeletal system and its partners, biomechanics and physics; the sensory system and its role as the messenger to and from the brain; the emotional system, which can change our entire postural and movement presentation in an instant; and the brain itself, from the effect of our beliefs to the extraordinary daily opportunity we have to construct new pathways and possibilities for ourselves.

Simplicity of communication is a sophisticated and powerful agent of change and empowerment, giving people ownership of their experience and inspiring them to become fascinated in their own movement process. This is fundamental to the JEMS® approach, a method that emerged from dynamical systems theory in the 1990s and has evolved to support thousands of professionals and their clients in a diverse array of contexts, from rehabilitation to high performance, children to the elderly, disability to dance.

Within every person is the potential for their own expression of the power and the grace. Discovering it is an adventure that everyone can participate in, and a path we can walk for a lifetime.

I am light, color, and endlessly shifting pattern, my fragments dancing with the kaleidoscope's turn...

Imagine for a moment that your movement fits you like your favorite sweater. It is completely comfortable and completely expresses "you." You feel that you can do anything in it: dress it up or dress it down, climb a mountain, or turn a cartwheel in it. You push your arms out into its sleeves and you are ready to go.

For movement to feel like this, many factors must play with one another. There is no single element that can transform a person's movement into this very personal, harmonious, and effective expression of their intentions, drives, and desires. The body and brain together need a balanced diet of "movement nutrition" in order to flourish, and to explore the many physical and functional possibilities that we have as humans.

This integration of mind and body systems functions much like a kaleidoscope. Kaleidoscopes, humble sealed tubes containing a cascade of tiny glass pieces, create integrated and complex designs from the multicolored collection within it. A tiny twist of the kaleidoscope's barrel changes the conditions, and a whole new design emerges that is as harmonious and coherent as the previous one. With another twist, the elements are reorganized again – the same elements are present, yet they offer a multitude of solutions. So it is with movement, where multiple processes within us work together to produce endless possibilities, ranging from extravagant forcefulness to dynamic stillness.

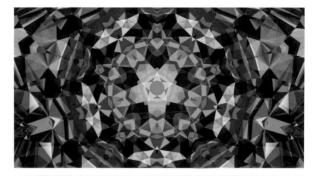

Figure 1.1

The kaleidoscope achieves a wide array of harmonious patterns in response to a change in stimulus

Instead of pieces of glass in a tube, we blend aspects of our thinking and emotional brains, our sensory and wider nervous system, and our musculoskeletal system to create patterns of movement to meet our daily needs and aspirations. We have a vast array of options available to us, but most of us display a mere fraction of our possible movement strategies. We are only turning our kaleidoscope through a few settings. As we shall see in later chapters, this is partly because our efficiency-driven brains streamline their activity by creating movement templates based on prediction and expectation. These become the habitual strategies that we reproduce in our daily lives, which saves on energy but narrows the variety and adaptability of our movement. This not only decreases our options, but tends to load our bodies in repetitive ways, and can contribute to eventual injury.

We don't realize that we are using ourselves in repetitive patterns. In fact, most of us are unaware of how we move at all, unless stopped by pain or injury. We tend to assume that the way in which we move is a preprogrammed inevitability, but the strategies that we develop don't just arise from our own physical warehouse of possibilities: they can be influenced by our environment, our jobs, our emotional state, and even the habits and posture of the people around us. Our histories are written in our movement and posture, but we can choose what our future holds when we become aware of the flexibility of the nervous system and our body's capacity for change.

To achieve this, we need a change in attitude. When our movement strategies aren't meeting our needs, we tend to think of them as errors to be corrected. This assumes only two options: right or wrong. This is not only incredibly limiting but highly inaccurate. You have many possibilities available, but you are expressing an edited version that has been pruned and shaped over time. If your movement habits aren't what you would like them to be, the answer lies in unearthing and reconnecting with some of the other possibilities that have been dormant. People who move well have more settings on their kaleidoscope: they are able to access more combinations of factors, giving them many options and allowing them to respond and adapt to a wider range of movement challenges. Fundamentally, people who don't move well have fewer options – they are often locked into their habits, which reduces their adaptability and loads their body's structures more repetitively. If our bodies are able to move in different ways, they can choose the best one for the job.

It's not about corrective exercise; it's about opening up new options and making new choices.

For health throughout our life span, therefore, our focus for exercise, training, and movement is to develop a wider range of effective, sustainable, and adaptable movement strategies. We want to maintain the integrity of our body over a wide variety of activities and contexts, to be able to create and control forces efficiently, to readily adapt to the new or unexpected, and to do so with confidence and spontaneity. In other words, we want not only to access more settings on our kaleidoscope but to see more colors inside it. This is clearly going to demand more than mere muscle activation – it will involve the seamless integration of multiple factors.

This doesn't have to be complicated. When we think of our daily diet, we understand that good health is supported by variety and balance. We are simply going to take the same approach to our movement.

The wheel of interdependence

The wheel of interdependence shown in Figure 1.2 is a simplified diagram, but it serves to illustrate just some of the many factors that influence and modify one another in the production of effective movement. At this point, some of the terms shown will be more familiar than others, but over the next few chapters, you will become comfortable with each one.

If you are willing to challenge yourself, look at this collection of factors and note whether you feel more attracted to some than others, or secretly believe that some hold greater significance. If you find that this is the case, it is a wonderful start, because if we can identify our biases, we can set about overcoming them. More rewarding results and a deeper understanding for both you and your clients become possible.

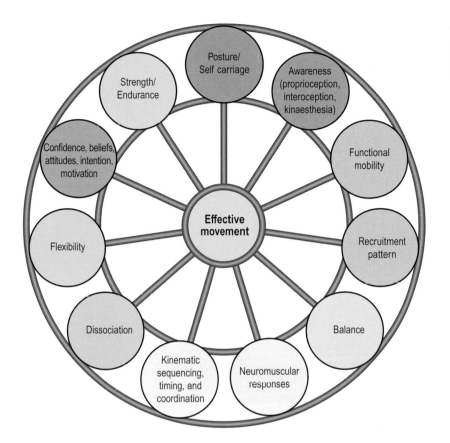

Figure 1.2

The wheel of interdependence. Effective movement results from a constantly adjusting blend of many contributing factors

To appreciate the interplay of factors on the wheel, let's select *functional mobility*[G] as an example. Functional mobility is the ability to move freely and with control through the full range of motion required as you perform a dynamic activity. Functional mobility is only possible if you already have *flexibility*[G], as this is what gives us the potential for a range of motion. Having a potential range of motion, however, doesn't mean that we can actually use it during movement, nor that we can control any flexibility gains that we achieve.

In order to meaningfully integrate the flexibility potential, we must have *dissociation*[G], which is the ability to move our body segments[G] independently of one another. Keeping the pelvis in place as the rib cage turns into rotation is an example of this.

Dissociation requires an appropriate pattern and level of *muscle recruitment*. If there is too much overall muscle recruitment, you cannot easily move one body segment away from another; instead they become fixed together, which makes you feel restricted.

Excessive muscle recruitment may be due to a number of physical or psychological factors. Selecting a task that is too advanced or heavy, trying too hard, or lacking confidence can all provoke this response. Let's say, for example, that muscle tension is a reaction to a *balance* challenge. You start to wobble, and your senses tell you that there is too much movement, so you respond reflexively by contracting many muscles at once in an attempt to control the situation. This relatively immobilizes you, gluing your body parts together. If you attempt to move a limb with this process in play, you are thrown further off balance, as your muscles are working to resist the motion as you are trying to create it. You are pulling against yourself. You respond to this uncontrolled feeling by further increasing muscle tension, limiting your mobility even more. Your confidence becomes affected, your beliefs about your balance capability are reinforced, and above all you think to yourself that you really must do more stretching, because you don't seem to be very flexible!

> When the level of difficulty is too great, the "kaleidoscope" can become distorted, and effective, beautiful movement moves further from reach. Steady progression teaches the nervous system mastery rather than struggle.

We bounce from one part of the wheel to another as factors connect, either working for us or against us. It is easy for us to fixate on one factor, without realizing that it is a relationship between factors that we need to develop instead. Our preferences come into play very readily, exposing our own biases. Most people, for example, will select flexibility rather than balance to work on, because improvements in it are so much more easily perceived, and this in turn feeds our motivation – although it doesn't necessarily improve our overall performance.

What if you selected balance to work on? Balance is often considered as a single entity, yet it both influences and is influenced by many factors. Its direct influences come from three main contributing systems: visual, vestibular, and proprioceptive. The *vestibular system*^{G}, located in your inner ear, is intimately connected with your upper cervical spine as part of a neural network, so if you are compressing the small joints at the top of the spine with a forward head

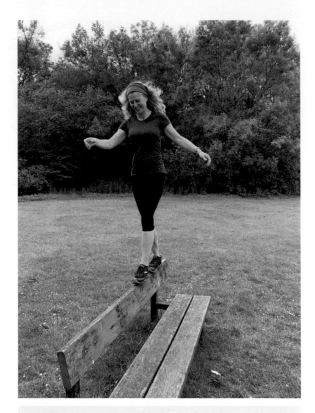

Figure 1.3

Adaptable balance is the result of multiple factors

posture, you could be creating interference within this sensitive relationship.

The feedback from your feet is also critical, but if you lack the functional mobility for your lower leg and foot to accommodate to an uneven surface, you will not receive the accurate feedback that you need for balance. The other factors involved may depend upon the activity you are performing. If you unexpectedly trip, slip, or are bumped, or land from a jump not quite in control of yourself, do your *neuromuscular responses*^{G} enable you to quickly adjust your body to recover your equilibrium? They are often slower yet stronger than necessary, and the resulting overall body stiffening can block functional mobility or interfere with timing and coordination. The more tense you are, the worse your balance tends to be – just ask any novice skier or paddleboarder! Alternatively, your balance might be quite good early in your activity, but because fatigue can erode *proprioception*[G], *endurance* may be the most influential factor.

This process of connection can seem overwhelming, but it doesn't have to be complicated. Just think of it as simply having many more tools to play with to improve physical capability.

> Think of the wheel as opportunity, rather than as complexity.

But, you might say, what about strength? Surely this is an entity unto itself and not subject to the influences of other factors? Certainly, if you looked at a muscle's performance in isolation, this might be the case. You can look at repetitions and sets, and how these create the necessary physiological stress to change how that muscle performs. This is potential-building, but the ability to actually utilize that strength during a dynamic movement may be dependent upon other factors, for example, the timing and coordination of your body parts. This in turn may be influenced by functional mobility, which, as we have already seen, can be influenced by a number of other factors. It may also depend upon your balance, your awareness of body position, your confidence, and your intention. Even endurance is subject to the wheel – you may have physiological capacity, but if you over-recruit muscles or have poor timing and coordination, it will cost you more energy over time as you move. There is no escaping the wheel!

The prime example: stability

You might note that *stability*[G] is significantly missing as a factor on the wheel. This is because stable functional movement is the result of the interaction between multiple factors, including psychological and emotional attributes such as confidence and *self-efficacy*[G], to meet the variety of demands of a normal life. Each factor on the wheel provides potential, and the degree to which it is involved is dependent upon the activity you are engaged in. No matter who you are and what you do in your life, all of the factors shown are required for stability in movement.

Where, then, do we start?

Setting our intentions

Let us agree that our overall intention is to help people to move with ease, effectiveness, and enjoyment; to overcome physical limitations and injury; to expand their capabilities; and to look forward to a healthy active future. This can be encapsulated in a single statement.

We intend to help people to move beautifully.

It doesn't matter whether a person is learning to walk again, to compete as a weightlifter, to play the violin, or to spend fun time with their children. "Moving beautifully" is simply a term that captures a person's effectiveness, efficiency, spontaneity, and confidence.

Most professionals in the health and fitness industry would say that they are broadly working toward that aim. However, do common training practices promote movement, or *anti-movement*[G]? When it comes down to what actually happens in a training environment, is our input facilitating natural movement or unintentionally blocking it?

We need to be clear about the intention of our cues, and recognize contradictions between our aims and our actions. For example, when you ask someone to brace, set, or hold, you are asking them to prevent something from happening. You are cueing for anti-movement.

Sometimes this is entirely appropriate. If you are going to be tackled in a fast multidirectional sport, for example, you want to prevent your joints from being suddenly forced beyond their normal safe range. If you are going to rotate your whole body quickly in a ballet pirouette, you similarly must maintain a consistent trunk position to enable your body to control this rapid motion.

However, these are specific tasks, and represent only one aspect of movement. The problem comes when we apply this principle in a generalized way, in the form of rules that are applied regardless of the task. Engagement of abdominal muscles to counter excessive lumbar motion, or contracting gluteals for a knee falling inwards are common examples of this. These actions increase muscle tension and create a "stop point" in the moving kinetic chain.[G] When we constrain movement in a body region, the brain performs some rapid calculations, and works out how to bypass the blockage to achieve the objective of the movement. Although the overall alignment might look better, this may not necessarily result in effective movement, and may increase stress elsewhere in the body as forces are redirected.[1]

Movement exploration

Take a moment to imagine that you are standing in a library, surrounded by shelves filled with books.

You want a book on a shelf above you, but it is a high one and you will have to reach for it. Let's imagine that you have been told that for the sake of your back, you must pre-activate, or "set" your abdominals before movement. You may even have been taught to maintain a consistent distance between your ribs and pelvis throughout the movement. To emphasize this experience, place the fingers of one hand on the top of your pelvis and your thumb on the bottom of your ribs.

Now reach for the book, without the distance between your ribs and pelvis changing. Does that feel natural? This is unlikely, because you have interrupted the movement impulse[G] that would otherwise run from your feet through your body to your hand. Your lumbar spine may not be excessively extending, but your spine as a whole is now not moving as it normally would. You have not so much improved your spinal mechanics as stopped them. The movement is different, but not better (see Fig. 1.4).

Now abandon the need to set the abdominals, and just reach up for the imaginary book. Feel how the body would normally lengthen when unconstrained. You may even notice that your body weight has shifted subtly under the reaching arm to support the movement, connecting your arm to your foot. These are natural responses, but cueing anti-movement through abdominal bracing or setting will block them (see Fig. 1.5).

Although we do need to pay attention to movement quality, it is how we address it that is in question here. Consciously holding a body part in place may create a theoretically correct position, but yield a prescriptive, constrained movement. Simultaneously processing conflicting stop and go messages makes fluent, coordinated, and efficient movement very difficult.

This concept will provoke considerable conflict in the professional mind, because the prevalent approach of teaching a conscious form of muscular pre-setting is framed as "control," and is therefore associated with safety and movement proficiency. In emphasizing

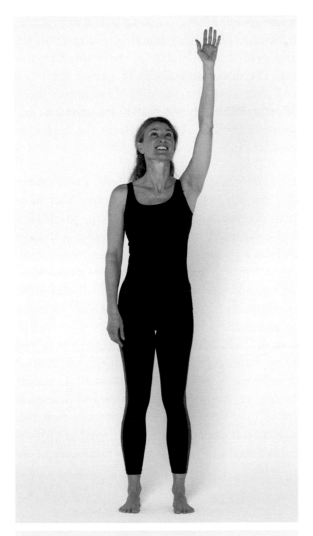

Figure 1.4

Reaching up with preset abdominal muscles

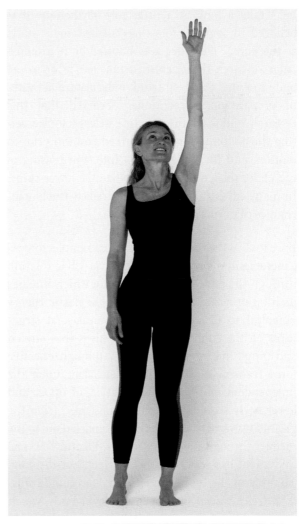

Figure 1.5

Making a connection from the foot to the hand by allowing the body to naturally lengthen on the reaching side

this, however, are we moving toward or away from normal movement?

The control conundrum

The control concept has exploded in popularity over recent decades, and has developed a language and discourse that has gained widespread acceptance in the health and fitness industries. Unfortunately, it carries with it assumptions that do not necessarily match the research into its effectiveness, nor do they necessarily support the performance of normal movement. This has led to increasing controversy and conflict between professions.

Let's take a look at a little core mythology. It is believed in some sectors that "all movement starts at the core." This idea was boosted by neuromuscular research that identified that just prior to the body moving, the deep trunk musculature activates in preparation.[2] Practitioners believed that this research endorsed the practice of consciously setting the abdominal wall in a fixed position prior to motion, and (in some sectors) into firm tensing of the abdominal wall to immobilize the lower spine. In many cases, however, this contradicts the biomechanics of normal movement.

If we look at the tennis forehand for example, force is generated in the legs, transferring via pelvic rotation through the torso to the upper body, which initiates its rotation just slightly later to allow elastic energy potential to develop across the myofascial structures on the front of the body. This is the "stretch and ping" that creates efficiency through effective force transmission, and it is dependent upon the independent motion, or dissociation, of upper and lower body segments. Having transferred from the ground upward, forces are finally funneled out to the racquet through the arm (see Figs. 1.6 and 1.7). The movement has started from the floor, not the core. The role of the "core" here is to *connect and transfer forces* between the upper and lower body, which requires an ability to move these segments relative to each other. The abdominals are not acting at a fixed length – instead they maintain connection while lengthening and shortening. This has very little relationship to the "preset and hold" approach taken in most gym classes.

Nevertheless, this practice continues, especially in the arena of low back pain rehabilitation.

The theory was simple: in the presence of pain, key muscles that contributed to control of joint segments were found to change their behavior.[3]

It was assumed that an ensuing lack of control contributed to ongoing dysfunction, and therefore the area needed to be "stabilized" with specific training. The discourse was one of damage limitation and protection, carrying with it a subtext of threat of recurrence. This was easy to communicate and seemed very logical, especially to the frightened person in pain.

If we fast-forward to the present time, it now appears that our conceptualization was naive. Analysis of years of research indicates that reducing people's fear and catastrophic thoughts (*catastrophizing*[G]) about their back pain has been shown to have more consistent influence on low back pain outcomes than transversus abdominis muscle activation.[4] Taking active responsibility for one's own personal health, learning to understand and interpret a range of new sensations in the body, overcoming unhelpful beliefs,[5] and being challenged while supported with reassurance[6] can all contribute to reducing helplessness, increasing confidence, and equipping a person with independent self-management tools. It is possible, then, that stability training may have a positive effect early on, but not necessarily for the reasons that its practitioners believe.

> If you want to be evidence based, aim for confidence development.

Mind the gap

In the case of low back pain, it would be a misinterpretation to say that stability training is of no benefit. The research does not indicate any lack of benefit, merely that specific stabilizing training is similarly effective to other forms of general exercise in the short term, and that none of these approaches holds the answers for long-term recovery.[7,8] Rather than succumb to petty battles over whether control

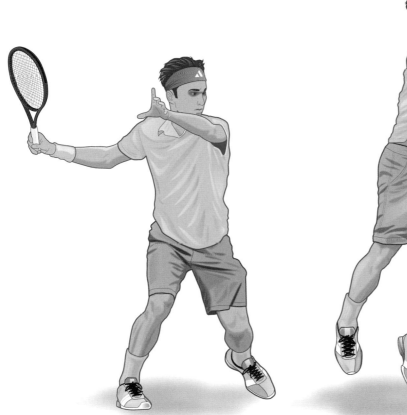

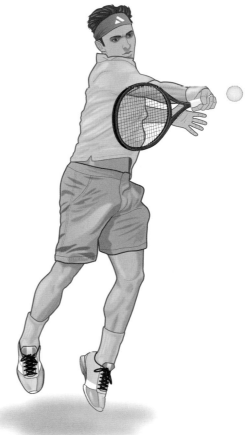

Figure 1.6

Generating the movement impulse in the legs

Figure 1.7

The movement impulse has transmitted from the legs and out to the hand via rotation in the body

exercises have a role, we need to recognize global body control not as an entity trainable by "stability exercises" but as something that develops as the result of multisystem interplay. It requires a range of inputs, and these will vary and progress based on the functional, physiological, and contextual requirements of the individual. In other words, we need a variety of experiences and challenges in our training.

Once we understand this interconnectivity of factors, our personal perspective on training and rehabilitation starts to become more inclusive and elastic. We start to step out of our own boxes, expand our vision, and work with greater creativity, curiosity, and accuracy for each individual.

In appreciating the intelligence and responsiveness of our system, we can grasp that our personal movement kaleidoscope will put together muscular responses in different ways depending upon what we are doing. This helps to make sense of apparently conflicting research regarding whether there is a single correct solution for training the abdominals. The bracing strategy, which involves an anti-movement, *co-contraction*[G] technique using high levels of trunk muscle activation, was more effective than other alternatives for stabilizing the spine against a heavy load.[9] The abdominal hollowing strategy, however, which involves lower levels of muscular activity to draw the abdominal wall inwards and upward, was found to improve the timing of the muscles around the spine to provide stability in response to a sudden disturbance of our center of gravity.[10]

It is not so much a case of which strategy is right, but which is relevant to the task. We have many roles to fulfill. Sometimes we need greater stiffening around our joints to withstand a load, and sometimes we need coordinated and quick responses.

> We need more than one strategy to control our joints.

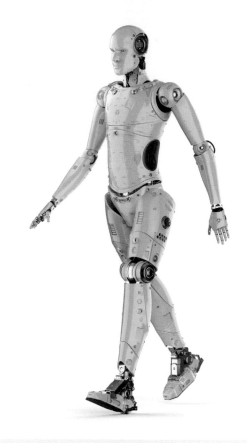

Figure 1.8

Overcontrolling can interfere with spontaneous natural movement

It is tempting to think that the exercises that provoke the most muscle activity in target muscles are going to be the most effective. The philosophy is that more must be better, but is this always the case?

More is not necessarily better

Research on lower back, neck,[11] knee,[12] and hip injury indicates that too much muscular activity is associated with ongoing dysfunction. In other words, *over-controlling* is emerging as a problem (see Fig. 1.8).

Individuals with acute back pain actually demonstrate an increase in spinal stability, using more, rather than less muscle activity.[13] This is a very natural initial response to protect an injured area, as you will know if you have ever experienced back pain. It is not helpful as an ongoing strategy, however. Constantly maintaining a protective activation pattern around the spine can compromise normal neuromuscular responses including the ability to make the small, sudden adjustments necessary in order to regain balance. Such adjustments require rapid but coordinated relaxation of the spinal muscles.[14] The longer the delay in someone's ability to relax these spinal muscles, the greater the risk of low back injury.[15] Similar findings have been shown for knee and hip patients – too much muscle activity around the joints changes the way we use ourselves, compromising normal movement.

It is alarmingly easy to amplify this response in an injured person. People seek safety and reassurance when injured, and an explanation that promises protection of the injured part seems like a good idea. *Co-contraction*, the simultaneous activation of opposing muscles around a joint, has been promoted as the antidote to the threat of "uncontrolled movement." Although it does initially provide a degree of functionality, co contraction also creates an ongoing barrier to recovery; in fact, it may lead to recurrence later due to altered trunk dynamics.[16] The "functional frozen" vigilantly control their previously injured area with various learned muscular setting behaviors. They come to believe that these behaviors protect them, but they actually end up preventing their bodies from regaining natural spontaneous movement responses. People trapped in this cycle have lost the overall goal of recovery, and instead make control their holy grail.

Can't we just get stronger?

Strength is vitally important in maintaining musculoskeletal health across our lifespan.[17] However, more strength cannot compensate for deficits in other systems, any more than increasing the size of a single jigsaw puzzle piece will create a complete picture by simply covering an empty space.

It is a fundamental error to assume that if you have enough strength to meet high load demands, you will cope with lower load situations competently. This is not the case: each should be viewed as having differing requirements. Strengthening involves high load tasks that demand commensurately high levels of muscle contraction, and this provides plenty of sensory feedback to let you know where your body parts are relative to one another. This doesn't necessarily carry over to low load tasks, where you need a more finely tuned ability to process sensory feedback. For full-spectrum function your brain needs to be able to hear the body's whispers as well as its shouts. It is not unusual for people who struggle with body awareness to be attracted to high load training, as the strong feedback feels reassuring and pleasurable. To optimize their overall physical capability in the wider context of life, however, they need to improve their ability to sense themselves.

To develop strength in order to manage high loads, the complexity of the exercise is usually reduced in order to optimize force output. Common techniques requiring a very stable, bilateral foot position, such as squat and deadlift exercises, do not necessarily equip a person for a lower load task requiring speed, balance, proprioception, timing, and coordination for each leg separately.

For example, gluteal strength is not the sole determining influence on pelvic and knee control, but gluteal strengthening is nevertheless the most common approach for addressing it. This demonstrates the gap between what we are aiming for, and what we actually achieve. Studies on gluteal strength have demonstrated, first, that strength and knee control are not necessarily consistently correlated,[18] and, second, that training of gluteal strength may not transfer to improved functional knee control.[19] Gluteal muscle *timing* has been found to be an important factor in knee control for runners,[20] and studies that have emphasized *awareness* of knee position during dynamic functional movements have yielded positive results,[21,22] as did a neuromuscular program of mixed movement activities.[23] This opens up many exciting possibilities for improving movement in simple ways, as we shall see in later chapters.

Having more strength is universally beneficial, but strength alone will not necessarily confer the power and the grace of effective, adaptable functional movement.

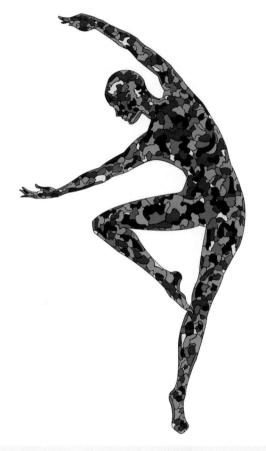

Figure 1.9

Movement is the embodied expression of constantly changing shapes and patterns

Biases and beliefs

Contemporary research continues to demonstrate how much more we have to learn about this extraordinary, sophisticated body that we inhabit. Accordingly, we must evolve our thinking, although every movement, rehabilitation, or training discipline has biases and beliefs that can impede this progress.

It is a position of integrity and strength when a discipline can look at itself objectively to see what is outdated, misunderstood, or limiting. Without this, our growth as practitioners and students of movement learning and teaching is constrained. Only when we can identify the gaps in our understanding, and respect the role of factors with which we are perhaps not so comfortable, can we progress.

Your profession may have a specific emphasis, for example, strength, control, or flexibility. Each has much to offer, but none provides a comprehensive solution for improving functional movement in the real world. Appreciating the wheel of interdependence allows us to reflect upon our approaches, and to creatively balance what we offer while still maintaining the spirit of our background and training.

When we look at the roots and meanings of kaleidoscope (*kalos* from Greek, meaning beautiful, *eidos* meaning shape, and scope "to view"), it can literally mean "to see beautiful shapes." Lord Byron himself in 1819 attested that the word should mean "constantly changing pattern."[24]

What better metaphor could we use for the magnificent and complex, yet so responsive and malleable entities that are our moving selves?

Movement is usually considered to be an activity of the body, but could more accurately be seen as the brain visibly expressing itself.

Whether our movement is fluent, effective, and pleasing, or labored, painful, and difficult, it is telling the story of how our brains are meeting the challenges that they encounter. Understanding how to influence this process is one of the most powerful ways to open new movement possibilities. This is where the art and the science of movement truly intersect.

Plastic fantastic

The bleak perception that our brains and bodies are inexorably deteriorating over time is persistent in our society; yet, as it turns out, our bodies, including our nervous systems, are constantly remodeling in response to the input and experiences to which they are exposed.[1] This is called *plasticity*, and the term *neuroplasticity*[G] is used to represent the nervous system's constant reorganization of its structure, function, and connections in response to the stimuli that it encounters. Whatever you are thinking, feeling, or experiencing, change is taking place in your brain via the process of neuroplasticity. This process is inevitable, but whether it is adaptive, in that it helps you to function, or maladaptive, where your functioning is compromised, depends upon an interplay of factors.

For example, research has demonstrated that the amount of space relating to each body part in your brain can change depending upon how, or how much, you use it.[1-3] The actual volume of the thinking and processing part of your brain, known as the *grey matter*[G], can be increased depending upon your activities and how you learn to use your brain.[4] From dancing to learning to drive a London taxi, what we set our minds to learning shapes the structure of our brains.[5,6] The brain is therefore dynamic and changeable. It isn't just a case of "use it or lose it," but "use it and shape it."[7]

Only a few years ago, researchers discovered that when exposed to chronic stress, the part of our brain that best helps us to cope with it actually shrinks, and this in turn compromises our response to stress still further.[8-10] This apparent downward spiral seemed like pretty bad news, until more recent research revealed that in as little as eight weeks of mindfulness practice, we can rethicken that part of the brain again. This has been investigated with mindfulness-based yoga and tai chi, as well as in more formal meditation and mindfulness practice.[11] Just imagine that – you actually increase your brain volume by doing something that is well within your power and capability.

> How extraordinary that we can literally increase the amount of brain we have to work with, and how effectively it works, through the humble means of a regular mindful commitment to the practice of our choosing.

This journey that we are making into movement begins with the nervous system. It is time to acquaint ourselves with some of the intriguing and deeply enriching insights that brain science has to offer us.

Brain economics

In recent years our understanding of brain function has radically altered, and with each piece of new research, we can find relevance for our work as movement practitioners.

To appreciate the cleverness and complexity of our brain, we need first to consider it in terms of economics. Relative to the size of our bodies, the brain is a metabolically very costly organ for us to use. When we learn something new, or change the way in which we use our brain, a process of neuronal connection rewiring takes place, which requires a high investment of energy. As such, we have evolved to conserve our resources by operating a trade-off between the cost of neuronal activity and the development of valuable new patterns of activity and connectivity.[12] Daily, our brains are pruning away unused connections and buffing up new ones, so there's a lot of background activity going on. To perform their function well, brains have to have compelling efficiency strategies.

The predictive brain

Way back in the Industrial Revolution, we learned that the quickest way to make a process more efficient is to make it predictable and repeatable. Developing a process involves an investment of time and energy, but if a template for the process can then be generated, it can be repeated with less effort and fewer resources. Our brains are natural experts at this.

Until relatively recently, it was assumed that sensory information flowed into our brains, where it was then processed and used to form an action response. This seemed logical but meant that every action would have to be freshly generated, which would be both slow and expensive from an energy point of view. As it turns out, the brain actually makes predictions based on its existing database of previous experiences and then uses incoming sensory information to either confirm or contradict those predictions. When the sensations confirm the prediction, the behavior continues, but a contradiction will stimulate the nervous system to respond with a new possibility. This is much faster and more efficient, because instead of creating a stream of new solutions, it is editing and tweaking a pre-prepared template.

The cerebellum (meaning "little brain") has a major role to play in this process. Located at the back of the brain underneath the cerebrum (the main body of the brain), this small but mighty structure only occupies about 10 percent of the brain's volume yet contains more than 50 percent of the total number of neurons. Modern research is starting to reveal why this is the case: the cerebellum appears to be involved in a remarkable number of processes, including vision,[13] hearing,[14,15] proprioception, motor coordination,[16] language,[17] and even emotion,[18] communicating with multiple areas of the brain and processing large amounts of sensory information from the entire body.[19-21]

Among its many roles, the cerebellum is the master of prediction. When you read and understand the meaning of a sentence despite a missing word, or finish someone's sentence for them in a conversation, it is a demonstration of your cerebellum's ability to calculate the most likely solution. It is not waiting for all the information to come in – it is talking to many other parts of your brain to harvest associations from which it can construct a prediction.[22]

> Your cerebellum uses your past to predict your immediate future.

This predictive ability is necessary to be able to act in real time. Processing incoming sensory feedback and then creating an appropriate motor response is just too slow to be effective. This applies not just for fast movements but also during slow ones. The cerebellum makes continuous calculations and modifications a fraction of a second in front of the movement's point of progress to ensure a smooth motion. Without this mechanism, there would be a time lag between the feedback from the body being received and processed by the brain, and the next motor command executed. This would result in the movement having a juddering, stop/start quality.

This is all good news until you try to change or improve a movement. To perform a movement, a motor command is generated in the brain that is then linked to all of the sensory information associated with that movement experience. This creates a template for the movement, an internal loop between the cerebellum and other parts of the brain, such as the motor and prefrontal cortex (see Fig. 2.1). When we intend to perform this movement again, our brains are triggered to run a simulation of it based on this template. In simple terms, it is like pushing a button on a switchboard that runs a specified program. This is far more efficient than creating a new solution every time. What is most profound, however, is that this automatic response is so fast, *the brain has actually completed the movement before your body has even begun it.*

Just take a moment to digest that; it cuts right to the core of movement training. How do we change a movement that the brain has completed before the movement has even begun?

It suddenly becomes clear as to why it can be so frustratingly difficult to change a movement, despite understanding cognitively what should be happening. Many people practice diligently for little reward in terms of change, and become understandably

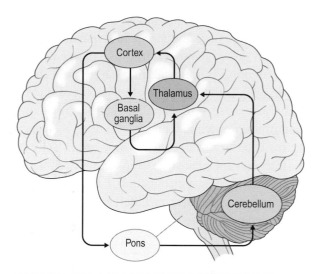

Figure 2.1

The impulse to move activates the cerebellum to trigger a predictive loop involving an array of brain structures

despondent and demotivated. If something doesn't disrupt the predictive movement template triggered in the brain, the same old pattern will continue to be reproduced.

Changing the game

Fortunately, we are not trapped in a cycle of unmodifiable simulations, because the system is highly adaptive. If you decide to lift a box from the ground, your cerebellum will generate computations based on an expectation of the weight of that box. If it is much lighter or much heavier than expected, you will experience a movement error. However, the new sensory input generated by that experience will be used to adjust your movement for your next attempt, and for any further encounters with boxes.

Altering the expected sensory feedback associated with a movement causes the motor loop to adapt, making change possible. Our aim, then, is to surprise the system, and the key we use is sensation.

To play with this, we need to be aware of the inputs we are giving. If we give mechanical instructions (the "what to do" of the movement), we engage the person's cognitive processes. This means we are choosing to work with the prefrontal cortex, the area of the brain associated with planning, memory, reasoning, and problem solving. Using this strategy, the person learns what to *think* about the movement. However, to interrupt the predictive template, we need not so much mind over matter, but mind *in* matter – the person needs to feel something different. We need to talk to the cerebellum.

Say, for example, that you want to help someone to be able to drop their center of gravity. They have always struggled to squat, and it has never improved with practice. Their brain's "squat template" locks their hips and pelvis together, dragging their spine into a poor position, and their ankle mobility seems to be severely restricted, blocking their motion. Knowing a little neuroscience, you understand that further instructions on where to put their knees/pelvis/spine is unlikely to achieve tangible change, because this is talking to the thinking brain rather than to the sensory processing brain that can really impact on this habitual movement strategy.

You decide to change the person's focus from "achieving" a better squat to noticing what happens to their balance point. You redirect their attention away from whatever they think "squatting" is to what they are feeling in their feet. They notice that as soon as they start to move in a downward direction, their weight shifts into their heels, causing the body to tense in response to this change in balance. The increased muscle tension locks the ankles and hips, limiting their motion. You invite them

to play with this: is it necessary to have the weight in the heels? You take them by the hands to offer a little support, and invite them to explore moving the weight forward from the heels to make contact with more of the foot, and then back again. They are greatly surprised to find that they have a choice in where to put their weight and, furthermore, that with a more secure balance point, their muscle tension reduces, opening up a greater ability to move the joints in their legs. You invite them to return to their former movement habit, and then compare this sense to that of the new strategy, to more clearly perceive the difference (see Fig. 2.2).

Meanwhile, the cerebellum is speedily encoding this new experience, logging the sensorimotor relationship for future use. It expands its catalog of squat-related associations to incorporate the new experience.

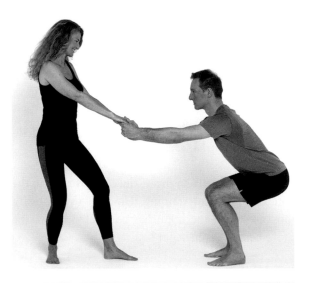

Figure 2.2

Supporting an exploration of balance point

Change can happen surprisingly quickly when someone is offered the skilled guidance and space to learn to sense themselves, because it is novel sensory input that makes the nervous system sit up and take notice. The traditional instruction/correction dynamic can inhibit this; in other words, more thinking can get in the way of better sensing.

This training method doesn't actually take more time – it just requires a different dialog. It is a matter of choosing which part of the brain to talk to.

> Changing the sensory experience associated with a movement lights up the nervous system to facilitate change.

The functional blur

For us to be able to move well, our brains need to be able to distinguish movement in one body part from another. As a teacher of movement, there will be many times when it is evident that the person in front of you cannot do this. The hip, pelvis, and lumbar spine region is a common example: in hip-bending tasks, people will often skip the hip and fold in the lumbar spine, because, as far as the brain is concerned, the whole area is an indistinct functional blur.

Cleaning up the functional blur in the brain requires the fundamental building block of dissociation. This is not necessarily a question of cognitively learning the technique but of the nervous system needing a new piece of information. In this example, the question asked by the brain is: "Where is my hip?"

Your objective is to help the brain to answer this question. For example, during a basic supine heel slide along the floor in a Pilates class, most people are so busy focusing on lumbar spine and pelvic control

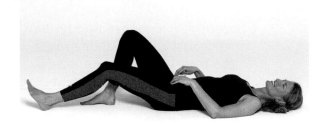

Figure 2.3

Feeling where the motion occurs

that they have only a vague impression of the moving leg above the knee, and rarely any awareness of the hip itself. However, if you ask them to use their own hands to identify the exact spot where their hips bend, then, while sliding a heel away and back again they are able to feel the joint motion under their fingertips. This discovery can help them to distinguish between the motion of the hip and that of the pelvis, which in turn encourages easier hip movement (see Fig. 2.3).

Similarly, in a yoga class, you might observe an experienced practitioner carrying their trunk into their triangle pose by effortlessly side tilting their pelvis over their front hip joint. In doing so, they share the total motion experience between their hip and spine. A novice frequently misses this hip/pelvis motion and begins the movement at the spine, which must side bend more deeply. The movement proportions are very different: the spine is now experiencing far more motion than the hip.

To bring the pose into balance, the brain needs to clarify the blur between the hip, pelvis, and spine, and we can do this by uncovering the missing element.

Once the feet have been placed in the starting position, invite the person to place their hands on each side of their pelvis. Next, suggest they visualize their pelvis as a teapot between their hands with the spout facing their front leg. Ask them to pour water down their front leg by tipping the teapot, and then to right the teapot again (see Fig. 2.4). With their fingers falling into the crease of the front hip, can they feel it bending? Do they notice that the pelvis moves toward the thigh, closing that space? Once they have explored this motion, it can be integrated into the full pose.

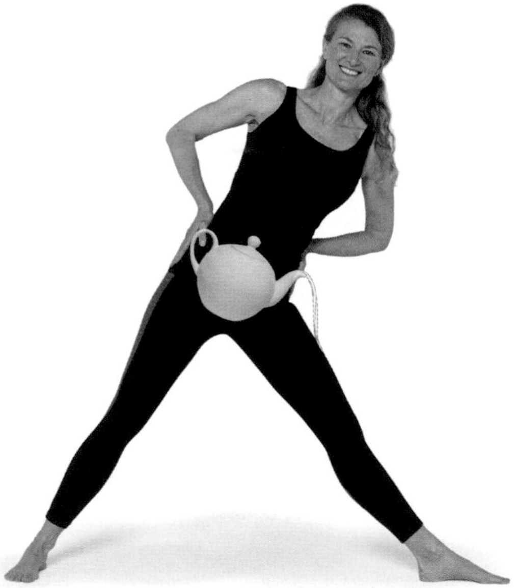

This process is an example of more clearly defining hip bending for the brain, creating a transferable asset that can be drawn on in other poses. You might follow that thread through the class, so that as people change positions or tasks, the brain learns to apply its new understanding, and each person identifies the sensation of hip bending compared with spine bending in a variety of ways.

You are teaching people how to feel in a way that changes their relationship with themselves, rather than just how to perform the pose or exercise. The experience of sensing and understanding the self is priceless, not just for the progression and deepening of the practice but beyond, into everyday life.

This is process focus, rather than outcome focus. Whether it is through yoga, Pilates, or any other form of movement training, process is what keeps us securely rooted in the present. It deepens our understanding of ourselves and ensures that we are truly working mindfully for, and within, ourselves, rather than chasing the shiny prizes of increasingly extravagant poses or exercises. In doing so, those outcomes will come, but from a stronger foundation.

As we move more deeply into the book, we will explore other common functional blurs, and learn how, by clarifying them, apparent mobility and stability problems can be resolved.

Figure 2.4

Visualizing the teapot to clarify the motion of the pelvis over the leg

When the body parts don't seem to be able to move independently of one another, it constitutes a functional blur. If you help someone to clarify these movement relationships, you gift them with a transferable sense of body connection that will enrich their practice.

Respect the cost

Because the energetic cost of rewiring the brain is so high, it is important as a practitioner to know how to optimize the process. Just as a sprinter would train with short bursts of intensity requiring recovery before the next drill, so it is with the brain.

When your client is learning something new, you will find they achieve much better results and can maintain their form over a longer duration if the movements are performed in short sets of limited repetitions, with brief periods of complete rest in between each one. Imagine what is happening in those pauses as the brain engages in rapidly sorting and filing the new information. If you allow the pauses, the learning process can be much more efficient. The movement develops over the session.

If you attempt the same number of repetitions without these pauses, you will notice that the form begins to erode. This is rarely muscular fatigue – it is neural fatigue. There is no time for the brain to do its sorting. It is like being interrupted constantly when you are trying to get something done. The person often ends the session quite disconsolate, as they had started to improve and then suddenly lost the thread.

> The learning happens in the pauses.

The art of movement teaching

The science of movement is powerful and compelling, but the science of *teaching* movement is the art of translating knowledge into meaningful change.

Mirror mirror

How you present yourself and your own movement to someone is an extraordinary means of deeply influencing a person's ability to learn and produce a movement.

One of our brain's remarkable efficiency strategies is the activation of mirror neurons. Although the exact mechanism for these is still controversial, it appears that when we observe someone else performing a movement, our own brains activate in the same areas as if we were performing the movement ourselves. An observer's brain is harvesting a whole lot more information than you realize, and activating different parts of itself accordingly. Research has demonstrated that observing someone else performing an action at a certain rate spontaneously alters the observer's own rate of movement execution.[23] Perception of load and effort is also absorbed, so if you want to communicate a sense of effortless, fluent movement, then you should be aware that your own effort is being read by your client and their brain is responding accordingly.[24]

> A person's mind might be engaged by the words you are saying, but their brain is paying attention to the rhythm, rate, and effort that they observe, which in turn can influence their own motor output. Knowledge alone then does not create great teachers. Deepening your own practice and becoming increasingly authentic in your own movement will strengthen and deepen your communication and enhance the learning of your clients.

Observation and movement imagery both activate similar brain regions to those involved in movement execution, and, acting together, they generate a form of movement simulation. It seems that combining imagery with action observation is even more effective than simply observing a movement. It is thought that by watching a movement, the need to generate a mental visual image, including the rate of movement and other visual cues, is removed, creating more

Along with creating a visualization to light up helpful associations, the rhythm and timing of your words will provide even greater levels of unconscious information for your client's brain to read. Modulating the pitch of your voice, and matching it to a change in the rhythm of your speech, can focus the person for either an excitatory or calming effect. Timing your vocal cues accurately can iron out motor control difficulties, reining back those who are rushing, pausing them for a moment of increased awareness, or enhancing the clarity of intention in those people who are struggling with coordination or movement fluency. This is an invaluable skill to develop – you can change movement quality rapidly, keeping people grounded in their bodies and learning through the sensing brain rather than being thrown back into their thinking brain with more instructions.

> Just as an actor would, work on your range of vocal options, and play with varying your pitch, rhythm, and timing. Many instructors use a single pleasant "instructor voice," without realizing the huge opportunity that they are missing through honing their vocal skills.

Relaxed faces, happier minds

When greeting a client or facing a class, your friendly welcoming expression is likely to encourage a reciprocal positive facial response from them. This happens through the mimicry that we naturally use to decode others' expressions.[26] It's an automatic response for most people, and it is part of what helps us to function socially. If you can induce people to relax their facial tension, or even manage to provoke them into a smile, it turns out that from a brain perspective, you are doing powerful invisible work before your session even begins.

The link between our facial muscle postures and our formation of emotion is known as emotional

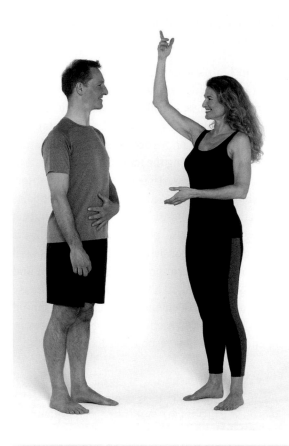

Figure 2.5

The brain harvests movement information from multiple sources, including your body, vocal tone, rhythm, and imagery

attentional space for a person to focus on the kinesthetic elements of the movement.[25] It seems, therefore, that involving your client in imagery as they observe you demonstrate will stimulate more comprehensive firing in more regions of their brains (see Fig. 2.5).

> To help people reproduce what you are doing, paint a picture with your words as you demonstrate a movement.

proprioception. Investigation into the association between facial expression and activation of the limbic system (a group of brain structures that are involved in emotion processing) have found that even intentional changes in facial expression can alter the activity in these brain areas.[27] In other words, you can bias your emotions in a certain way just by placing your face in a particular expression, even if you don't feel that emotion to begin with. Pulling the edges of your mouth upward, clenching your jaw, or pushing your eyebrows together is sufficient to activate your brain to respond with emotional associations, so you really can manipulate your emotions into happiness, anger, and sadness.[28–30]

This is powerful knowledge: rather than just hoping that someone enjoys the class, you can more deeply affect their mood through what you express facially, and by gently encouraging them to find the expression that best represents how they want to feel.

> Your impact and effectiveness as a teacher lies not just in the information you impart but with the emotion you project.

This is really starting to touch on the art of movement teaching. Master teachers often instinctively influence their students and clients through these means. You can use the neuroscience of learning to decode their methods and apply them with intention.

Priming

Priming[G] is a way for us to activate particular associations and disrupt others, in this case, for the performance of a movement. It has been found that priming young adults with related action words before performing a task significantly improved their upper limb movements.[31] Older women improved their learning after being told that the task that they were about to

attempt was usually performed well by their peers.[32] They were primed to expect success, and their brains arranged their family of associations accordingly.

Over-thinking, self-generated pressure and fear of failure prime the brain for a negative result. They freeze the potential for change better than any roadblock, and this needs to be disrupted if change is to occur. A little laughter is a wonderful disrupter, and is a reminder that it isn't necessary to take ourselves too seriously to take our practice seriously.

Setting an intention for the session is a positive priming strategy that lends itself well to groups and classes as well as individuals. Adapt your wording to your audience, but present an intention that will lift their sense of pressure, lighten the mood, and focus them on non-judgmental exploration. For example, an intention for the session may simply be to discover where they are, right now, today. Or perhaps it might be to inhabit every movement in the class from the top of the head to the tips of the toes. Or maybe it will be to work with a sense of lightness throughout every movement. Prime for an attitude or intention that will free people of their barriers and help them to access new associations before they begin.

Whatever suits your clients, just remember the power of priming at the beginning of each session.

Mind your language

Do you cue or command?

Imagine the difference between a command to control a movement and an invitation to explore a movement to find out what happens. Using "control" as a key word when instructing can make your job much harder. The word control is often associated with *preventing* something from happening, and is highly likely to induce tension, which in turn diminishes movement fluency. If, however, you cue in a way that shows how to positively advance into the movement, you encourage the coordinated balance of tensions in the muscles.

For example, rather than telling someone to control their speed, invite them to choose the speed of their movement. How slowly would they like to go? How slowly *can* they go? Introducing choice powerfully changes the brain's perceived objective. A flexible, exploratory space opens up to offer a range of possibilities.

Ask your clients to note whether the speed is the same throughout the movement. Is it faster at some times and slower at others? Can they smooth out that rhythm? This type of supportive cueing focuses the brain on different qualities of the movement, and really engages the cerebellum, which has to make the necessary calculations to smooth out the movement.

Rather than asking someone to control their spine in supine as their arm moves overhead, invite them to leave their trunk behind on the floor. Leaving it on the floor is very different to keeping it on the floor. One implies a reduction of effort, and the other triggers an increase in tension.

Take care also with the insidious and confidence eroding "try to ...," which precedes so many instructions. This automatically implies that there is some uncertainty about the outcome. Doubt creeps in. To counter the doubt, the person prepares to make a bigger effort, which, in turn, amplifies their tension.

The most devastating combination is, "Try to control your ..." This set phrase reflects the conventional model of physical development, which is founded on an assumption of necessary struggle to succeed.

When beginning with this mindset, it is hard to evolve toward freedom of motion. Make it easier by dropping this phrase from your vocabulary.

Giving up these terms asks for a higher level of skill as a practitioner – it requires a deeper understanding of the movement itself, and a more creative and insightful approach to expressing the intention of the movement.

In the words of Yoda, "Do, or do not. There is no try."

Clarity of intention

Ideally, we would like to strengthen associations within the brain that help a person to more easily execute a movement in a certain way. The primary motor and premotor cortex respond with greater excitation to positive cues ("do") than negative ones ("don't do").[33] This should make many professionals pause – how many times might we use a cue that involves what *not* to do in a movement?

Clarifying the intention of a movement is one of the most liberating things you can do for a person. Many of the people I encounter begin an exercise with their heads full of movements that they are trying to prevent and no clear vision of the movement impulse that they actually want to perform. Rather than committing to the movement, they resist it in an attempt to maintain control. There is no joy and no richness to this as a movement experience.

For example, a young violinist with significant wrist and arm pain told me that she struggled to stop the bow from moving sideways on the strings. She was very clear about what she didn't want to happen, and the resulting tension was increasing her problems. I was curious to find out where she actually wanted the bow to go. This required a pause, as this wasn't usually the way she thought about the movement.

For the two weeks between appointments, this is all I wanted her to do: to simply clarify in her mind where she wanted the bow to go, and follow it.

The result? Everything improved greatly. As she said herself, it seems so obvious, and yet so completely counter to how she had been approaching her movement. The lesson for her was simple: instead of fighting what you don't want, how about focusing on what you do want?

Your brain is capable of extraordinary feats of calculation and calibration if you learn how to work with it. It responds to intention, but frequently our intentions are not as defined as we think they are, at least from the brain's perspective.

> Cue for what you do want, rather than focusing the mind on what you don't.

There are several key elements that can refine intention.

1. If you want to move, then move! Frequently, people don't realize that their approach to movement is like dipping one toe into a warm bath but never actually stepping in. They hold back or fight the movement, mistaking this for control. They need help to let the handbrake off, by understanding that movement is something to go forward into, not something to hold back from. When you push your arms through your sweater sleeves, your intention is channeling forward into the motion. Your mind and body are positively and purposefully committing to the movement. You are not afraid of losing control, nor even aware of controlling the movement – you just have a clear intention.

    If someone has pain, caution is understandable, so it is important to choose the right level of challenge to encourage them to psychologically and emotionally move forward into exploration.

2. Clearly see the line of motion. One of my clients was tall, hypermobile, and struggling with chronic anterior knee pain. Stairs were very challenging for her, so we decided to investigate this together. Unsurprisingly, as she attempted to step up, her knee fell inwards, her foot rolled flat, and the rest of her body more or less crumpled over the leg as a result. Although we had already awakened some of the reflexive connections necessary, the step-up movement had not yet responded.

    With her foot on a step placed in front of a mirror, I asked her to begin by visualizing a colored line of light running up through her leg from foot to hip. Her job was to follow this line of light straight forward and upward. She realized that prior to this, she hadn't had a clear understanding of the movement intention for this task – she had rules for where her body parts should be, and her efforts had mostly been directed at trying to control her hip and knee with great determination, but this had not translated into the idea of a movement itself. In her next step up, she followed the imaginary colored line in her mind's eye, identifying when it was pushed out of shape, and then being delighted that she could change the shape of the line during the movement to move cleanly forward and upward onto the step. Seeing and sensing a direction of motion rather than fighting for specific knee or hip joint position allowed something to change in her nervous system.

3. Invoke movement quality when crafting intention. The brain doesn't so much work on the question, "What is this?" but on the basis of, "What is this like?" so that it can find an existing comparison within its vast libraries.[34] Use this knowledge to enrich intention. Does the

movement invite the sinuous lightness of quicksilver, or the rich fullness of hot toffee? Are you like mist upon the ground, or an ancient boulder filled with the wisdom of the ages? Does the impulse move through you like a tumbling river, or settle as effortlessly as a still mountain lake?

Be as relevant as you can. One of my musician clients played much better when thinking of water cascading down her arm to wash away her tension, but another violinist was not visual at all. Wait … this is a musician. What if an auditory association made a more effective connection? She was quick to identify that her bowing arm felt like it was full of a loud, discordant piece, played with lots of brass and percussion, but when she then imagined a sonata that represented qualities of smoothness and harmony, her movement quality changed completely. The associations triggered motor change.

In my athlete clients, I might choose to ask whether they channel a rhinoceros or a panther. Each has distinctive qualities to their movement, each effective in their own way. However, so many of my clients are training like rhinos but hoping to move like panthers. Focusing the image harvests associations from across the brain, linking together qualities that clarify intention and can aid movement execution.

4. Make it look easy. When movement has always been a struggle, people think that they have to fight hard to move. Sometimes people want to please you by making their effort visible. These thoughts trigger a neural pattern based on tension, and no matter how much you instruct, the movement fails to improve. Expose that thought and replace it with this single sentence. Make it look easy.

Power points

- The brain is responsive, malleable, and versatile. Learning how it functions helps you as a teacher of movement to communicate with a person's nervous system more effectively.

- Our brains are predicting the future based on our past. Change is made in the present. If you want to help someone to make change, we need to ground them in the present by learning to sense themselves.

- Don't be satisfied with just finding a different mechanical cue – enrich the learning, and help people to really own that movement by guiding them in how to feel it. Right from the beginning, you have the opportunity to move the brain.

Dancing with forces 3

Physics: it isn't just rocket science.

In high school and at university, I struggled with physics. I just didn't connect with calculating trajectories of bullets, strain on inanimate objects, and relative velocities between cars. It wasn't until much later into my career that I realized that I worked with physics every single day, and it was not just easy, it was fun! It isn't all rocket science after all – it is the fundamental common sense that underpins our human movement, and it has allowed me to explain things to clients in ways that make simple sense to them. Let me show you how …

Movement is a constant dance with forces. Every movement, no matter how small, involves a process that both creates and controls forces. From the simple act of quiet breathing right through to high-performance activities, our strategies for managing forces will determine the effectiveness of our movement, and the influence of that movement on our body structures.

Just to walk around, we encounter not only the downward press of gravity but the upward ground reaction force on our body with every foot strike. We withstand force when it is applied from the outside, for example, when we are bumped or jostled in a crowd. We understand how to exert a force upon an object in order to open a door, lift a grocery bag, or throw a ball. In fact, most of us are actually pretty successful on a day-to-day basis at working with forces, and although they are often looked upon as something to battle against, they are actually needed to stimulate positive adaptation and efficiency in the body.

Varying in their magnitude and direction, forces get our bodies moving. When we see powerful, expressive movement, we unconsciously discern the use of just the right amount of force – neither too much nor too little – applied in a clearly directed path. The first key to analyzing the effectiveness of a person's movement is therefore simple yet richly nuanced: do they create enough or too much force, and is it moving in the right direction?

When force is applied to our body structures, they experience load. Depending upon our movement habits, certain body structures will experience more load than others. Our clever brains send resources to wherever in the body they are most needed, and will also withdraw them from areas that are not regularly stressed. If the body detects that load is applied to it regularly in certain places, it will act to better support them.[1-5] Therefore, if your muscles are pulling on your bones, and your skeleton is experiencing regular demands in terms of weight-bearing exercise, your body responds by increasing bone density where it is most needed. This is positive adaptation.

In terms of ageing, this has very interesting implications. By now, we have all grasped that too much sitting creates a host of problems, and that we need to get onto our feet and experience gravity for bone health. However, we also need to keep lifting, pulling, and pushing to stimulate the bones of our spines and upper bodies. A balance of guided loading experiences for the upper body is invaluable.

It isn't just our bones that change through positive adaptation: recent research has identified thicker, more robust intervertebral discs in regular runners than non-runners,[6] which overturns the old assumption that repetitive impact hastens degeneration. Research on not just elite athletes but also elderly people has demonstrated that our tendons achieve greater structural integrity in response to regular loading.[7,8]

To build muscle, the body must be exposed to some form of stress beyond what it is accustomed to. To improve our cardiovascular fitness, we need to move sufficiently beyond our normal rate to provoke our hearts to beat faster. Clearly, our bodies are designed to need a degree of moderate but regular stress in order to adapt in a positive, healthy manner.

> What an extraordinarily encouraging message: our bodies are constantly listening to our needs, and doing their best to meet them.

Forces propel us through our environment, and allow us to exert our will upon the objects around us. Our ability to manage and direct forces by moving effectively determines whether they are a source of physical ease or daily challenge in our lives. When we don't manage forces effectively, we can experience too much load, too frequently for the body to adequately adapt and repair, and this can create musculoskeletal stress. We begin to experience load as a threat: a source of potential injury.

However, if we learn to create, move, control, and disperse forces effectively, we can positively influence the experience of load on our body structures.

> Our bodies need to experience load to flourish. Forces apply load to the body. How well we manage these loading forces influences their positive or negative potential on our body structures.

To achieve this, we must understand where a movement should begin in the body to most effectively create force, and how to use the coordinated and beautifully timed motion of one body segment upon another throughout our kinetic chain to transmit this energy with clear directional intent through the body.

Functional Force Management

The implications of force on a person's body is determined by how they use themselves.

To reveal this, the concept of *Functional Force Management*®[G] provides a simple outline for individual movement analysis that can be applied to people at any level of function.

We want to know:

1. How effectively is the movement created?

2. How effectively are forces shared over a large surface area?

3. How effectively are forces transmitted through the body?

4. How effectively are forces released from the body?

Creating movement

When looking at a movement, the first thing to identify is where in the body it begins. There are multiple ways to begin any given movement, and these variations will influence how that movement unfolds.

This involves not just the biomechanics of the movement, but also the conceptualization that someone has of the movement. For example, to throw a ball effectively, the force is initiated from the ground upward, by stepping forward and engaging the legs to create a pulse of energy. This pulse is transmitted up from the lower body to the central torso as the pelvis turns, which facilitates our rib cage to revolve, until finally, the force is channeled out through the arm to propel the ball. Some people do this naturally – they understand intuitively where the movement starts, and allow it to progress through their whole body.

Others, however, identify throwing a ball as an arm movement. Their body is left behind, and the movement begins and ends in the shoulder itself, amplifying the load this joint must bear as it attempts to create and control a whole body's worth of force on its own. The person's perception of the movement drives their biomechanics. The biomechanical problem will not resolve into fluency until the person understands that the arm is the end of a whole body movement, and that their hand as it releases the ball is the very tip of a ringmaster's whip when it cracks. The movement begins in the legs, and is completed from the hand.

Ask yourself, either when you are teaching another or practicing yourself: where should the impulse for this movement spring from? It seems too obvious, too simplistic a question, and yet … when you really think about it, sometimes you realize that a secure beginning point is not quite clear. We may be focusing on the control of the movement, or the joints and muscles involved, but these aspects change entirely depending upon where the movement begins.

Movement exploration

In standing, lift both arms toward the ceiling. Note how this feels in your body, and what body parts you are aware of. Become aware of the rhythm of the movement.

Now, think about the movement beginning in your feet, and draw the impulse up through your body and out through your fingertips as they stretch toward the ceiling. What is that like? Can you feel a change in the rhythm of the movement as it passes through your body?

Return your focus to simply lifting your arms. It should be easier to feel now that this movement holds within it a sense of restriction that is focused in the shoulders and upper back.

Now start the movement from your feet again. Can you feel that the restriction is removed, the load in the shoulders reduced, and the need for resistance diminished?

Can you feel that one movement is, well … workmanlike, while the other is elegant?

In most movements, drawing the impulse through the body from a clear start point creates greater connection, smoother transmission, and improved efficiency. It may be the most powerful key for some people to find both their power and their grace.

For a movement to be fluent, powerful, and effective, we must clearly understand where it needs to begin in order to initiate the energy that will drive the motion. Everything that manifests in the movement after that moment is a response to that choice.

Point of preparation

In the space between our decision to move and the actual movement, is a preparation phase. The brain sends lightning-fast messages to different muscle groups to prepare for the moment of movement, a phenomenon called feedforward activation.[9]

If all is well, this automatic response primes the body transiently, the muscles holding no longer nor more strongly than is necessary as they coordinate their roles with the wider cast of players as the movement progresses.

However, sometimes our system is not so well calibrated, and it develops a "persistent *point of preparation*[G]" in the body. This is the area that reacts first to the impulse to move, and remains active throughout the movement, indicating that it is a key strategy for achieving stabilization. These points tend to keep holding on, often strongly even after the movement has been completed. As they are usually not physiologically suited to sustain this level of contraction, the involved muscles soon become sore and tight.

Common persistent points of preparation include the jaw or mouth, which tighten with tension; the upper neck, which shortens and compresses itself below the skull; the shoulders, which can either lift upward using upper trapezius or hunch forward using the pectorals; the shoulder blades pinning back with the rhomboids; the lower back contracting into a deeper lordosis; the hips closing into fixed flexion; or the inner thighs pulling inward. You might observe it as a catching of the breath. You will even see it in the feet, which tighten and claw at the ground as if trying to dig holes with the toes to gain purchase. All of these strategies indicate the body's attempt to create a platform of stability, but they are actually immobilization strategies. Once locked in, it is very hard to let them go as the movement proceeds, which limits

> **Common persistent points of preparation**
>
> - Suboccipital muscles
> - Upper trapezius
> - Shoulder blades: rhomboids
> - Facial/jaw muscles
> - Lumbar muscles
> - Hip flexors
> - Hip adductors
> - Toe and foot muscles
> - Breath

the fluency of the movement, and loads these muscles and the structures they connect to. Their action is that of compression, the pulling together of joints.

These are the muscles and joints that people seek to relieve through massage, stretching, and manipulation. However, passive treatments can only ever offer temporary relief – the person must learn a more dynamic strategy for movement preparation if they are to overcome this pattern and alleviate their discomfort.

> Is a repeatedly identified tight, sore area signaling a persistent point of preparation that needs attention?

As we learned in Chapter 2, disrupting a person's habitual preparation movement opens the door for something new to occur. If the person is prevented from locking down their system with their customary strategy, the nervous system is stimulated to find a new solution. So how do we address unhelpful points of preparation?

You can address a dysfunctional point of preparation by introducing a specific awareness cue prior to the movement, and emphasizing this focus throughout the movement. It is important to understand that this is a releasing cue, not a counter-lock with an opposing muscle group.

For example, teaching someone to tuck their chin in to address a poked chin or compressed neck is quite common. However, this is a counter-lock, which is simply replacing one lock with another (see Figs. 3.1 and 3.2). The chin tuck may change the position of the head on the neck, but it is a cosmetic rather than a functional change because it is just a new fixed control point. This doesn't demand change elsewhere in the wider landscape of the body. If, however, you cue to release the lock at the back of the neck, the brain is encouraged to find a new neuromuscular solution for control. If you are not locking in the neck, then the wider body must reorganize itself for stability. Neurons fire like crazy, new sensations emerge, and the exercise experience changes.

> Releasing a persistent point of preparation asks the body to seek a new neuromuscular possibility. Replacing one fixed point with another may create a more pleasing alignment, but have no wider impact on the efficiency of the performance.

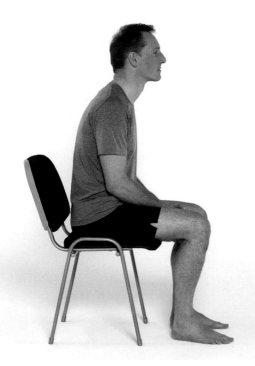

Figure 3.1

Forward head or "poke chin" posture locks at the back of the upper neck

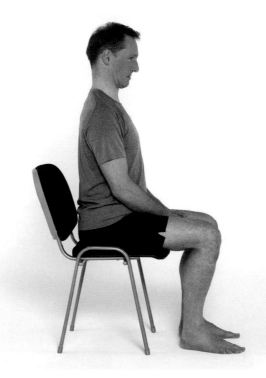

Figure 3.2

Overcorrected "chin in" posture locks the front of the upper neck

How might we address this issue then? Perhaps, if we take face-down postures as an example, we might encourage opening the neck and shoulders by imagining being lifted by the scruff of the neck as a cat will pick up a kitten (see Fig. 3.3). It is a cue of kindness and support, an encouragement to let go of the lock to change the entire neuromuscular landscape for the movement. Relieving the tight shortening in the back of the neck and the upper shoulder muscles has a global effect, allowing the scapular stabilizers, rotator cuff, and abdominal muscles to become more available (see Figs. 3.4 and 3.5).

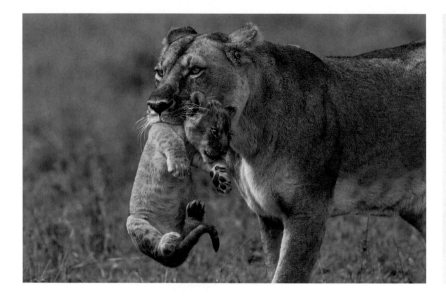

Figure 3.3

Imagine being lifted by the scruff of your neck

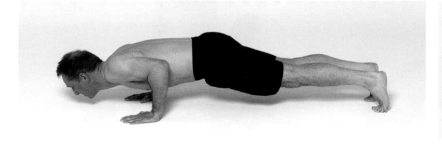

Figure 3.4

Compressed neck compromising trunk and shoulder function

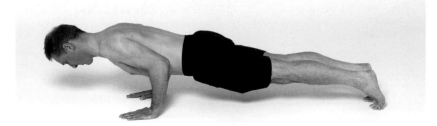

Figure 3.5

Decompressed neck allowing the body to open and lengthen

It may be simpler still. The locking at the back of the neck is often associated with looking forward. Imagine looking at the floor instead as if gazing at your reflection in a pool of water. "Looking at the floor" can increase neck tension, but the image of seeing your whole face in the water creates a softer and subtler change to the carriage of the head on the neck.

> Run a little scan through your familiar instructions. Are there any counter-lock cues lurking there? Can you instead think of images or metaphors that invite the release, spreading, lengthening, or opening of the compressed body parts? Play with these, and feel how the body pays attention and starts to adjust.

Look for the common points of preparation, and when you see them, pause the movement before continuing, draw the person's awareness to the tightened area, and invite them to see how they can open and release it for themselves. A simple smile, a sigh to release a held breath, and an invitation to find some space in that area may be sufficient to make the difference.

Allow time and space for experiencing this new movement set up by minimizing the distraction of other instructions, at least for the first repetitions. Then you can offer a nudge of extra input, a little at a time, if necessary.

Sometimes we do this beautifully, but then forget our brain science and fall into the old habit of engaging the cognitive brain with too many instructions that tangle the mind. But how do we instruct without too many instructions?

Having given a person a sense of where the movement originates, we can cue using a further aspect of creating the movement, which is the expression of movement impulse in the body. Look at this picture of children performing a reach and balance exercise (see Fig. 3.6). Can you see that every child except one is

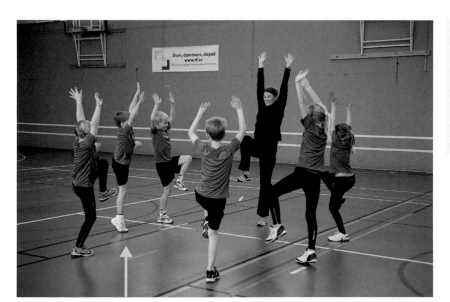

Figure 3.6

The child indicated demonstrates the "up" impulse

From Elphinston J. Basträning för barn, 2011. Sweden: SISU Idrottsböcker. With permisssion

exhibiting a downward impulse? Their hips and knees are bent and their bodies are moving toward the floor even though the task is to reach up high. One child, however, has nailed it. Everything about his movement emphatically says "up." He is the only one to automatically fire up the coordinative pattern that has created extension from his feet all the way up through his body. Even in a still frame, you can clearly see the difference between the two movement impulses.

Just because our mind has an idea of where it wants to go, it doesn't mean that the body knows how to express that idea. In fact, we frequently and very effectively get in our own way, sometimes naturally but sometimes due to a coaching cue that has interfered with the natural movement strategy.

Let's take walking, for example. If you ask someone which way they want to move as they walk, they will answer "forward" very easily. Yet many people do not exhibit that impulse at all: some lurch from side to side while others collapse their sternum, which compresses them at the waist and dumps their weight into their heels. As they walk, gravity is falling toward the back of their bodies. They are actually exhibiting a backward impulse, and they move as if having to pull themselves against an invisible bungee cord around their middles.

Yet if we introduce a forward impulse, we can change this gait entirely. First, we need to release the invisible handbrake, by floating the head upward to decompress the spine, unload the hips, and lift the sternum. Then we instruct the person to simply lean their whole body forward a little until they roll toward the front of their feet to trigger themselves to step. To a normally compressive walker, this feels as though they are falling forward, and everything seems to move much faster. In reality, they are simply upright and moving more efficiently, having lost the backward tug. Using a forward impulse, they are surprised to find that they can walk much faster without trying.

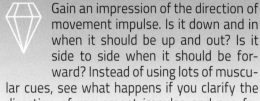
Gain an impression of the direction of movement impulse. Is it down and in when it should be up and out? Is it side to side when it should be forward? Instead of using lots of muscular cues, see what happens if you clarify the direction of movement impulse and cue for this instead.

Rotation is another prime example. When thinking about rotation, many people strain to turn their upper body, or turn their torso as a single block. They comprehend the concept of rotation, but are caught in the idea of trying to turn their shoulders and chest. It becomes much easier when they think of a spiral that radiates outwards from deep in the pelvis toward the head, the enlarging rings of the spiral shape reflecting the increasing rotational availability in the joints. The impulse experience is then "out of the pelvis," rather than "around in the upper body." The same would apply in seated positions, whether sitting on the floor or on a chair for a seated rotational stretch: if a person thinks upward through the crown of the head, with a spiral starting at the base of the spine, they create an axis to more easily rotate around (see Fig. 3.7).

Working with movement impulse is a sophisticated and streamlined approach to teaching. Learning to see and cue it effectively allows our clients' marvelous brains to make the necessary calculations for coordinating a new neuromuscular pattern. Teaching the overarching sense of the movement allows the cerebellum to make its complex adjustments unimpeded by the sluggish interference of too much conscious thought.

The brain is far smarter and more sophisticated than our conscious self. Our job is to set up the conditions for it to be able to do what it does best, and get out of the way.

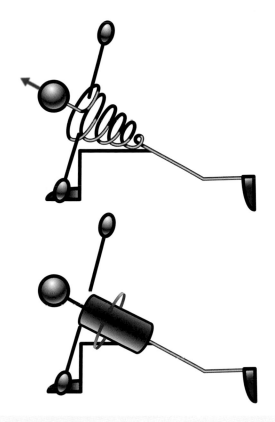

Figure 3.7

To overcome a blocked sensation in the spine when rotating (lower image), imagine the motion emerging from the base of the spine (top image)

Sharing forces

Whether we talk about bridges, buildings, or bodies, the principle of sharing forces is the same. The bigger the surface area you can share a force over, the less load you apply to any one area.

The formula is simple: Stress = Force/Area.

That's physics again, isn't it? Yes it sure is, and you are going to become a master of it, because it is the route to power production in movement, and the key to understanding overload and over-use in the body, which is a common source of pain and injury.

Let's take an example in just one area of the body. If you were to lift a heavy load with your upper limb, you would need to transfer forces between the central body and the arm. The central body must support the muscle pull needed to create a movement. There are, however, a number of different possibilities for doing this. We could choose to support the load of the arm by using the muscles linking the scapula to the relatively small structures of the neck, as happens when we elevate or "hunch" the shoulder. Long, strap-like muscles such as levator scapulae are not suited to sustained loading, and the structures of the neck offer only a small surface area to bear a load, so it is not surprising that people with this strategy experience neck and upper back pain as well as the painful muscle knots that arise when a muscle is asked to perform a role for which it is not well designed (see Fig. 3.8).

Fortunately, we have alternatives.

The attachments offered by the middle and lower fibers of the trapezius and the serratus anterior give us access to our robust rib cage and more substantial segments of the spine. This is a huge area, and if we understand how to access this strategy, we bring the forces to structures that are not only more substantial themselves but also allow connection to the rest of the body below via a network of myofascial connections. Now we can lift a load with support from the whole body, not just the neck – that really is using Stress = Force/Area! (see Fig. 3.9).

Were you wondering about upper trapezius in this example? It can contribute in both strategies, but it can choose how it wants to play, and that choice will determine its action. If it chooses to play with levator scapulae as it draws the scapula upward, upper trapezius will tend to exert a downward pull on the base

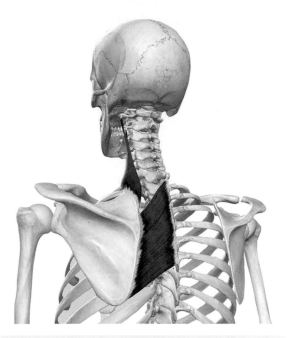

Figure 3.8

Load being supported by the relatively small surface area provided by the smaller vertebrae of the neck and upper back

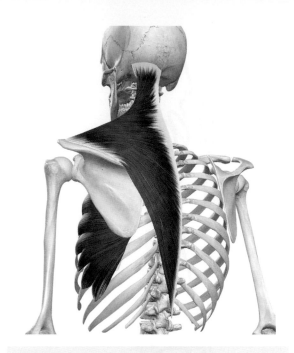

Figure 3.9

Load being supported over the large surface provided by the rib cage and more robust mid-back vertebrae

of the skull, amplifying the compression of the neck structures as the upper neck extends. If, however, it decides to play with the muscles connecting to the thorax, it helps to upwardly rotate the scapula as the arm lifts, increasing the biomechanical efficiency of the shoulder movement and helping to avoid impingement. Our bodies always have choices.

Transmitting forces through the body

One of the ways that we can share forces over an even larger surface area is to transmit them through the body.

We experience less load on any specific body structure or area if we can reduce the amount of time that force is being applied to it. Moving forces through the body is one of the ways that we can do this, and,

even better, it is also one of the ways that we can be more efficient, as it allows us to utilize our myofascial system.

Force transmission allows us to use bigger, stronger parts of our body to initiate a movement impulse and then to move this force through the body to other areas. This gives the biggest role to the region most suited to bear it, and reduces the muscle effort needed in any specific area. For example, to hit an effective tennis forehand with good technique, the energy is created in the powerful legs, and via the spiraling action of first the pelvis and then the thorax, that energy is transmitted all the way out through the arm, from which it is released. The robustly muscled legs are well designed to perform this role. If the player has poor force transmission, however, perhaps due to inadequate pelvic or thoracic rotation, they have no alternative but to make up the deficit by using their hitting arm more. Now the arm must withstand much higher loading relative to the size of its smaller muscles, ligaments, and tendons. Injury risk rises for no performance benefit, as the arm alone cannot generate the power that the legs are capable of.

When you are making up your bed with clean linen and need to shake out that sheet to cover the mattress, you can use the same principle: if you stiffen your body, you will use the muscles of your shoulders and neck to create the force, but if you softly bend your hips and knees a little, you will create a push from the feet that transmits up through your body and out through your hands, releasing the force to float that sheet out in front of you with ease (see Fig. 3.10)

It is not just the light and easy movements where this applies: the same principles apply using battle ropes

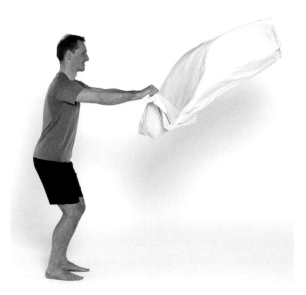

Figure 3.10

Forces transmitting through the body and releasing out through the hands

in the gym. Many people brace their bodies against the load of the ropes, eliminating the potential offered by their legs, and thereby increasing the demand on their shoulders. Some even bob up and down with their knees, assuming that this energy will somehow make it past their rigid midsection. Ultimately, though, the ropes should mirror the ripple of energy moving up through the body, and this can only be achieved by sinking the body into the feet, transforming the legs from tense to elastic, and allowing their energy to transmit up and out through the hands.

> Force transmission allows us to use the bigger body parts to do the most work, and to reduce the stress on the smaller body parts.

To transmit this energy with clear directional intention through the body requires the coordinated and beautifully timed motion of one body segment upon another throughout our kinetic chain. If we block the motion somewhere in this chain, it will cause trouble nearby.

Think of the force that moves through your body as being like a river, and that each joint in your body represents a solid gate in the river that must open to allow the water to flow through. Each gate must open at just the right time after the one before it to let the river continue to flow smoothly. Imagine then, in the case of an actual river, that one of these gates gets stuck. What happens to the water? The river keeps flowing, so the water keeps accumulating, throwing itself at the gate until – under the strain – either the gate gives way or the river diverts to find another route.

This is not so different to the effect of force on the human body. If one of our body segments doesn't move enough, or at the right time, we block force transmission. Our clever brain wants to solve whatever movement objective we have decided upon, so it tries to find a way to get around the problem, often diverting forces or amplifying them on certain structures. This works for a while, but rarely as efficiently, and, eventually, the body structures that have had to cope with the diverted force start to complain.

It could be a simple problem, perhaps one of joint stiffness or muscle flexibility. The person may simply not have enough mobility to move that body part adequately. This is the relatively easy problem to fix, and most health and fitness professionals have a collection of potential solutions for this.

However, sometimes the mobility could be available, but the person cannot access it. They feel stiff and look stiff, but the issue is not so much in their tissues as in their nervous system. The culprit is *held tension*[G]. Held tension causes holding or blocking of forces in the body instead of allowing them to move freely. It also prevents us from both transmitting and releasing forces from the body, and when forces stop moving, they stop working for us and start working against us.

Sometimes held tension is naturally occurring. It may arise due to stress, for example, or for basic physical reasons. Poor balance and inadequate sensory feedback cause the muscles to contract strongly in multiple sites in the body as it seeks a way to sense itself and maintain control.

Three tips for held tension:

Create the opportunity for improved mobility of each body part relative to the next by lightly scanning the body for areas that may be holding tension. This kind of activity often happens lying down at the end of a class, but if introduced in standing or sitting at the beginning instead, along with a little relaxed breathing, it will enhance the potential for better movement within the session.

Stimulate sensation with brisk rubbing of the feet and body in a warm up. When the brain can better detect where the body is in space, and in relationship to itself, it does not need the noisy muscular feedback created by muscle tension. It also dependably triggers a smile.

Aim to make it look easy. Setting the intention for each movement to be effortless, regardless of the level of load or challenge, actively encourages a release of held tension. Less held tension leads to smoother muscle length change, which in turn achieves a freer flow of force between body segments.

Releasing forces

Releasing held tension not only unlocks our ability to transmit force but also to release it from our body. This is the fourth principle of Functional Force Management, and it is essential for both performance and health.

Excessive muscle tension holds forces in the body tissues, exposing them to greater stress. When landing from a jump, for example, allowing the hips, knees, and ankles to shock absorb releases the landing force into the ground. If we block this action, the full impact is either stored in the lower body, usually the knees, or it is pushed up into the spine.

Similarly, arm or hand tension can block the outward flow of force through the upper limb in a full body movement, whether you are throwing, punching, or hitting a ball. Your power potential is reduced when that force is trapped in the arm tissues instead of releasing it out through the wrist and hand, and the tendons, ligaments, and muscles of the arm are placed under greater stress.

> Create the force, and then unleash it. There's no need to hold it in your body.

Trained tension

Although held tension is often a naturally occurring response, sometimes it has been consciously learned. This is what happens when posture is seen simply as alignment, and the principles of normal movement are not fully understood. Actively maintaining the scapulae in a retracted position interferes with the biomechanical relationship between the shoulder and the thorax. Holding tension in the quadriceps or gluteals deeply affects the mobility relationship between hip and pelvis. Too much tension held in the core is

one of the biggest blocks to natural movement, as it affects the relative motion between two of our biggest body segments, the pelvis and the thorax. Far from being protective, sustained active abdominal setting is fundamentally disruptive to the restoration or expression of normal movement.

This is the troubled interface between natural movement and many training methods. Over the next few chapters, we will reconcile this potential conflict, because within each movement discipline lies the seeds for natural movement that with a little additional knowledge, can bear exceptional fruit.

Power points

- Every day we dance with forces. Using them as resources rather than viewing them as threats opens the opportunity to save energy and prevent stress on the body.

- For power and for grace, we must be masters at creating, controlling, directing, and releasing forces.

By design we have power and resilience beyond our imagining ...

Visualize your entire body encased in a stretchy superhero suit: a suit made of strong yet supple superfine threads that penetrate through every layer of your body. The threads reach between each bone, muscle, and organ, such that your internal body is suspended in a web of supportive tension that is as finely balanced as a spider's web yet as strong as the slender wires securing a ship's mast in the wind.

*Fascia*G is this web of connective tissue that envelops us, connecting, reinforcing, and supporting our muscles and organs. It is both protective and performance enhancing, buffering the effects of forces on the body, reducing the muscular effort required to carry ourselves,[1] and a key factor in producing power beyond what our muscles could achieve alone. It is remarkably responsive to our activities, becoming less elastic and mobile if we do not move sufficiently, yet as with our other body structures, willing to improve when exposed to regular movement and loading through exercise.[2]

Our myofascial web adheres to the principles of Functional Force Management. When our muscles contract, the force created is communicated out into the surrounding fascia, distributing that pressure over a larger surface area.[3] This not only shares and disperses force to minimize tissue stress[4] but positively influences the balance of supportive tension in the system. The resulting dance of coordinated pulls between our muscles, fascia, and the skeleton embedded within them is called *tensegrity*G.

Fascia is highly involved in the principle of force transmission through the body, via our elastic energy mechanism. This mechanism is another demonstration of our body's design for efficiency: if we have gone to the trouble of creating force potential, we want to be sure that we make the most of it. As body parts move away from one another, the tissues connecting them start to stretch and the entire myofascial relationship stores energy in the same way as an elastic band does when we pull on it. Once we have stored this elastic energy, then we can release it to move the body part back in the opposite direction swiftly and smoothly, with less requirement for muscular effort.[5,6]

You have experienced this: brisk walking feels far more invigorating and much less tiring than ambling idly around a shopping center. This is because your body segments are moving through larger ranges of motion, creating greater pulls on your myofascial structures and allowing them to store and release elastic energy to propel you forward. Without the benefit of this elastic mechanism, greater muscle effort is required, and the body experiences more overall load.

If, due to held tension, our body parts cannot move relative to one another sufficiently, this capacity for elastic energy and force transmission is lost. In our classes and programs, we have the opportunity to balance and enhance the possibilities for force transmission by addressing this. To improve the fluency, flow, and power output of our bodies, we need to understand the principles of Functional Force Management.[7]

One body, many solutions

A great place to start the exploration of Functional Force Management is the central body, the so-called core, which offers multiple options for force management. It is an area subject to significant conflict between the various movement ideologies, and ideas about the "right way" to train this area are often at odds with the expression of natural movement itself. To unpick the tangle of arguments, we must first understand that there is no single correct way for us to use our central body.

Just considering the abdominal muscles alone, it is obvious that there is no single general-purpose solution. When bumped or jostled in a crowd, or standing on a moving, swaying bus or train, we need to allow the rapid, unexpected forces acting upon us to be able to move through us like wind through long grass if we are to regain our equilibrium. This requires finely tuned, intricately timed adjustments in multiple parts of our bodies, including rapid, coordinated, low-level activation in our abdominal wall. If we are running a marathon, however, our abdominal wall is engaged in continuously transmitting forces between our lower and upper body, requiring the endurance to repeatedly lengthen and shorten in alternating diagonal patterns. In contrast, if we need to push a heavy load, our abdominal wall will activate more strongly with little or no abdominal muscle length change. This ensures that our rib cage is securely connected to our pelvis, forming a firm foundation for our arms and legs to pull from.

It is not one solution at varying strength levels. These are different neuromuscular patterns arising through different mechanisms.

Setting the stage

To understand these functional possibilities, we need to consider the planes of movement that the body uses in a seemingly infinite variety of combinations.

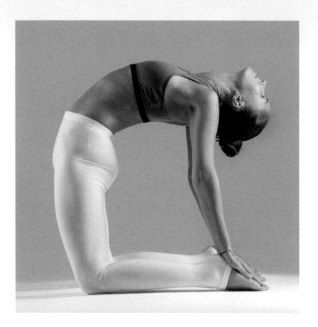

Figure 4.1

Sagittal plane

The sagittal plane is the plane of our flexion and extension actions, allowing us to bend forward and backward, to reach high with our arms, and drop low through our legs (see Fig. 4.1).

The frontal or coronal plane represents our side-bending actions as well as abduction and adduction of the limbs (see Fig. 4.2). It is a challenging plane: when we control it, it is exceptionally graceful, yet it is also the plane into which we most easily collapse.

The transverse plane is the plane of rotation (see Fig. 4.3). From our feet all the way up through our kinetic chain, our body uses rotation for stability, balance, and force transmission. We are deeply rotational creatures: even the act of walking involves rotation at every joint from the midfoot all the way up to the neck and shoulders. Our freedom to rotate throughout our body like this is uniquely human – no other creature has so many rotational possibilities – and we cannot move efficiently without it.

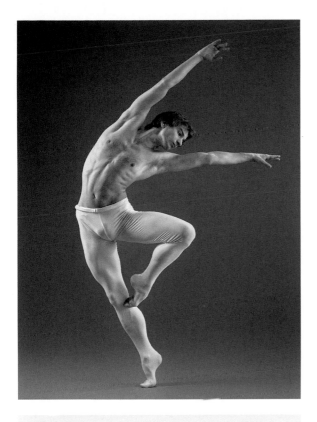

Figure 4.2

Frontal (coronal) plane

We blend these planes, varying both the proportion that each one contributes and the timing with which they are used, to allow a proliferation of possibilities. It is virtually impossible to comprehensively define what human movement is when we display such vast creativity and adaptability.

Getting in the zone

With the planes of movement under our belt, we can add the zone concept to build our understanding of central body force management. Imagine for a moment three large cylindrical building blocks resting on a platform where your legs meet your body (see Fig. 4.4). In this image, these blocks are firm but flexible, and a sticky, stretchy substance connects each to the next. The first of these blocks represents the lower zone, which encompasses your pelvis and hips. This creates a foundation of support for the body above it. Sitting upon the lower zone is the central zone, located between the top of the pelvis and the ribs. This acts as a connector between the upper and lower torso. Sitting on top of these two zones is the upper zone, which incorporates the structures of our shoulder girdle. These are our force management zones, but

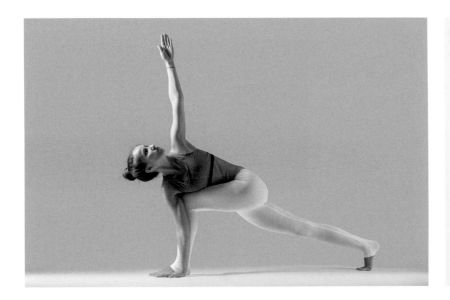

Figure 4.3

Transverse (rotational) plane

could as easily be referred to as control zones or power zones, depending upon the wording that resonates most with the person you are working with.

For force transmission over the wide range of activities that we can perform, we need to be able to maintain a connection between these zones, while allowing them to move independently of one another in a variety of planar combinations.

The most familiar of the central zone force management strategies is *zone stacking*. From dead bug exercises to planks, this is the concept most strongly

associated with core stability training and it has been the linchpin of low back pain rehabilitation for many years. Its purpose is to keep the zones connected in a consistent position, neither moving toward one another nor apart, and not turning relative to one another.

We use zone stacking, along with other force management strategies, in a wide variety of functions because it is particularly useful for establishing a consistent foundation from which to push or pull. For example, a cyclist who maintains his ribs and pelvis in a consistent, secure relationship ensures that his powerful legs channel downward pressure into the pedal, containing that energy between the hip and the foot rather than losing it up through his spine. Zone stacking will make pushing a load more effective by preventing the force created by the legs from escaping in any direction other than straight through the body and out through the arms. Whether we are pushing a shopping trolley, a car, a lawnmower, or just a heavy door, this is the most effective strategy to use (see Fig. 4.5).

We also use zone stacking transiently, as in a ballet pirouette where, after the initial momentum is created, the upper and lower body must be securely connected if the dancer is to turn quickly and accurately. In the same way, a discus thrower must move their trunk and pelvis as a single unit around a central axis in order

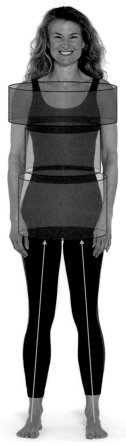

Figure 4.4

Force management zones

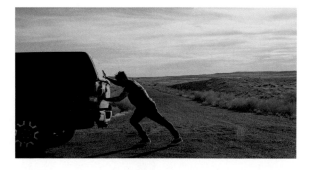

Figure 4.5

Zone stacking provides a direct line for force transfer from feet to hands in pushing tasks

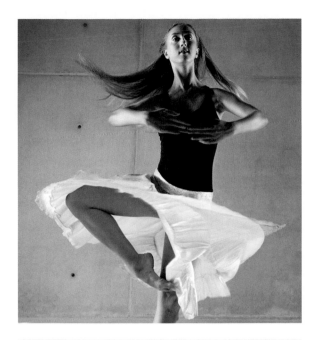

Figure 4.6

Zone stacking is essential for fast, efficient turning

to generate speed and power. In these cases, the zone stacking does not initiate the energy for the motion but helps to retain it for maximal efficiency (see Fig. 4.6).

When the loading demand is too high for the ability level of the person to control it, they find themselves pushed into the "suit of armor" strategy. In normal function, we use this strategy for body protection, rapidly increasing our central muscle tension to compress our zones together as we prepare to withstand a blow. The purpose of this strategy is to prevent excessive and potentially harmful joint motion, so it not only braces and compresses the trunk and neck but also tightens the flexor muscles of the vulnerable hips and shoulders, pulling them inwards. It is a normal response to threat, but should be transient. You may recognize that some people display the defensive, protective suit of armor strategy as their normal posture: they have become stuck in a threat response.

Due to the high energy cost of the muscle force it engages, and its purpose to restrict movement, the suit of armor should appear rapidly, and dissipate easily.

For those people who struggle to improve their flexibility despite dedicated practice, persistent use of the suit of armor strategy can be a key issue. It could be a physical response to exercise choices that are too highly loaded, an attitude of "trying hard" that induces excessive muscle activation, or stress-induced held tension that creates it. No amount of stretching, self-mobilizing, and massage will overcome this regular, sustained, habit of muscle shortening.

On the gym floor and in Pilates and yoga classes, a prolonged usage of the suit of armor can be seen when someone's body reacts defensively to a demand beyond their current control capabilities. The instructor may be aiming for an open, uncompressed posture in the trunk with full range of motion in the joints, but instead the person's torso seems to shorten, their neck pulls in, their shoulders, hips, and knees cannot release, and their abdominal wall may even tensely protrude. It is important to recognize this as a survival strategy rather than simply weakness. If we modify the task to marginally reduce the load, the brain can drop back out of defensive struggle mode and reach fully into the challenge to allow the person to improve more quickly. We are not teaching someone to simply withstand a position but to acquire mastery of a new neuromuscular pattern.

Take a load off

To reduce load, we need to apply a little more physics. Consider whether you are using a long lever or a short lever to apply force to the body. Not familiar with the concept? In closed chain work, this is the distance between the points where the body makes contact for support. For example, a full body plank, perhaps preparing for chaturanga or a press-up, has a relatively long distance between the two points of contact with the floor, the hands and the feet. Beginner exercisers experience this as high abdominal load, and it frequently provokes a suit of armor response.

Developing movement capability, however, is not simply trying to withstand a poor position for a longer duration. If we drop the knees to the floor, the distance between the hands and the knees is far less, reducing the load experienced in the shoulders and trunk. The person can then expand out, allowing their hips to straighten, their neck and spine to lengthen, and their shoulders and scapulae to settle into a supportive position. They experience the feeling of an efficient posture from which to move, and establish an excellent platform from which to progress (see Figs. 4.7 and 4.8).

In an open chain technique, the arms and legs act as levers against a stable trunk and pelvis. To either increase or decrease load on the body, note how far

the end of the moving body part is from the center of the body. When it is farther away, the load increases, and when it is closer, the load decreases. So, if you are lying on the floor and straighten one leg out, you are moving your foot away from your body. If you lift this straight leg, the lever arm is longer and therefore the load on the central body will be greater than if you were lifting with a bent knee.

For the same reason, hands at shoulder height applies less challenge to the trunk than extending them overhead. You can feel this for yourself: if you are working on back extensor strength while lying face down on a mat, compare the load when your hands are held level with your shoulders with your elbows bent, and then with your arms outstretched (see Figs. 4.9 and 4.10). When your hands are farther from your body, the load is magnified. For beginner exercisers, a shorter lever will make it possible to improve the quality of both

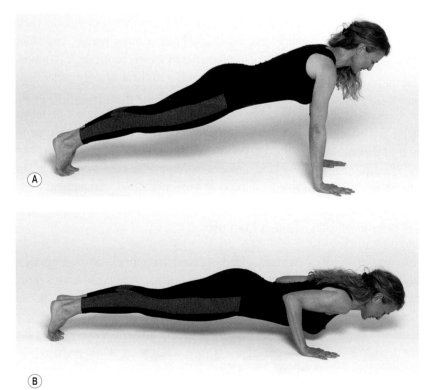

(A)

(B)

Figure 4.7

Long lever position applies high load to the abdominal muscles. *A.* Press-up start position. *B.* Finish position

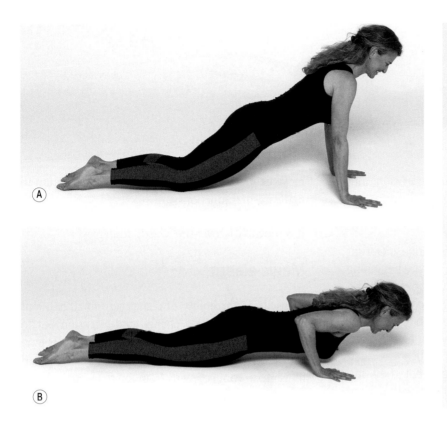

Figure 4.8

Shorter lever position reduces the load and allows the body to release its "suit of armor." response. *A.* Press-up start position. *B.* Finish position

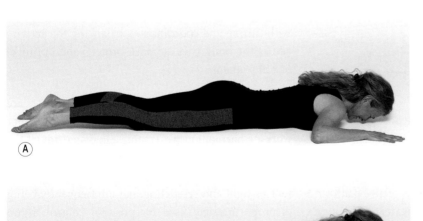

Figure 4.9

Prone extension. *A.* Start position. *B.* Short lever arms reduce the load

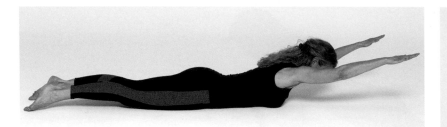

Figure 4.10

Long lever arms apply greater load to the shoulders and posterior surface of the body

their movement and their endurance before moving on to higher loading.

> To open the possibility for change, interrupt the suit of armor program before beginning by inviting an attitude of open, relaxed readiness prior to starting each movement or sequence. If you see someone caught in the suit of armor strategy during the task, adapt the technique to reduce the load on their body just enough that they can safely expand their capabilities with a more effective pattern.

> Cue the intention to make it look easy – this will allow the cerebellum to calculate the most efficient program for the task.

Suit of armor and zone stacking are both non-elastic strategies that limit joint motion. Suit of armor uses a transient burst of high muscle force for protection, while zone stacking uses a lower, more sustainable level of muscle activity to provide a secure platform for the limbs to push and pull against. Although zone stacking is often presented as the generic trunk stability solution, especially in low back rehabilitation, maintaining the spine in a single consistent "neutral" position simply isn't reflective of the array of movements that we perform in our normal lives. Zone stacking will actively inhibit effective, efficient

movement and limit full hip and shoulder motion in many normal functions.

It is time to discover the "elastic strategies."

Magic elastic

Elasticity is the ability of a structure to stretch and recoil – to undergo a change under tension but to return to its original state when released. This behavior actually underpins the majority of our human movement, connecting us from top to toe as we use it to move with natural efficiency.

We have diagonal, spiral, and linear myofascial relationships throughout our bodies, and when we move with timing and coordination, balancing the activity across the body, they support, protect, and optimize our movement.

There are certain stereotypical patterns that are commonly seen when these relationships are not working harmoniously.[8] Tracing a line up through the front of the body, rectus femoris, the hip flexors, upper rectus abdominis, pectorals, and scalenes often present as tight and restricting, but are frequently being disproportionately used for postural control. If we consider the entire anterior chain of muscles and fascia as one long, wide elastic band from the upper surface of our feet all the way up to deep in the throat, this will appear as though there are various pinch points of tension separated by areas of relative laxity or underactivity. To facilitate efficient movement, we must balance the forces across the entire chain, not by strengthening and stretching isolated muscles, but by altering the entire pattern of activation that we choose.

Similarly in the posterior chain, tight gastrocnemius, hamstrings, lumbar, and cervical erector spinae are common, with the hip extensors often struggling to participate. Again, it is not a simple case of stretching and strengthening: the way in which we use ourselves will determine the neuromuscular strategy we employ. If we don't coordinate our body segments adequately, some muscles will take on more of a role, and others less. Although this will eventually lead to weakness in muscles that don't get the opportunity to activate properly, and tightness in those required to hang on to provide support, these are secondary issues. If we don't get to the cause, the same stretch/strengthen/massage regimen will provide symptomatic relief but continue indefinitely. This is managing the problem, not transcending it.

As we move through the book from here on, we will discover a variety of similar relationships in function and dysfunction. To address them, we will be using natural movement principles to balance the myofascial relationships throughout the body.

The diagonal elastic strategy

This strategy involves rotating the lower zone in the opposite direction to the upper one, and it is the key to efficient walking and running. As we step forward with our left foot, the pelvis on the same side follows the foot forward, which turns the face of the pelvis to the right. We would call this rotation of the pelvis in the transverse plane. The upper body counter-rotates in the opposite direction to maintain our central balance point, and, in doing so, creates a diagonal stretch on the myofascial structures connecting the rib cage to the pelvis on both the front and the back of the body. This stores energy in the central zone that

can then be released for the next step. Forces are able to flow efficiently between the lower and upper body (see Fig. 4.11).

This mechanism enables us to involve myofascial relationships crossing multiple joints in long chains – ideal for storing and releasing energy. Considering the front of the body, you can appreciate the diagonal stretch created across the abdominal wall as the thorax and pelvis rotate against each other. Centrally, this is predominantly through the external and internal obliques

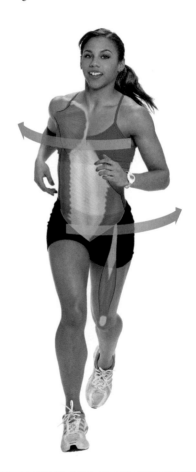

Figure 4.11

Counter-rotation of thorax and pelvis, setting up a diagonal myofascial relationship across the front of the body

working on opposite sides, and the stretch is further amplified both down the front of the thigh as the hip extends in push-off and across the pectorals and biceps on the opposite side as the chest and shoulder open.

Looking at the back of the body, the posterior oblique myofascial relationship is created between latissimus dorsi inserting into the strong, supportive thoracolumbar fascia on one side, and gluteus maximus (Gmax) connecting into it from the opposite side.[9] With such significant tensioning influences acting upon it, the diamond-shaped thoracolumbar fascia plays a key role in transferring forces between the legs, pelvis, spine, and upper body. It is tensioned in many directions by means of a range of other muscular connections; these include the deep abdominal layer of transversus abdominis, the erector spinae, and the short-fibred multifidus nestling in close to each vertebra. Even the hamstrings contribute, with fibers from biceps femoris merging with the sacrotuberous ligament, which ultimately blends with the broader fascial web across the pelvis (see Fig. 4.12).[10]

It is possible to appreciate from Figure 4.12 that, as the upper torso is turning left, and the left side of the pelvis is moving forward in counter-rotation, a diagonal stretch is set up across the back from the right shoulder across to the left hip, and extends still further down the back of the left leg to effectively store elastic energy for the next stride.

It is sometimes helpful to think of it as an alternating forward motion, rather than as a turning motion. One side of the pelvis advances forward with the foot on that side, while the shoulder of the opposite side also moves in the forward direction as your arm swings. This creates a mild twist in your middle. Then as you take your next step, the pelvis on that side is carried onward with the foot, while your opposite shoulder catches up and passes the other shoulder. On each step, the twisting action between your upper and lower body sends your body forward.

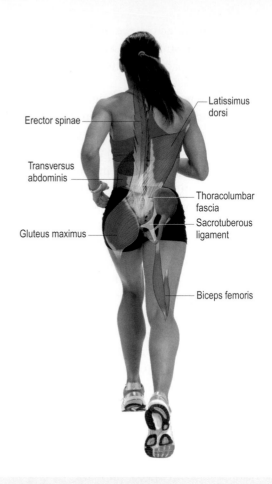

Figure 4.12

Diagonal myofascial relationship created by counter-body rotation

Movement exploration

Thigh Slide

A simple diagonal elastic preparation exercise, and one of my clients' absolute favorites, is the Thigh Slide, an easy technique to achieve independent movement of the upper zone on the lower zone while remaining connected. Begin in a relaxed upright position, seated on a chair with your hands resting on your thighs.

With your head facing forward, slide one hand away from you, allowing your chest to follow it into rotation. Notice how this draws the other hand back, with the shoulder following. Continue to alternate smoothly from side to side, letting the upper body turn easily in one direction and then the other. Feel how one side moves forward and then the other as the ribs turn (see Fig. 4.13). It is wise to check your movement in the mirror at first – you might be surprised to find that it is trickier than you think to separate your head and neck from your shoulder movement!

Real life study

A story of blocked diagonal elastic movement

My client, a runner, was struggling with Achilles problems. She ran with her shoulders pinned back and abdomen tense, and the overall quality of her movement was clipped and choppy. She did not counter-rotate at all, which made it impossible for her to transmit forces between her upper and lower body. Without this capability she could not access her elastic mechanisms, thus increasing the need for more muscular effort. In this case, it was the calves having to work harder to push her along. Stretching those tight calves did not alleviate her symptoms because she needed to relieve them of the need to over-work – by getting those forces to flow.

Think simply. What did this runner need? Simple rotational movements like the Thigh Slide enabled her to find the freedom between her upper and lower body, and to release the postural tension that was blocking her movement. Following on from this, the experience of carrying herself with postural ease allowed her to integrate her new rotation potential into her running, restoring a fluency and freedom to her gait. This increased efficiency meant the loading

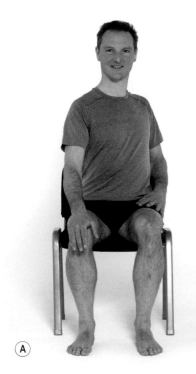
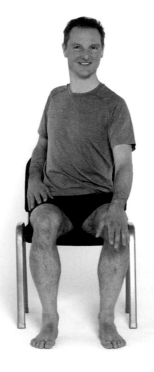

(A) (B)

Figure 4.13

A. Right thigh slide. *B.* Left thigh slide

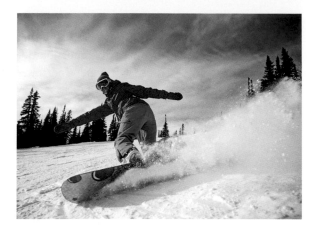

Figure 4.14

Snowboarder using the spiral elastic strategy

on her Achilles was reduced, and after a few sessions she observed with a sigh, "This is what it felt like when I used to enjoy running."

The spiral elastic strategy

This is the strategy that supports throwing a ball, swinging a golf club, or initiating a turn on a snowboard (see Fig. 4.14). It involves turning the upper and lower zones in the same direction, but with slightly different timing.

To feel this, stand with relaxed joints in your legs, and start to loosely move your whole body into rhythmic rotation, turning your body to first look around to the left, and then to the right. Allow your arms to swing naturally as you turn one way and then the other. Initially, you might turn as a block, but as you relax into the motion, feel for an increased awareness of the separation between your pelvis and your rib cage. Can you notice that the motion is initiated by your pelvis turning, which pulls your rib cage around

and creates the momentum that causes your arms to swing?

The timing separation comes *just as the direction changes*, where the pelvis starts to initiate the return movement while the upper body momentarily keeps going in the original direction. This creates a stretch between the two, which stores energy to be released for a faster, more efficient movement as the upper body then follows the pelvis in the new direction. This connection can be extended further across the abdominal fascia and down into the adductor group, as shown in the golf back swing (see Fig. 4.15). Can you see that if the left knee fell inwards, it would reduce the stretch potential of the entire chain?

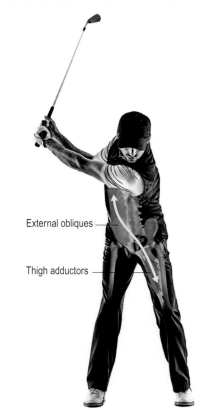

External obliques

Thigh adductors

Figure 4.15

Myofascial relationships lengthening in the golf back swing

Movement exploration

Rotational independence

To enable us to access the spiral elastic mechanism, we need to be able to turn our upper and lower body independently of each other.

To do this in standing, soften your hips and knees, and melt your feet into the floor. If you check yourself in the mirror from the side, your body should be vertical. Imagine a car headlight on the front of each side of your pelvis. These will stay shining straight ahead. Place your hands around each side of your rib cage. Leaving your pelvis and legs facing forward, turn your rib cage smoothly to the right. Briefly check whether your pelvis and knees are still facing forward before returning and continuing around to left (see Fig. 4.16).

> Notice that the instruction is to leave the pelvis and legs behind as you move the rib cage, rather than to "keep them in position," which is an anti-movement cue. Can you feel a difference in effort? Telling the brain to leave something behind often greatly reduces the effort involved in movement control.

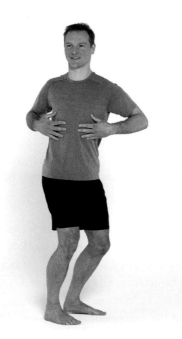

Figure 4.16

Can you turn your upper body while leaving your pelvis and knees in place?

Real life study

A story of blocked spiral elastic movement

My client, a young tennis player, was experiencing forearm and elbow pain when hitting forehands. His arm was tense, stiff, and heavily muscled, which was an early indicator that the efficiency of his technique should be examined.

He had been told that he must develop a strong core to hit well, so he regularly included extensive core conditioning in his training program. He was good at holding his core still while moving his arms and legs but was completely unable to rotate his pelvis on his hips, or to separate his upper body from his lower body. This prevented force transmission through his body, so he could not use the energy potential of his strong legs. This in turn meant that he needed to create the majority of his force with his arm.

Learning to turn his pelvis with simple movements and to experience his thorax rotating freely allowed the player to discover a new fluency in his forehand movement. The movement of one body segment on another reduced his need for muscular effort, because he could now access his elastic mechanisms and use the power of his legs. The arm symptoms simply disappeared.

Exercises that emphasize a rotational separation between the upper and lower body, either by actively turning the upper body on the lower body or vice versa, contribute to the Spiral Elastic strategy. Rather than thinking of turning the shoulders, consider directing the focus either toward turning the rib cage if moving the upper body on the lower body, or leaving it behind if turning the lower body on the upper body. This can give a richer motion deeper into the trunk, and a greater connection into the oblique abdominals.

The linear elastic strategy

At this point, a simple audit of your common exercise choices can reveal whether you have a balance between zone stacking and rotational exercises. The next strategy, however, may test your beliefs – a far more challenging proposition.

In the previous two elastic strategies, the body parts have moved relative to each other, but the distance between them has remained the same. The linear elastic strategy involves lengthening the body and results in the zones moving away from each other.

The support and feedback from the myofascial relationships across our entire body are made available through this strategy, allowing us to move fully into our available range with control and connection. It allows us to freely move our shoulders and hips for more efficient limb movement, and supports the spine into smooth, coordinated curves.

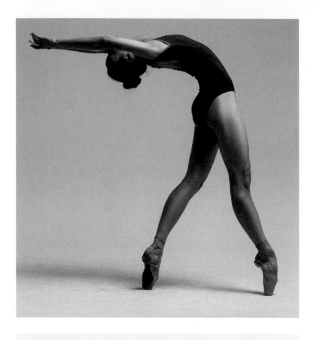

Figure 4.17

The linear elastic strategy supports the back bend

The high jumper arching backward over the bar, your child executing a cartwheel, and a swimmer stretching to catch the water for his next stroke all exhibit the linear elastic strategy. It is the key to safely and enjoyably reaching into our potential range, and restoring confidence if there has been a history of injury (see Fig. 4.17).

The key to the linear elastic strategy is that it is actively connected throughout the entire motion, at whatever speed and level of muscle contraction is appropriate. There is no passive, empty moment – we carry our intention to the very end of the motion. It involves a sense of the movement as an occupied space from start to finish, whether it is light and graceful or explosively powerful. When we achieve this, we are aware that the movement engages full connection through the body, and the sharing of forces across a wide area.

Pan-tastic

When you yawn and stretch in the morning, experiencing that delicious feeling when every muscle seems to be contracting as you press your limbs and body into the far corners of their range, you are engaged in a behavior called *pandiculation*[G].

Pandiculation is a process of vibrant, active lengthening in the body, and is utilized in our linear elastic strategy. Every creature does it, from fish to birds to cheetahs. It enhances proprioception with a burst of sensory feedback from muscles and fascia, and subsides into a relieving sense of simultaneous relaxation and readiness for action.

Pandiculation is thought to be a mechanism for regulating our nervous system and balancing the tension in our myofascial structures.[11] Our joints move into their full range against finely calibrated resistance generated by our own muscles. Although it is considered to be an involuntary response, with yawning being our most obvious example, we can facilitate a similar effect of muscle-engaged active lengthening from the body with three main cues: *pressing, filling,* and *reaching*. These cues actively direct us forward into movement, instead of bracing for control against

it. In doing so, we connect to our elastic selves, and bring our movements to life.

For example, the familiar quadruped Bird Dog exercise is frequently taught as a zone stacking task, a spinal static posture maintained against the moving levers of the limbs. The abdomen is pre-tensioned, and the arm and leg are lifted in an upward direction. When the brain reads the movement impulse of the limbs as upward, the natural countermovement in the spine will be downward into extension. To prevent this, the abdominal muscles must actively resist the downward spinal motion. The front and back of the body act against each other. This is anti-movement training, a non-elastic task (see Fig. 4.18).

We can transform this movement into the more dynamic, elastic Superman with two simple adjustments. First, it is not necessary to pre-tension the abdominal wall to find a neutral spinal position when supported on hands and knees: it is proprioception rather than strength that we need. Imagine a laser pointer on the very tip of your tailbone, and experiment with pointing it upward, then downward, and even using it to trace an imaginary circle on the wall behind you. Settle in a position where the laser beam

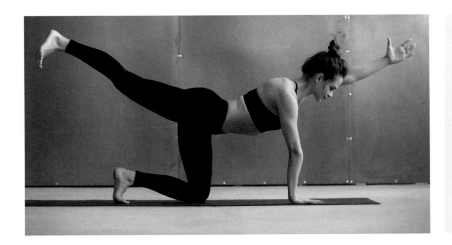

Figure 4.18

The upward movement impulse of Bird Dog, performed with consciously pre-tensioned abdominals to control the spine, is an anti-movement task

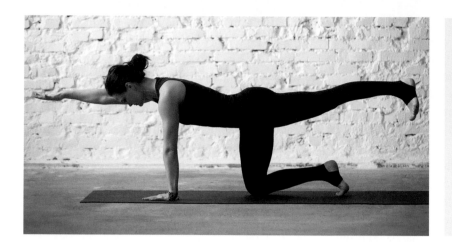

Figure 4.19

Superman, performed with a lengthening impulse, facilitates an automatic abdominal response and becomes an elastic experience

aims straight behind you. This requires very little muscle activity.

Now we can trigger a global elastic response by changing the movement impulse. Instead of thinking "lift," press your heel straight out until the hip and knee are straight (see Fig. 4.19). Pressing creates a co-contraction response throughout the leg, which regulates speed and timing as well as engaging coordinated muscle activity along the limb. Reach the opposite fingertips away from that heel. The simultaneous pressing and reaching intention stimulates a lengthening response through the body, triggering the abdomen to lift upward involuntarily. Now we are balancing the anterior and posterior surfaces of the body so they work together, rather than fighting each other. This lumbopelvic–hip action is that of the sprinter exploding out of the blocks, the swimmer pushing off the wall – the impulse of forward propulsion. It teaches the hip to extend smoothly from the pelvis without creating compressive force on the spine. The timing and balance between erector spinae, gluteals, and hamstrings are calibrated as one smooth coordinated movement, stretching out through the entire posterior chain. The movement has become elastic.

Many people overuse the muscles of their lower back in hip extension tasks instead of coordinating the movement with their gluteals and hamstrings. Actively contracting the gluteals rarely helps in this situation because it usually just increases the total tension. The pressing cue establishes balance between the posterior chain muscles by encouraging the spine to maintain its length as the hip extends. The movement experience is redirected from the spine to the hip, which encourages the gluteals to activate.

If you teach an airplane pose, you can also experiment with this pressing concept. When the cue is to look slightly ahead as the trunk tilts forward and leg lifts behind, you will initiate an extension response triggered by your neck. This emphasizes the posterior musculature but inhibits the anterior muscles (see Fig. 4.20). Alternatively, if you cue to press out from the very top of the head, all the way out to the heel behind you, the anterior and posterior muscles synchronize, creating a more balanced position (see Fig. 4.21).

Pressing can even bring an elastic impulse into a zone stacking exercise, to trigger greater myofascial support. If we take the plank, think about pressing the heels away from the crown of the head – this tensions the myoelastic structures all the way down the

posterior surface of the body, triggers an abdominal lift, and, in doing so, overcomes the suit of armor response.

For any muscularly active lengthening to occur, there must be an awareness of a reference point at each end of the movement. Sense the difference when you aim to move each point away from the other. A yoga pose such as the extended side angle pose shown

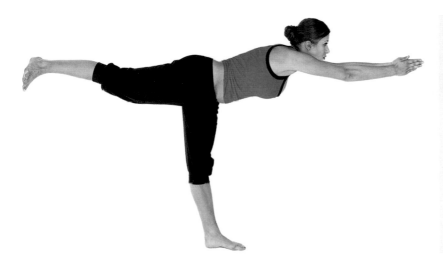

Figure 4.20

Closing the back of the neck facilitates the muscles down the back of the body, but disengages the front surface of the body

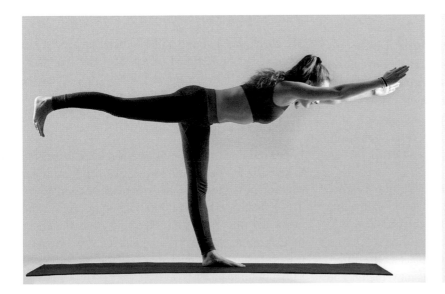

Figure 4.21

Pressing the top of the head out away from the foot engages both front and back of the body

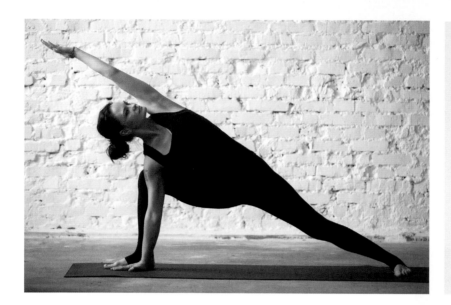

Figure 4.22

A two way expansion creates a sense of elasticity

in Figure 4.22 comes to life elastically if it is cued as a two-way expansion, pressing out from the outer border of the foot through to the fingertips, rather than a stretch from the arm and chest.

> If you want something to lengthen, it must have a secure point to lengthen from.

Filling a movement is more subtle, but can be just as effective. Let's compare two similar movements to feel this. In standing, move your arms straight out away from you at shoulder height, ending with your palms facing away from you. Repeat this, and feel the effect in your body. Not much going on, is there?

Now soften your hips and knees a little, and visualize every part of your body as a soft hollow tube. Imagine drawing pressurized air up through your feet, into your trunk, filling these tubes before directing it out to fill your arms and hands. Can you detect the difference between this and the previous movement? The feeling of filling a movement engages a neuromuscular pattern that creates connection and control (see Fig. 4.23).

Real life study

A story of blocked linear elastic movement

My client was a young ballet dancer, poised on the verge of her professional career. She was experiencing sharp pain in her upper lumbar spine when she performed any kind of back bending movement, and, in fact, had developed a small stress fracture in the vertebra at the site of her pain.

In her training to this point, she had been instructed to stabilize her pelvis and lower back firmly with her abdomen and then draw her scapulae back and down. This effectively immobilized her spine above and below the site of her pain. Her injury site, the upper lumbar spine, was the focal point of stress because it was the only remaining area available for the extension motion to occur.

back bend. First, she needed to relax the strong abdominal and scapular stabilizing action at the beginning of the motion. Without this release, her spine could not move at each successive segment, which it needed to do if it were to share the load. The "setting" of her abdominals also cued them to maintain a fixed length, but in a back bend, her muscles needed the ability to be continuously active *while lengthening* in order to relieve pressure from the injured vertebra. It was therefore necessary to help this dancer to establish a more relaxed, buoyant starting posture that enabled more coordinated and supported movement.

> Far from enhancing spinal control, firm abdominal tension actually reduced this dancer's stability as she moved into an extension movement of the spine.

Having addressed the initial barriers to the movement, we needed to replace the movement impulse of "back" to "up and out" so as to achieve better support and a more even distribution of extension demand throughout her spine.

I asked her to rest the fingertips of one hand on her lower abdomen, just above her pubic bone as a point of reference, and to reach upward through the fingertips of her other hand so that she felt herself moving her hands away from each other, lifting up and out of her pelvis. This action stimulates an automatic abdominal contraction that shifts the load bearing from the back to the front of the body. You can try this yourself.

I invited her to continue to follow the "up and out" impulse with her fingertips along the ceiling behind her into whatever pain-free range was available. She felt the supportive stretch between the anchor point just above her pubic bones and her reaching hand, and, indeed, all the way down the front of her legs, and up through her upper arm. Having opened out into a stretch from the anchor point, I invited her to return to it again like a rubber band returning to its original shape.

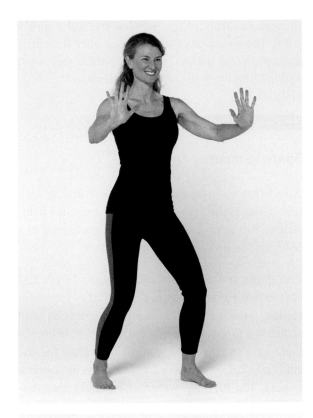

Figure 4.23

Filling a movement to establish connection

In terms of intention, when performing a back bend, "back" was indeed all that she was thinking. Back, and further back. Her hips slid forward to counterbalance the backward intention, switching off the myofascial connections down the front of her body. The abdominal wall had only been trained to contract at a fixed length, so when asked to work eccentrically to support the spinal extension movement, it simply switched off. Without anterior support, the painful spinal joints rapidly became loaded, and this passive, empty, stressful movement effectively left the dancer resting on her delicate spinal structures.

In order to address this injury, we needed to teach the dancer how to use herself more effectively in a

The result was a deeper, more elegant, and most importantly, pain-free back bend, which allowed the dancer to return to function in a short space of time. The "reach" cue created global muscle activity, which shared the load over a large surface area through the myofascial system, enhanced sensory feedback, and also replaced the empty feeling of leaning on the spinal joints with a sense of fullness and connection throughout the whole movement. The blocked movement was transformed into a natural, sustainable elastic solution.

The impulse of "out" can similarly be used in arabesque or backward leg lift to reduce spinal compression and improve the balance of muscle activation down the posterior surface of the body. Many dancers strive to lift the leg from the back of the body, but this can create rapid lower back extension without fully engaged hip extension, even when mentally focusing on the gluteals.

Movement exploration

Choose a leg to stand upon, and softly raise one arm. Lift your other leg up behind you, feeling where the motion and effort is most noticeable. This is the "up" impulse. Now let's explore a different option. Place the fingers of your free hand on the abdominals just above the pubic bone again. This will be your imaginary center point to extend from. Visualize your movement impulse as moving out from here, along the front of your leg all the way to your pointing toes. Feel the front of the leg stretching away from your imaginary center point, carrying your leg up for you. You might suddenly feel that you want to lengthen up through your body as well as out through your toes. This is global engagement (see Fig. 4.24).

Take a moment to compare the impulse of "up" from the back of the leg with "out" from the center

through the front of the leg. Can you feel a difference? The direction of impulse can alter the entire neuromuscular pattern, reducing joint compression and lighting up elastic support throughout the entire body.

Space to move

Alleviating the sensation of tightness and restriction in our bodies, especially in focal areas like hamstrings, hip flexors, and pectorals, is something of a holy grail for many people.

Prominent fascia experts like Thomas Myers and Robert Schleip hypothesize that activities like foam rolling, which apply localized compression and squeezing forces, achieve a greater sense of movement ease by decreasing congestion within the tissues and inviting rehydration.[2,12] This in essence reduces the pressure within the muscle compartment by creating more space, which in turn allows for more fascial mobility. Lymph drainage and compression garments (which aid fluid return) can have a similar effect.

This makes sense: we don't actually want long loose fascia – it would compromise our body's stability, proprioception, and force management. However, ensuring that our fascia has space to move in response to the pulls of the muscles upon it will decrease the resistance that it must move against. Less resistance permits the speed of movement that is associated with the stretch-shortening involved in elasticity.

Wearing our emotions

If we expand our thinking beyond fascia itself and consider the myofascial web, we remember that it is made up of the contractile elements in

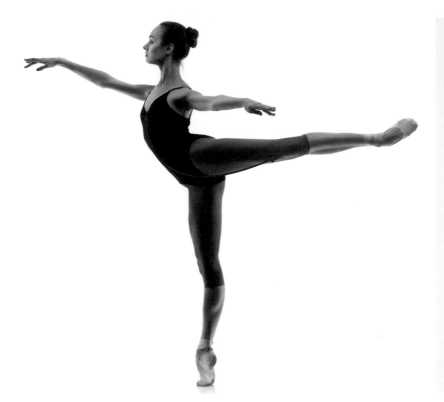

Figure 4.24

To reduce spinal compression and improve the balance of muscle activation through the posterior trunk and leg muscles, shift your focus from the back to the front of your body, imagining support radiating out from the pubic bone to float the leg upward

the muscle fibers interwoven with the fascial fibers. Muscle fibers are capable of lengthening, but can also shorten in response not just to mechanical demands but also to emotional or psychological stress. This shortening will place widespread tension on the fascial component of the web. Have you ever noticed that you seem to be more flexible when relaxed, and less flexible when busy, rushed, and under pressure?

Thinking functionally, if you release held tension in the contractile muscle component of the web, you establish more space within it, such that the body segments can start to move independently of one another while maintaining their connection. If this becomes possible, we can move into positions that foster elastic energy transfer, allowing our myofascial system to function beautifully to share, transmit, and disperse force.

Power points

- Our myofascial network works hand in hand with our biomechanics to maximize our efficiency.

- The cues that we choose can transform an exercise from a struggle to a challenge, from static to dynamic, from rigid to elastic.

- Training activities can be balanced to prepare us for a range of force management strategies, to better meet the demands of our lives with power and fluency.

Vibrant self-carriage

Posture is not a battle with gravity but a dance with the forces around us.

The P-word, *posture*, comes loaded with associations and assumptions. For some people it represents an insurmountable struggle in their fight to hold themselves up against gravity and is a continuous source of low self-esteem. To others, it is an oversimplified business of simply lining up body parts and training for sufficient endurance to retain this position.

In reality, our posture is the result of an intricate interplay of structure and function, emotion and communication, biology and biography. Posture is so much more than a plumb line from ear to ankle; it is an honest and visible expression not only of our state of being but of the way we interact with the world.

Changing the narrative

The common conceptualization of perfect posture as a constantly maintained single state of alignment is a myth of our own devising. Our posture responds and adapts to our thoughts and feelings, the quality of sensory feedback from our body structures, and the demands of our daily lives. We move in and out of shapes constantly, and it is how well our choices respond to gravity, and how easily we can access our deep reflexive neurological responses that determines the quality and effectiveness of our posture.

Posture is dynamic, in motion and also in stillness. Even the concept of "our" posture is tenuous, as we can change it instantly if we change the narrative

behind it. If I asked you to assume the posture of a self-conscious teenager, you could fold yourself into that shape. If I asked you to show me Superman or Wonderwoman, you would expand in the reverse direction. For the fun of it, you could strike a pose like a supermodel at the end of the catwalk, shrink under the burden of hard life experience as a very elderly person, or draw yourself into the upright rigidity of a Marine on parade. You would laugh and say that it is just acting, but you will have demonstrated the extraordinary range of possibilities available to you right now with your current resources.

> Posture is a story that you are telling rather than a position that you are holding.

Even without portraying a character, our emotions are there for all to see, written in the way that we arrange our frames. We wear our simmering habitual anger with our shoulders tensely held up and forward and our legs stiff with indignation; when provoked into acute anger, we thrust our head forward to press our point.[1]

Sometimes we become stuck in the posture of go-go-go! as we race around, trying to muster the capability we need to cope with the multitude of demands upon us. With our heads up, our shoulders pinned back, and our spines rigid this posture speaks of withstanding what is coming at us, and of trying hard to be good enough. Like standing in the face of buffeting winds, it can be exhausting, and, over time, it can become rigidity and resistance.

Sometimes we are so overwhelmed that the sense of motion grinds to a halt. We fold in on ourselves – the front of our bodies closing and compressing with flexion, internal rotation, and adduction of our limbs. Whereas the previous posture was like having a foot stuck on the accelerator, in this state, you have run out of fuel and come to a stop. This posture speaks of emotional energy at a standstill and is associated with both submission[2] and depression.[3] The narrative for this posture may be visible in the musculoskeletal system, but its driver is emotional.

Yet, conversely, our posture can also shape our emotions. Simply making the effort to sit more upright has been shown to influence the symptoms of depression and anxiety in a positive way,[4–6] just as expansive postures can decrease anxiety and tip our hormonal profile in the direction of confidence.[7] Even arranging our facial muscles in mimicry of an emotion can alter our brain response so it aligns how we feel with our facial expression.[8–10]

This fascinating field of research is opening up our understanding of body posture as a resource that can change how we feel in ourselves, how we perceive the world, and how we communicate with others. For the health and fitness professional, this is powerful knowledge.

> People don't just want to get fitter, but to *feel better.*

Could it be that the most sophisticated postural technique available is to activate the associative networks in the brain and their motor responses, by cueing someone to portray what happy, confident, or ready for action might look like?

Relief from rigidity

A message of relaxed readiness from the body assures your nervous system that all is well. Ideally then, your posture should be achieved with the least amount of muscle effort necessary to meet your functional challenges most efficiently and effectively. If you ask most people what "good" posture might involve, however, many will think it represents quite the opposite. Most will mention standing up straight, pulling shoulders back, and maybe also drawing the stomach in. In some quarters a squeezing of the gluteals is encouraged as well. It takes effort to hold yourself in place, and no matter how much you try to use only a little muscle, you will find that you will interfere with your normal function.

> Ideal posture is that which requires the least amount of muscle effort to arrange the body for efficient and effective performance.

Every breath we take creates displacement in the body, and this influences our natural postural sway. When we breathe more deeply, our body sways more in response, but as it is designed to accommodate this, balance is not compromised. Multiple joints in the legs and in the natural curves of our spine absorb a small amount of the motion,[11] and the lumbopelvic and hip joints are key contributors in this natural process of managing postural stability. Compromising the mobility in these areas makes a difference: research has shown that people with low back pain exhibit reduced hip motion and greater postural sway than those without pain.[12] Low back pain sufferers also appear to use more global co-contraction as a control response, which further inhibits multi-joint absorption of displacement.[13] It seems that in order to be stable, we must also be mobile.

This explains why traditional postural cues can feel so unnatural. When you hold body segments in place to prevent them from moving, you inadvertently compromise postural stability by preventing the normal absorption of postural sway. Just think about the implications of so many people being taught not only to stabilize at the lumbar spine with an active abdominal contraction but also to tighten the gluteals, which blocks the fine-tuned mobility response of the hips to our breath. If we also hold our scapulae in place, the thoracic spine contribution is compromised as well. The body starts to run out of options but has to find a way to compensate in order to maintain postural control. The most likely strategy is to change the way we breathe, either reducing depth of breath or moving the breathing higher in the body. No amount of breathing practice while lying down in a class is going to transfer to standing if postural cues prevent this most fundamental of normal movement strategies.

> It is time to let go of old postural holding cues. No more squeezing, tightening, or tucking. These anti-movement actions oppose normal effortless whole-body function at the most fundamental level.

It seemed logical to simply stretch and strengthen enough structures to achieve alignment along a vertical plumb line, and if we were machines, perhaps it would work. However, we are far from mechanical.

Less plumbing, more wiring

The concept of the plumb line – the theoretical alignment of ear, shoulder, hip, knee, and ankle – has long provided a reference point for assessing postural types. Deviations from this line are often seen as indications of weakness or tightness in various muscle groups. However, the plumb line and postural typing have also been the source of much

misunderstanding, and they have frequently led to simplistic mechanical solutions that fail to account for the sophisticated neurosensory processes that underpin our posture. They marginalize the people whose skeletons do not fit the model, such as those with scoliosis, ankylosing spondylitis, osteoporosis, and Scheuermann's disease, and label those who deviate from the tyrannical line.

Conventionally, it is thought that strengthening certain muscles brings better posture by holding the skeleton in place, but changing your posture can switch muscles on or off regardless of their strength. Sliding your pelvis into a sway back posture, for example, will decrease your trunk muscle activity, while resuming a more neutral position encourages activation.[14,15] Using a visualization cue to change the head and neck posture changes the postural neuromuscular pattern in a positive direction.[16] Changing the body position to alter the muscle behavior instead of the other way around hints at how dynamically we are wired.

Could there be another way to approach our views on posture and how we present them?

The central longitudinal axis

From the field of biomechanics comes the concept of the central longitudinal axis (CLA). This is a conceptual line that passes vertically through the very center of the body, giving us a deep internal balance point about which our body movement is most efficient. From lifting to throwing, a secure axis has been found to be associated with greater adaptability and effectiveness.

The CLA is not a rigid position, rather a firm yet flexible central reference point for movement. Importantly, it does not run through the spine but through the middle of the body itself, thus creating a more substantial sense of location in the body.

It represents buoyancy against gravity and a power board for your limbs to plug into. Imagine it as a long elastic tube, like a bicycle inner tube or a long party balloon, inflating from deep in the center of your pelvis all the way up through the middle of your body until it touches the underside of your skull. As an inflatable tube, it can bend in all directions yet maintain its structural integrity as we flex, extend, and side bend. However, if you let some air out of the tube and press down upon it from the top end, it will buckle, displacing forward or backward, and even perhaps sideways, depending on where the resistance is least. The load is no longer shared evenly throughout the tube, so areas of higher and lower pressure are created.

You might attempt to gather these collapse points back into a straight line with conventional postural cues, but they will sag back out as soon as the attention is drawn elsewhere. This becomes a cycle of repetitive effort. To break the cycle, you will need to re-establish the integrity of the central axis by reinflating the tube again.

In body terms, we can achieve this not by forcing disparate parts forward or backward onto a rigid hypothetical line but by thinking about removing the compressing hand of gravity pressing down from above. If we allow the body to decompress by expanding upward, it can start to pull its own kinks out (see Fig. 5.1).

To achieve this upward impulse without effortful straining, we need to recover our sense of buoyancy. For this, we must dive into our nervous system.

Do what turns you on

Our postural development begins with the progressive appearance and integration of a wide range of reflexes throughout our early childhood. As adults, reflexes continue to play their part in how we orientate ourselves in space and against gravity. This

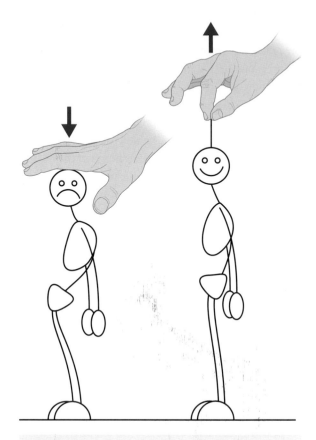

Figure 5.1

Expand upward and outwards into buoyant posture

involves multiple structures and neural pathways working together in a complex dance of lightning-fast communication.

Our balance system, for example, involves the integration of our vision, the proprioceptive feedback coming from our bodies, and our vestibular system – the delicate, curling structure located in our inner ear. This triad of sensory sources is also intimately involved in our postural control, influencing the brain's rapid calculations through a network of connections between the vestibular system and multiple parts of the brain, including the cerebellum. The vestibulospinal reflex, which is highly sensitive to head position, not only stabilizes the head with respect to the body as it moves but activates the antigravity muscles throughout our body.[17] Vestibular influences even help us to adjust our blood pressure in response to a change of body position. This means that both our head position and our freedom to make finely tuned adjustments to it are of utmost significance when we consider posture and movement.

Neck posture is automatically implicated in head positioning. The upper cervical spine is intimately connected to the neurology of our balance system, and altering its position affects postural control (see Fig. 5.2).[18–20] Extension of the upper neck, that very familiar position adopted when gazing into computer screens or adopting a forward head posture, has been shown to decrease postural control, for example (see Fig. 5.3).[21]

Given this understanding, our aim will be to decompress the spinal structures of the neck and achieve a fluid, gyroscopic quality to the relationship between our head and neck. When our head is free to move rather than being held in a fixed relationship to our neck, the sensitive structures in our brains and upper spine are able to accurately detect our position in space and organize us – through reflex activity – to achieve balance and postural control.

How do we influence our head position?

Let's investigate an old familiar approach first. Looking straight ahead and keeping your eyes level, let your head glide forward on your body into the forward head posture. This is a common posture, and people are frequently cued to draw their chin back in to bring the head into line with the body to address it (see Figs. 5.4 and 5.5). If you try this for yourself, however, you will realize that you are actually putting a direct stress on the spine by asking it to reverse its curves. It is uncomfortable and takes away the gentle inwards curve of the natural cervical spine lordosis. This is not moving us toward normal posture.

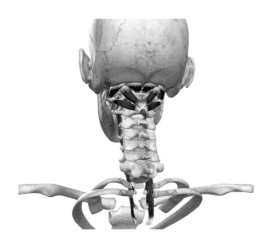

Figure 5.2

The deep upper cervical muscles contribute sensory information for postural control

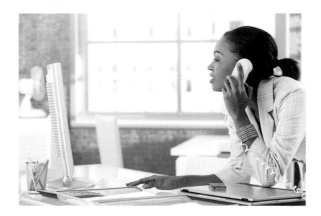

Figure 5.3

Compressed neck posture is common in daily tasks

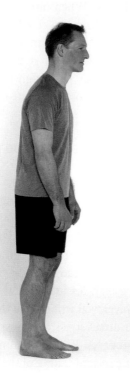

Figure 5.4

Forward head posture

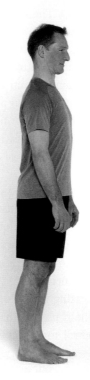

Figure 5.5

Retracted head posture. Over-correction of the head position creates compression in the throat area and fixed tension in the muscles in the anterior upper neck

Movement exploration

To discover another possibility, visualize your head sitting on top of your neck like a lightly oiled ball sitting on a cup. Place your hands on the sides of your head and rotate it forward and backward with your fingers, as if the ball is now spinning on the cup (see Figs. 5.6 and 5.7). Feel how your upper neck opens to flex as you rotate your head forward, and that it closes and extends as you rotate your head backward. You can move your head in any direction using this visualization – the frictionless ball can rotate in any direction with ease.

Now when considering the forward head posture, let go of the idea of this being a forward/backward issue, and use your new rotation awareness instead. As you move into this posture, can you feel that to keep your eyes level, the top of your neck compresses into extension? This happens because your head is subtly rotating backward on your neck, just as you explored previously. As you rotate it forward again, feel the back of the head lift. This unlocks the upper neck and opens the potential to reposition it directly over your body.

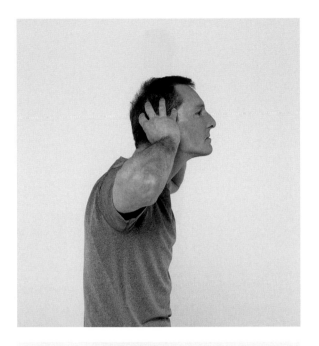

Figure 5.6

Rotating the head backward into forward head posture

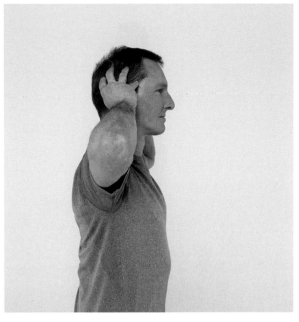

Figure 5.7

Returning to a neutral position by reversing the rotation

We therefore need a simple way to decompress the neck and neutralize this rotation. We will do this by cuing an impulse rather than a position in the body.

Cueing an impulse

Let us introduce a different direction of motion. In your forward head posture, imagine the top surface of your skull as having a front, back, and sides. In your mind's eye, attach a helium balloon to a spot on the back half of this surface. You can put a finger on this spot. Helium rises gently, so allow the balloon to softly lift the head, just enough to float it up over the spine itself. Did you notice the direction of movement? It is an upward motion while simultaneously rotating the head back to neutral. If you switch the balloon off, feel how your head slides down and forward as it rotates backward, closing the upper neck.

This time with your balloon on, feel how the head moves upward as it rotates forward, opening the back of the neck. This gives the head a way to balance itself over the body without having to be held in a fixed position. Test it out: the balloon's job is simply to take the weight of the head off the spinal structures, so you should be able to move your head easily and freely. With this freedom to make subtle gyroscopic motions in response to changes in the orientation of your head and body in space, the vestibular system can respond for finely tuned balance and postural control (see Figs. 5.8 and 5.9).

Facilitating posture from the head can engage the rest of the body due to this reflex activity. Your head is quite heavy, much like a ten-pin bowling ball, so use just enough balloon to float it off your spine, relieving its compressive action and allowing each segment

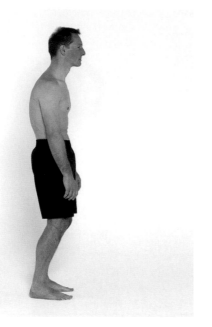

Figure 5.8

Collapsing under the hand of gravity

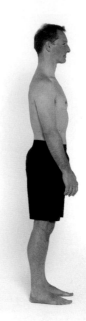

Figure 5.9

Expanding with the help of the helium balloon

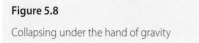

all the way to your tailbone to expand and breathe. In standing, practice a few repetitions of switching your balloon on and allowing it to switch off again. Notice the opening effect at the chest and shoulders, and the lifting effect in the abdomen with each repetition of the balloon. Instead of many body positions to think about, you can carry yourself with just one cue.

Appreciating the significance of the upper cervical spine to posture throughout the body helps us to unpick some other traditional cues. "Pull your neck back into your collar" facilitates a military-type posture that reverses the spinal curves in the same way as drawing your chin in does. "Head up" tends to provoke a lifting from the nose, which extends, or closes the upper neck. Both are tension-provoking positions. In understanding this, we can move away from positional cues and toward those that preserve a sense of motion, even in stillness.

The sense of being lifted suggests a movement impulse, but sometimes the point of reference for the cue needs to change. If someone cannot conceptualize the lifting motion of the balloon, it may be helpful to bring the visualization point to a more tangible part of the body: the ears. Think of growing the tops of the ears upward: they can be rabbit ears, elf ears … whatever kind of ears works! This works from a balance point that is slightly further forward on the head than the balloon cue, and it helps some people to stabilize the head in a level position more easily. This cue is useful for those who tend to overdo the balloon by pushing themselves into even greater spinal extension.

Ears hold even greater magic than this: to overcome a side-bent spine or a tendency to collapse laterally in motion, imagine one ear lengthening, and follow it upward to centralize the rib cage over the pelvis, correcting the balance point and equalizing the weight bearing.

Sometimes it is not a lifting but a dropping stimulus that is the key, especially in people who hold themselves tensely upright. These people often respond to the idea of being suspended, as if they were a wooden marionette puppet that has been picked up by their head string by a giant hand so that its body hangs loosely toward the floor. This allows them to explore the idea of their body dropping into alignment below this point of suspension, and that this support can move easily through space. Shoulders release, upper back muscles let go, and the body falls into a vertical alignment. It is an invitation to allow the body to experience the relief of letting go.

Sole magic

Our posture is not only driven from top down but also from bottom up. The soles of our feet work like pressure pads that are constantly mapping where the weight is being borne. They send information streaking upward to combine with visual and vestibular input, which then informs the brain about where to put our center of gravity.[22]

Our feet are also the initiators of the *positive support response*. As very young babies, we exhibit a positive support reflex, where the legs and trunk extend strongly if the balls of the feet are stimulated. This reflex fades at about two months of age, but it is integrated into a more mature form that responds to weight bearing through the feet by activating our antigravity muscles, particularly those that extend our hips and knees. Now we are equipped to develop our walking, running, and jumping.

> If you want well-functioning gluteals, you need to start a conversation with your feet.

We desensitize our feet from an early age, wrapping them in shoes and socks and rarely exposing them to sensory variation. If we don't receive enough high-quality feedback from our feet, we may increase tension in them to create more sensory noise, but this can rob us of foot and ankle mobility and suppleness, creating what is known as functional rigidity. This can manifest as the foot shortening and narrowing, the development of claw or hammer toes, the big toe digging downward into the floor with excessive flexor hallucis longus activation, restriction of ankle mobility due to excessive muscular co-contraction, or irritating compression of the nerves between our metatarsals. Difficulties then arise in adapting to balance fluctuations or changes in ground surface, and our postural control becomes further compromised.

Sometimes we fail to compensate, and the foot becomes passive and unresponsive, often sagging into excessive pronation. This is just as problematic as having too much tension – to have a viable positive support response, the foot needs to be "listening" to the floor and "talking" to you. If its response to weight bearing is to sink further into the floor and slumber there, it sure isn't lighting up the postural circuit boards with dynamic real-time communication.

A number of muscles can be implicated in this presentation. Tibialis posterior should be playing a part in supporting the arch, as its tendon passes behind the medial malleolus and divides to create a reinforcing sling by inserting into the medial tarsal bones of the navicular and cuneiforms, and the heads of metatarsals two to four (see Fig. 5.10). This is one of the muscles that we will need to awaken, along with small deep muscles within the foot called the lumbricals. These little muscles attach to the flexor tendons of your second to fifth toes, and they play a strong role in the internal stabilization of the foot (see Fig. 5.11). They strengthen and support your toes as you push off in gait, but, if they are weak, the common

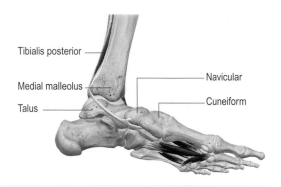

Tibialis posterior

Medial malleolus

Talus

Navicular

Cuneiform

Figure 5.10

Tibialis posterior cradling the bones of the medial ankle

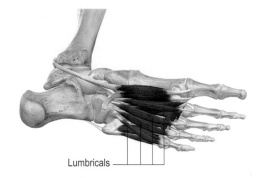

Lumbricals

Figure 5.11

The deep supportive lumbricals of the foot

compensations are increased toe flexor activity, leading back to those hammer and claw toes, and even increased calf tension.

Pedi-posture

To establish the foot connection for our posture, the first step is to increase the sensory connection to the brain.

This isn't complicated; anything that increases your sensation across the whole sole of your foot is good. You can rub your feet, massage underneath them, or roll them over a spiky ball before exercising, and practice walking barefoot over different surfaces whenever you get the opportunity. All of this gets you noticing how your feet feel and prepares your brain to connect with them actively.

Next, we need to teach your foot how to adapt to the floor. It needs to be strongly supportive for the body, yet fluidly responsive to its fluctuations – like an acrobat holding his partner overhead (see Fig. 5.12). To achieve this, we need to help the brain to rediscover the critical movement of tibiofemoral rotation, which will enable the foot to keep its connection to the ground while carrying the changeable body above it.

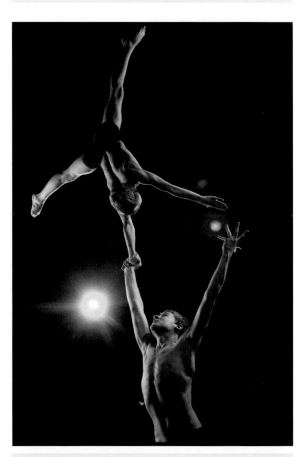

Figure 5.12

To effectively support the weight above, small balance fluctuations must be absorbed

The Listening Foot

Listening Foot is one of the most iconic of JEMS exercises. Perhaps because of the way we live our modern lives, it is rare to meet anyone who does not benefit from it!

Take your shoes and socks off and sit comfortably toward the front of a chair with knees at ninety degrees and your foot resting on the floor. Feel how your foot settles on the floor. Perhaps you feel more pressure in one part than another. Take a moment to play with changing this pressure, to become more aware of the sole of your foot.

Now rest your hands lightly on the skin just below your knee, making a circle around your leg with your fingers and thumbs (see Fig. 5.13A). Your hands are just there for feedback – you will not be using them to create movement.

As slowly, smoothly, and effortlessly as you can, move the pressure under your foot toward the outer part of your sole. You might notice that in doing so, your lower leg has rotated around its axis under your hands in response (see Fig. 5.13B). Reverse the procedure, and feel how you can move the pressure back across the foot, toward the inner border (see Fig. 5.13C). Notice again that your lower leg feels as though it turns under

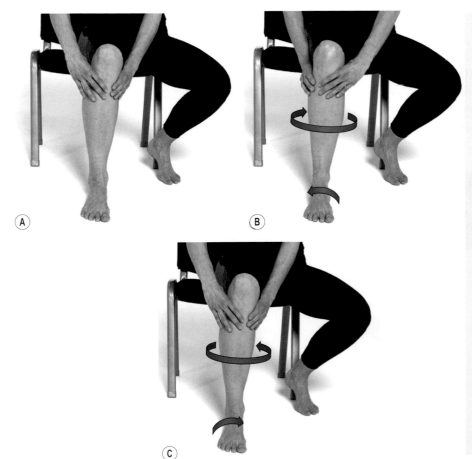

(A)

(B)

(C)

Figure 5.13

A. Place your hands lightly around the leg, and sense the pressure under your foot. *B.* As the pressure passes across the sole of the foot toward its outer border, the lower leg rotates laterally. *C.* As the pressure passes across the sole of the foot toward its inner border, the lower leg rotates medially

your hands. This is tibiofemoral rotation – the rotation of the tibia on the femur. You are making a sensory connection between your foot, ankle, and knee.

The important thing here is that the sole of the foot never lifts off the floor. Usually people begin by trying to force the movement, lifting one side of the foot and then the other off the floor, and even using toes to create the movement. This creates muscle tension that actually blocks the turning of the tibia, and is a good indicator that your brain isn't familiar with this critical movement!

If this is your experience, keep in mind that the body responds to persuasion much better than force. This isn't something that you need to make yourself do but something you allow yourself to do. When you take the pressure off and release the tension, the motor system is more willing to unlock.

If you are struggling to relax your foot, let's change the focus. Place your hands under your thigh, so that you can feel the tendons of the hamstrings (see Fig. 5.14). Imagine these as the reins on a horse, one connecting just below your knee to the inside of your

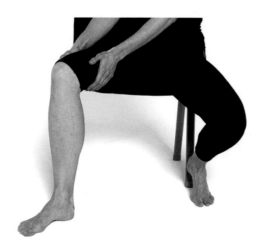

Figure 5.14

Connecting the brain to the hamstrings in Listening Foot

lower leg, and the other on the outside. As you move the pressure under your foot toward the outside, feel the hamstring on the outside pulling on your lower leg to turn it. When you reverse the movement, feel the inner hamstring "rein" pull to turn your lower leg as you move the pressure under the foot toward the inner sole under the big toe.

Once you get the motion going, really tune in to the surface of your foot, finding any gaps in connection to the floor and working on softening the foot so that the entire sole across the front of the foot becomes available to you. Then you can check in with your heel – can you notice how the pressure moves under the back of your foot as well?

Now that you have connected your foot to your knee, we can wake up those lumbricals to create a more self-supporting, springy, and resilient foot.

Foot tents

Getting your brain around these little muscles can be tricky to begin with, so it's easiest first to practice with your hand lumbricals to get the idea. Place one palm on your thigh, and keeping your fingers straight, slide the pads of your fingers inward to lift your knuckles, making a triangular tent shape with your hand (see Fig. 5.15). If this movement is happening in your foot, your palm would represent your arch lifting, and your fingers would of course be your toes dragging back toward your heel. Your finger pads are staying flat rather than curling under, and you will use your toes in the same way.

Now you are ready to start with the foot. Sitting on your chair, connect the sole of your foot with the floor, and wiggle and stretch out your toes before letting them rest on the floor (see Fig. 5.16). Keeping the underside of your toes long, drag them toward your heel, so that your knuckles lift (see Fig. 5.17).

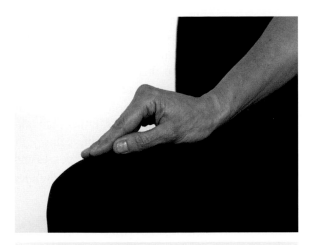

Figure 5.15

Finding the lumbricals with the hand tent

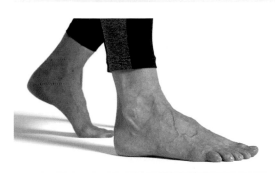

Figure 5.16

Foot tent start position

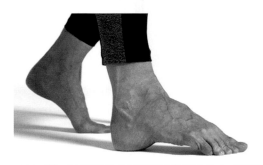

Figure 5.17

Finding the lumbricals with the foot tent

Sometimes it's helpful to put a finger on top of the joints to help your brain to recognize the lift. You will know that you have the right muscles working, because you will be able to pick up your big toe, which doesn't have a lumbrical attachment. Once you have created the foot tent, hold it for two breath cycles, before relaxing and repeating.

Finding your long lost lumbricals can be tricky at first, but with practice you will find that your feet become stronger and more balanced. You are making a great investment in decreasing stress on your foot joints.

So what about that tibialis posterior?

Whether you have an overactive or underactive foot, finding that dynamic balance point for optimal foot and ankle function can be tricky, as the muscles that should control this can initially be uncoordinated. The tibialis posterior muscle, for example, must contribute to the changing foot arch during the gait cycle. The foot naturally pronates for a short time, as part of our shock-absorption mechanism in weight bearing, before supinating to create a firm lever that is used in push-off. Tibialis posterior must therefore modulate its length with exquisite timing in order to control the arch as it makes these transitions, and also make fine, rapid adjustments to accommodate for fluctuations in our balance point. Too much or too little muscle activity will greatly affect our self-carriage in weight bearing. "Stack and reach" is a subtle functional technique that starts the process of training tibialis posterior in its postural role.

Movement exploration

Stack and reach

Stand with your feet hip width apart, and take a moment to visualize each bone resting perfectly upon the one below it, from pelvis to thigh, thigh to shin, and shin to ankle. Each segment is placed on the other like a set of children's building blocks, with your weight falling straight through their center. This is called being stacked. Now imagine that you have an oiled ball in one of your ankle joints. Allow your weight to slide off the inside of the ball, letting the ankle sag so that your foot flattens a little and the pressure moves across toward the ball of the foot. Feel how the whole leg follows it, turning the thigh inwards. Slide your ankle back into the vertically stacked position on top of the ball. The leg aligns itself on top of it again.

Now, bend an elbow, and then stretch your arm up and just slightly away from your head, letting your body follow it so that your weight floats up and over one of your legs (see Figs. 5.18 and 5.19). Maintain the stacked position of the ankle. If this feels quite stable, release the other foot so that you are now standing fully on one leg. Feel how the arch of your foot now starts to fluctuate. Your aim is to stay stacked on your ankle by making small adjustments, rather than falling off it to the inside or outside. To achieve this, your tibialis posterior learns to speed up its responses and make fine length adjustments, developing endurance at the same time.

With a foot that talks to the floor, and a balanced head and neck relationship, we have postural reflexes

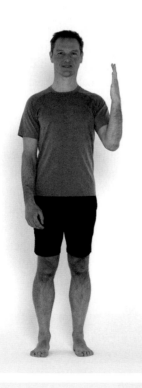

Figure 5.18

Stack and reach start position

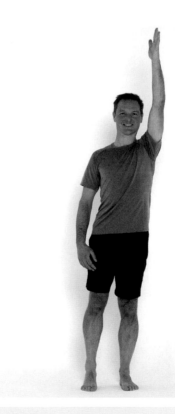

Figure 5.19

Lifting up and onto the stance leg as you reach

in place from bottom up and top down. However, we haven't completed the rewiring process yet. It's time to talk tone.

Tone and tensegrity

Our active postural subsystem arises from a fluctuating dance of postural tone – the deep low-threshold hum of muscle activation that gently tugs on our fascia. This is further supported by what is called human resting myofascial tone, which is a passive viscoelastic property of the tiny structures within each muscle fiber that makes them mildly resistant to stretch.[23] It is thought that our richly innervated fascial web is maintained in an optimal state of tension by this combination of actions in the muscle fibers attaching throughout it. In the same way that the perfectly tensioned threads of a spider's web transmit the disturbance of a blundering fly across the entire structure, our fascia is highly sensitive to changes in tension, and thus is a source of proprioception.[24] It is therefore fundamental to our postural control, not just mechanically through the support of tensegrity, but through the feedback that it contributes about our body position.

There is considerable variation in postural myofascial tone. It varies with age and sex,[23] but even within these subsets there are individual differences. We all know people whose bodies seem to be in a state of constant tension, or are habitually languid. Given the intimate feedback loops between the body and the brain, it is not surprising to observe correlations between these body states and the personality and attitudes that accompany them.

Developmentally, when a child with low tone moves into vertical postures, two compensatory strategies can emerge. An active compensation generates excessive tension in the superficial musculature.[25] These muscles usually cover more than one joint and have long lines of pull, so this strategy can limit joint motion, increase joint compression, and create functional shortening in some muscles. This pattern is carried into adulthood, manifesting in held tension, inflexibility, and difficulties with body part dissociation.

If a developing child comes to depend on their passive rather than active subsystem, they learn to hang on their ligaments and lean into the end of joint or muscle range to prop themselves up.[26] This is the switched-off look that is often associated with hypermobility. In adults with relatively low tone, pain can arise from joint loading, often in positions where the loading is unevenly applied and ligaments under constant strain. Tensegrity is compromised, which reduces structural stability, and, at the same time, proprioceptive information arising from the body is decreased, affecting postural control. Modifying tone is therefore a distinct priority when working on posture.

In both forms of compensation, "soft signs" are commonly seen. These indicate that some aspect of the postural control system is struggling, and they involve using other resources within the system to boost sensory information in order to compensate for what is lacking. Foot rigidity, as we have discussed, is one such mechanism. Eye fixing – the increased use of static visual feedback to maintain balance – is another. Generalized stiffening often shows itself through an oddly held arm or hand. Breath holding is common and facial fixing is prevalent. These are all messages from the body to the brain to help it to know where it is.

Facial fixing can include jaw clenching, repetitive chewing, lip biting, and grimacing. These strategies seem inconsequential, but they have a powerful effect on postural control because the jaw sensorimotor system is a strong source of proprioceptive information.[27] Even tongue positioning is significant. Although the familiar "tongue on the roof of the mouth" is cued to release the jaw, it is easy for *resting* the tongue to become *pressing* the tongue upward. When this happens, it feeds into our postural control system, providing a measurably effective compensatory strategy.[28]

> Recognize soft signs as coping mechanisms. If you allow them, the system learns to compensate more strongly but doesn't address its deficits. Smiling, speaking, whistling, or humming as you perform the movement keeps the face, jaw, diaphragm, and tongue from becoming fixed. Softening the gaze or moving the eyes diminishes their availability to compensate for poor proprioception. Wiggling the fingers and visualizing melting feet helps with the peripheral tension.

When you prevent the soft signs, the body and brain are compelled to work with the remaining systems, addressing the problems instead of masking them.

There is evidence to suggest that postural tone is sensitive and able to be modulated.[29,30] However, when tone is an issue, simply pulling body parts onto the plumb line simply creates a conscious compensation through the active global system. For those who have already adopted the active compensation mechanism, it will reinforce their tension and further compromise their mobility. These are those people who can stretch and stretch but never become more flexible. For those who have adopted the passive compensation mechanism, it is heavy work indeed to achieve and maintain active adherence to the plumb line. Without adequate sensory feedback, their muscles tend to over-contract, and then fatigue quickly. They may even become very painful, which is not at all motivating.

Don't worry – there is another way. The key is to use your wiring.

Sensation, followed by awareness, is key for regulating postural tone. The common problem, regardless of whether the compensation is active or passive, is that the person cannot sense themselves. This is remedied with surprisingly simple techniques, like vigorous slapping and rubbing of the body, starting in the legs, working up the body front and back, across the chest and out the arms (see Fig. 5.20).

Follow this up with high-frequency shaking. Stand on one leg and hold the other foot slightly in front of you. Bend your ankle and draw your toes back toward you so that you feel yourself pushing out with your heel. Maintaining the impulse of pressing out, shake that leg with the fastest vibration you can muster. Feel the

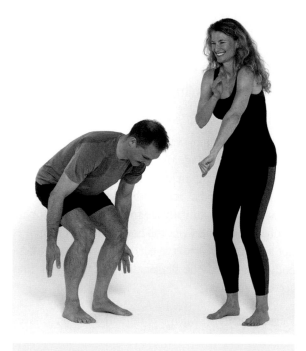

Figure 5.20

Slapping the limbs for sensory input

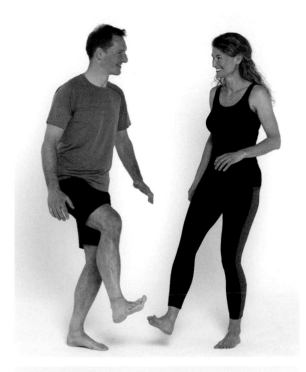

Figure 5.21

Creating a vibration by shaking out through the heel

vibration pass up your leg and into your body. After ten seconds, swap legs and repeat the process (see Fig. 5.21).

When you pause after doing both of these things, notice how alive your body feels, and how connected to the ground.

When you see someone struggling with an exercise that should be within their capabilities, pause, get them to boost their sensation, and then repeat. They are frequently surprised to find that an exercise that felt very heavy is suddenly quite easy. Even if someone does not have developmental tone issues, life stress and mood can affect the active postural tone, so this technique is relevant for many people.

Initially, you may find it necessary to do a little tone regulation at several points in the session, and even

between sets. Those who have been depending upon their passive system throughout their lives often need more boosts initially, as their system is not accustomed to processing low-threshold sensory input. They need that little extra sensory noise for their brain to hear their bodies to begin with, but, over time, the brain improves its ability to process with finer discrimination.

For the person who displays higher tension, the sensory boost encourages the muscles to relax into a state of readiness. By feeding in tactile and vibratory sensation, the brain is given alternative sources of postural information, allowing the high muscle "noise" of constant contraction to release. When a muscle can release effectively, it contracts more effectively, because more of the tiny cross-links within the muscle become available. More effective contraction means more power and speed potential.

> Regulating tone enhances both posture and performance, and it doesn't have to be complicated. This can be an amazingly empowering discovery.

Power points

- Posture is the visible manifestation of your emotions, your nervous system, and your developmental history.

- Working with the wiring instead of just the structure can result in more natural, meaningful change that recognizes the multidimensional nature of posture.

- Most importantly, it is time to cease teaching people how to hold themselves; instead, invite them to experience carrying themselves.

When presented with a lock, a key is mightier than a hammer.

Our posture should flow with ease through dynamically changing positions as we move, and so is constantly adapting. In healthy movement we select from a range of stabilizing possibilities, calibrating our neuromuscular pattern according to the task we are performing.[1] However, if our postural control is compromised in response to our emotional, behavioral, functional, or neurosensory landscape, our choices can narrow to adopt a habitual specific stabilizing strategy. This becomes a lock – the stereotypical immobilizing response in a part of the body that is used for stabilization regardless of the task demand.

Locks can be classified as being either foundation or functional. A foundation lock is one that is present in the person's posture whether they are in motion or at rest. It is a consistent postural feature and does not vary greatly in response to movement demands.

A functional lock appears in response to the impulse to move. In Chapter 3 we discussed the process by which our bodies prepare for movement: the feedforward response. This response ensures that our support musculature establishes the initial groundwork for our bodies to be able to accept load and generate force prior to the movement actually beginning. We have many possibilities for this, and muscles like transversus abdominis, multifidus, and the vastus medialis of the quadriceps have all been identified as behaving in this preparatory way.[2-4] However, in the presence of pain, a history of injury, or any one of the other postural influences that we discussed in Chapter 5, alternative feedforward responses can appear and become the primary preparatory strategy for the body. In Chapter 3 we also talked about looking for where a movement starts – the point of preparation. Persistent, habitual points of preparation that are used regardless of the movement challenge are in fact functional locks.

Distinguishing between foundation and functional locks helps us to identify how to address them. In the case of a foundation lock, there may be structural joint stiffening and soft tissue restriction that can benefit from direct treatment, mobilizing, or stretching. These techniques create movement potential, which must then be integrated using active movement to make the brain aware of how to access and use the new motion in the area.

Functional locks appear in response to movement, but subside at rest. Although a person will complain of tightness and stiffness in the lock area, this is the result of active muscle contraction rather than passive structural limitation. As such, stretching, massage, and mobilization can offer symptomatic relief and address the adaptive tissue shortening that may develop over time, but none of these treatments will make lasting change, because this is a motor program issue – it is in the wiring.

Working with functional locks therefore involves:

- making sure that the load or skill requirement of the exercise is within the person's capabilities, so that they aren't forced into the lock as a coping strategy

- using a cue that communicates the movement impulse clearly

- establishing an awareness of relaxation in the locking area prior to beginning the movement.

Sticky links

There are several common central body locks. Posteriorly, we have the upper (cervical) lock, the posterior rib lock, and the lower (lumbosacral) lock. Anteriorly, we have upper (throat) lock, the anterior rib lock (which we will look at in Chapter 9), and the anterior hip lock.

Although for ease of consideration we have identified the locks as separate entities, their biomechanical, structural, and neural relationships create significant interplay between them. Understanding these relationships can help us to avoid simply using forced muscle action to counter the locks, offering us, instead, the opportunity to uncover other neuromuscular possibilities, by gently unpicking them.

Upper lock

The first of the locks is already familiar to us: it is the *posterior upper lock*, sometimes referred to as the atlanto-occipital lock (see Fig. 6.1). This downward compression of the head on the upper neck, together with the accompanying backward rotation of the skull, influences global body reflexes, and as such it is the master key for the entire spine.

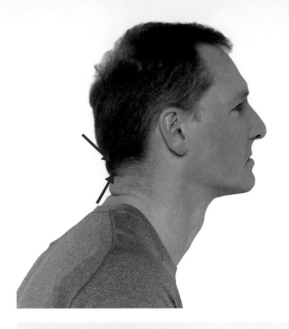

Figure 6.1

Posterior upper lock

In Chapter 3, we discussed the cues of being lifted from the scruff of the neck, looking into a pool of water, and projecting out from the very top, or crown of the head rather than looking forward. This was followed in Chapter 5 by the introduction of cues such as the balloon, the elongated ears, and the suspended puppet, which specifically address the upper lock. All of these cues modify the motor program. They don't just address the point of preparation but also introduce a sense of active intention to carry through the movement.

The posterior upper lock has an equally strong influence when working in supine. If the head is allowed to rest in backward rotation, the spine will be facilitated into extension via reflex activation. If you are hoping to relax the spine toward the floor, work with breathing or establish a neutral lumbar position from which to move the limbs, the upper lock will block it.

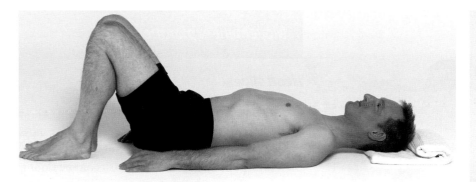

Taking the upper neck out of the extended position reduces extensor tone, which enables easier access to the back of the rib cage in breathing and diminishes the urge to force the spine toward the floor using the abdominal muscles. It should also make lumbopelvic mobility easier, as it will reduce the muscular resistance and joint compression caused by excessive spinal extensor tone.

Rather than forcing the head and neck into a counter lock, fold a towel to a thickness that will allow the person's head and neck to settle into a relaxed neutral position when placed under their occiput (see Fig. 6.2). There might be a need for many folds to begin with, but over time as this area of the body learns to open and lengthen, the thickness of the support can be reduced.

The *anterior upper lock*, or throat lock, is caused by a fixed contraction of the deep muscles on the front of the neck. Like an over-trained show pony, the chin is tucked down or pulled in at the front, immobilizing the head on the neck. This posture is just as responsible for neck pain as the posterior upper lock and can result from posture cues that encourage a person to pull their head back onto the plumb line. It is also prevalent in members of the health and fitness professions who have conscientiously attended to preventing the posterior upper lock, only to find themselves in a counter-lock (see Fig. 6.3).

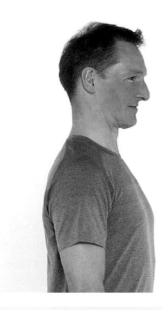

Figure 6.3

Anterior upper lock. The head is held in a fixed position on the neck. Note the skin creases under the jaw

Both the anterior and posterior upper locks alter the normal lordotic curve in the cervical spine and affect postural control by interfering with finely tuned head on neck movements. A neutral head carriage allows the head to float in balance over the spine and be able to move freely and smoothly in all directions

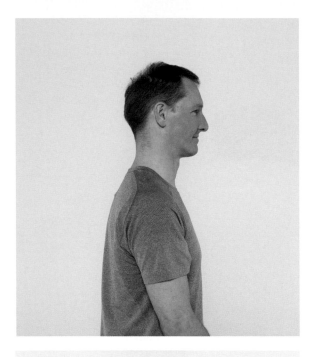

Figure 6.4

Neutral head carriage. The head floats in balance over the body, with an open throat angle

(see Fig. 6.4). To balance the muscle activity between the muscles at the front and back of the upper neck, "head slides" provide a low-stress opportunity for the brain to discover its mobility possibilities.

Movement exploration

Head slides

Lie comfortably on your back with knees bent. Allow your head to settle comfortably with your nose pointing toward the ceiling, placing a folded towel under the point where your head rests on the floor if necessary. Place a hand on the central bony projection that you can feel where your neck meets your body (see Fig. 6.5). This is your C7 spinous process. Become aware not only of the point of contact where your head rests on the floor but of its distance from the spinous process under your hand. Slowly slide the point of head contact along the floor toward your hand just a little, subtly deepening the curve of your neck to introduce a sense of motion awareness (see Fig. 6.6). This often persuades the neck muscles to release more easily as you then slide your head in the opposite direction, away from your hand. As you do this, feel how the back of your neck starts to open and that your chin tucks in a little. The muscles at the back of the neck start to stretch slightly, storing elastic energy (see Fig. 6.7). When you reach a comfortable end point, reverse the movement, allowing a sense of mild recoil until you move just a little past your original start point to emphasize the sensation

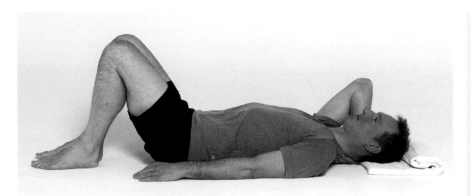

Figure 6.5

Head slide start position

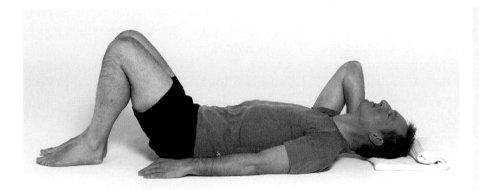

Figure 6.6

Gently sliding the head toward the hand initially

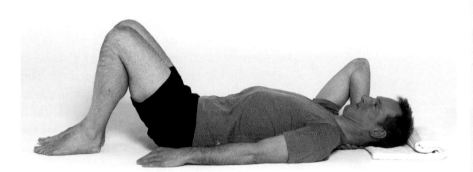

Figure 6.7

Lengthening and opening the back of the neck

of contrast. Slowly repeat this procedure, gliding smoothly and with minimal effort in each direction, feeling the mobility starting to become more available. Finally, allow your head to rest on the floor, and let that movement information assimilate in the nervous system.

A low-effort motion like this reminds the muscles on both the front and back of the upper neck that they can lengthen and shorten, rather than being caught in a single point of range. It mobilizes the joints and wakes up a connection to the deep upper cervical flexor muscles, key stabilizers of the neck (see Fig. 6.8).

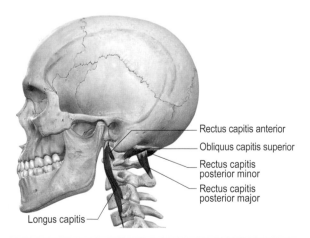

Rectus capitis anterior
Obliquus capitis superior
Rectus capitis posterior minor
Rectus capitis posterior major
Longus capitis

Figure 6.8

Flexors and extensors of the head on the neck

Lower lock

Deepening of the lumbar lordosis and tightening of the erector spinae in this area in response to movement creates what we will call the lower, or lumbosacral, lock (see Fig. 6.9).

Abdominal weakness is often blamed for this postural response. However, attempting to correct the lumbosacral position by increasing active abdominal tension creates excessive co-contraction, which – as we have discussed (see Chapter 1) – is a common neuromuscular dysfunction associated with chronic low back pain when used as a habitual postural strategy. Remember, co-contraction was seen as desirable in the 1990s, but now that we understand more about it,

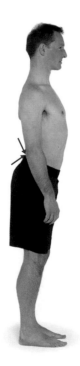

Figure 6.9

Lower, or lumbosacral, lock

we need to accept that more co-contraction isn't necessarily better, and constant co-contraction is definitely not normal.

Fighting back tension with front tension is energetically costly, and increasing total tension results in the natural movement associated with postural control being blocked.

> There's no need to fight tension with tension: it leads to immobility. Posture is a dance, not a battle.

If conscious correction isn't the answer, what are our other possibilities? When this postural lock is being driven by chronic muscle tension, we need to calm down the excessive activity in the erector spinae in order to make a deeper change. With the research indicating that the inability to effectively release the trunk muscles is strongly linked to the risk of low back pain,[5] unpicking the lumbar lock is of even greater significance.

At this point we need to issue an invitation to the lumbar spine to relax and decompress. When we down-regulate this habitual postural strategy, the brain must consider its other options. We open the door for the lower level autoactivation of the deep abdominals.

Movement exploration

Sacral rocks

To change the relationship between the lumbar spine and the pelvis, we need to develop an awareness of our sacrum. To perform a sacral rock, it is essential first to build the image of the sacrum as a curved bone that can be rolled over. Many people think it is flat, a misconception that creates a conflicting image for the movement that will be involved.

Cup your hand over your sacrum, with your fingertips pointing down toward your coccyx. Imagine the bone tapering down to that tip. Feel the curved shape under your palm, and rub it to let the brain know where it is and how it feels (see Fig. 6.10). Once you have made that connection, we can begin.

Lie on your back with your knees comfortably bent. If you naturally have a little upper lock, place a folded towel under your head at the point where you feel the skull curve outwards. If you don't neutralize the upper lock first, it will be very difficult to move the pelvis with ease. Finally, rest the palms of your hands on your ilia, the bones on either side of your pelvis (see Fig. 6.11).

Now notice where your body rests on the sacrum. Those with a habitual lower lock will normally rest toward the bottom tip of their sacrum. Those who have been trained to actively flatten the lumbar curve toward the floor in supine will want to assume a position at the top of their sacrum. It's important to recognize that this is just another form of lock, a point of immobilization that trains a lumbar posture that makes no sense once a person stands up.

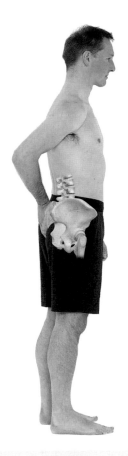

Figure 6.10

Discover the curved shape of the sacrum

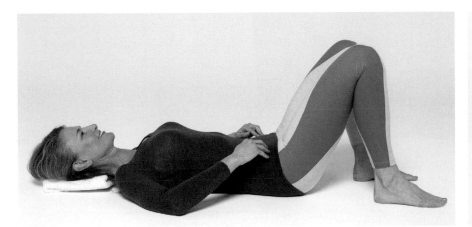

Figure 6.11

Sacral rock start position, with hands on front of pelvis

If you are training a spinal position lying down, make sure that it makes sense when standing up.

If we know what our habit is, we can play with it. With minimal effort, roll slowly over the sacrum toward the tip of your tailbone. This will accentuate the lumbar extension (see Fig. 6.12). But wait … isn't this the position that we are trying to avoid?

That's the old attitude sneaking through. We identify a position we aren't happy with and do the opposite, right? It's time to update our thinking. Our aim is not to avoid a position but to teach the lumbar spine to be able to move freely through its entire range. A lock occurs at a specific point in that range and the spine needs to be reminded how to move smoothly through it in both directions.

To unpick a lock, we first need to introduce some motion. Moving more deeply into extension is in essence moving into the direction of preference, which will require less effort than heading into the resistance of flexion. Think of it as your sock drawer

being stuck – you don't pull harder to open it, do you? You push the drawer inwards to release whatever is catching it, and then it pulls open easily.

By moving into extension, you remind the erector spinae muscles how to dynamically contract again, the microscopic cross-links within each muscle recalling how to shorten the muscle fibers into *inner range*^G. Instead of creating a lock by working continuously at a fixed point in their range, the muscles themselves are on the move.

Now that you have introduced some motion into the area by heading toward the tip of your tail, you can deepen your awareness of the soles of your feet connecting with the floor, and slowly roll back over your sacrum toward its upper margin (see Fig. 6.13). You are going to use as little effort as possible to do this, letting your abdominals fall toward the back of your pelvis. The erector spinae lengthen, allowing the lumbopelvic junction to open. You will only move as far as the top of the sacrum at this point – if you go farther, you might be tempted to start forcing the spine down into the floor by overusing your abdominals. Remember: we want the brain to discover that this is easy. This is an unlocking, not a forcing activity.

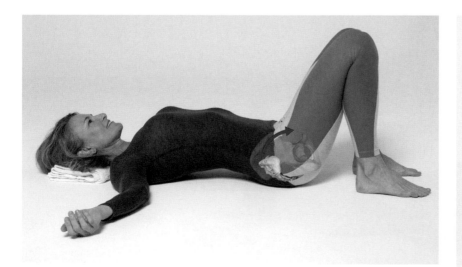

Figure 6.12

Sacral rock to the bottom tip of the sacrum. (Arms have been placed to illustrate the spinal position)

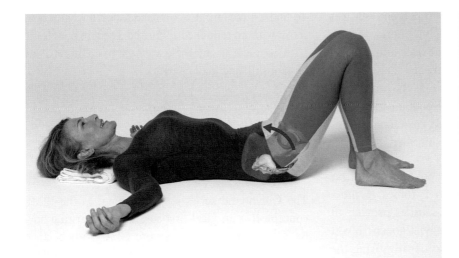

Figure 6.13

Sacral rock to the top of the sacrum, with the abdomen falling toward the spine

The sacral rock is much more specific to the lower lumbar spine than the more commonly used pelvic tilt, which often engages higher activity in the superficial abdominals. This increased abdominal activity actually blocks lower lumbar motion, shunting the movement farther up the lumbar spine and missing the opportunity to open the lumbosacral lock.

Allow yourself to freely, smoothly, and slowly move from the top of your sacrum toward the tip of your tailbone, feeling how this draws your hands up and away from you. As you reverse the direction, feel how your hands not only move toward you but also drop back toward your spine. After a few repetitions, just switch off, relax, and note where your body falls onto your sacrum. For most people, this will now be somewhere near the middle of the sacrum, the apex of the curve of the bone. This is your sacral support position.

You may still feel uncertain about the idea of relaxing into this position instead of creating it with conscious abdominal setting. Let's look at it logically: when supine, gravity is acting downward upon us. This should encourage our spine to drop toward the floor, so to imagine that an excessive curve is caused by abdominal weakness makes no sense! The only way it can be lifting off the floor into extension is if we are actively contracting the muscles of our back to push upward against gravity. It is primarily a tension problem of the back, rather than a weakness problem at the front.

In relaxed supine, there is no movement, neither is there any demand for postural control, so there is no reason for the erector spinae to be firing. If we cannot invite the spine to relax under these conditions, anything we teach to prepare for movement in this position is a coping strategy.

The sacral rock unpicks the erector spinae's fixed point of contraction, breaking the continuous neuromuscular holding pattern. When the sacrum can rest on a relaxed center point, the spine takes up a natural, unforced position. From this easy point of reference, a person can explore the relationship between limb movement and the central body. Proprioceptively, it is much simpler than trying to work out where your spinal position should be relative to the floor, and it allows for individual variation in structure and shape. Elastic limb movement becomes possible as the myofascial tissues throughout the front of the body are allowed to lengthen in the absence of the fixed, conscious abdominal contraction that is conventionally used.

Think of wiring instead of just positioning. As far as the brain is concerned when it comes to moving a limb, if the erector spinae muscles provide an adequate spinal stabilizing strategy, it doesn't invest more of the body's energy in additionally firing the abdominals. When we observe this, we conventionally interpret it as weakness and fight the tension in the back by ramping up abdominal activity. Although this might change the spinal position, it also initiates an unnecessary battle that blocks the muscle length change necessary to make myoelastic connections between the limbs and trunk.

If we take away the current stabilizing strategy, however, the brain is provoked into finding another solution. By inviting the back muscles to relax, we create the opportunity for the abdominals to come back online. It's like tuning a stereo system – if we turn down the base a little, we can hear the treble. If our approach is one of neuromuscular balance, we can progress the strength of the entire pattern systematically without compromising movement potential.

This understanding will form the foundation of any of the supine movements that follow.

Integrating the postural learning

We have altered the balance of muscle activity around the lumbopelvic area, but this is not enough to make a transferable functional change – it has simply opened a window of possibility.

To make it meaningful, we need to learn what it is to move with an unlocked spine and a secure but elastic CLA; to make it achievable, we need to do this at a low level of skill and load demand.

Movement exploration

Greyhound Hand Slide

The Greyhound series is fundamental to the JEMS concept. It is an ideal first step toward learning how to feel a responsive but secure CLA (with balance between the anterior and posterior chains) and establish the sense of elastic connection between the limbs and trunk. Why is it called the Greyhound? The inspiration came from the shape of the slender racing dogs: as their limbs extend away from their bodies, their abdomens tuck up toward their spines reflexively in order to enhance the stretch and recoil of the myofascial structures connecting forelimbs through the body to hind limbs (see Fig. 6.14). So it will be with you.

Take up the position of lying on your back with knees bent and head on the folded towel if necessary. Take a moment to find that relaxed central place on your sacrum, doing a few sacral rocks to remind yourself of what it is like to switch off and just let the body rest on the floor.

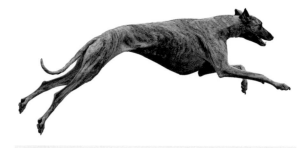

Figure 6.14

The greyhound's shape inspires this action

Place one hand on your belly just above your pubic bone. Lift the other and bend the elbow so that your fingertips trail toward the floor beside your head (see Fig. 6.15). Relax completely, and slide your hand along the floor until your arm has reached the end of its available range, allowing your spine to follow it (see Fig. 6.16). If you have accidentally held your breath, let it go, and feel how your back softens in response, dropping softly to the floor instead of arching upward. If you have remained relaxed, with no sign of bracing or setting your abdominals, you will find that your belly has sunk down toward your spine, just like the greyhound's. From here on, we will refer to this as the Greyhound abdomen, as it will apply in many techniques. This is often taught as a conscious contraction, referred to in the research as abdominal hollowing or caving in, but it should occur naturally as an automatic postural response.[6]

Wherever the belly has sunk to, you will simply maintain it there to provide an anchor point that supports the motion of your hand sliding back in. Initially, you may feel your belly pop upward into your hand as you bring your arm in. This is just your brain trying out the old strategy. There's no need to fight it. Just relax your spine again, repeat the sliding motion, and, this time, trust your body to support the movement without the need for so much effort.

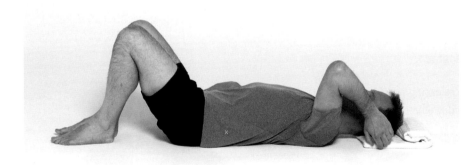

Figure 6.15

Greyhound Hand Slide start position

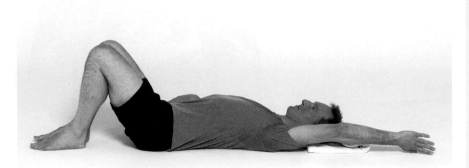

Figure 6.16

Greyhound Hand Slide lengthened position

From a JEMS perspective, breathing during movement should be natural and uncontrived. It is very tempting to cue action/breath matching (breathe in when you do this, and out when you do that), but at this low level of skill and load demand, you should be able to breathe independently of the movement, as you would in an everyday activity. We can, after all, walk and talk simultaneously without having to match our breathing to our steps. The easiest way to ensure this is to hum something simple to yourself, or speak out loud (complete nonsense is best) throughout the motion.

You will see the Greyhound shape appear in experienced practitioners in a wide variety of poses and movements, as it reduces tension and allows greater freedom in the hips and pelvis (see Fig. 6.17).

Erector spinae: release or strengthen?

With our emphasis so far on releasing tension in the erector spinae, you might wonder whether you should still be including direct strengthening of this group in your programs. The answer is an unequivocal yes. Erector spinae strength has been identified as a factor in spinal stability as well as in rehabilitation of lumbar spine injuries.

However, for safe, strong spinal extension, there needs to be a balance of forces around the spine to stabilize it throughout the motion. The erector spinae group is made up of relatively long fibers that cross many joints and – when unopposed – has a long line of pull, much like the string of an archer's bow. To prevent excessive stress at any one level, a collaboration of stabilizing muscles acting close to the spine (including psoas, multifidus, and transversus abdominis) control the alignment relationships between each spinal segment and ensure that each level participates appropriately in the motion created by the erector spinae (see Figs. 6.18–6.21). In this way, we preserve the CLA and create a foundation for strong, secure extension.

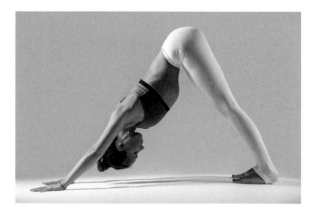

Figure 6.17

The Greyhound shape appears frequently in experienced movement practitioners

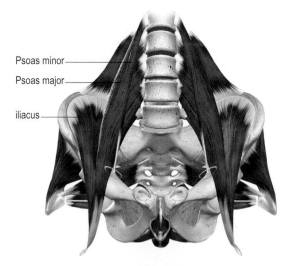

Psoas minor

Psoas major

iliacus

Figure 6.18

The significant spinal attachments of psoas

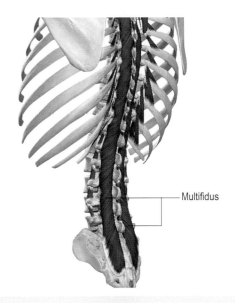

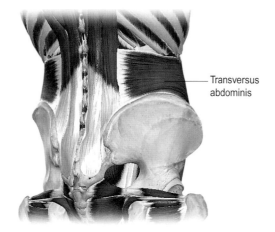

Figure 6.21

Transversus abdominis contributing to spinal support through its connections into the thoracolumbar fascia

Figure 6.19

The short fibers of multifidus sitting close to the spine

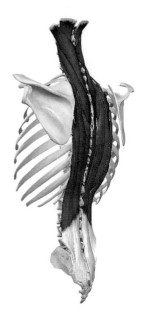

Figure 6.20

The long fibers of the muscles comprising the group known as the erector spinae

When the brain uses the lumbar lock as its primary stabilizing strategy, the cooperative partnership that should balance the forces applied to the spine becomes distorted. The altered ratio of erector spinae to transversus abdominis activity affects tensions in the thoracolumbar fascia.[7] Multifidus, the series of short, deep overlapping muscles lying adjacent to the spine, functions less effectively as a stabilizer in the shortened state that the lumbar lock imposes.[8] A fixed lumbar position will affect the healthy variable function of psoas, which changes its role in response to spinal position.[9] Easing the lumbar lock is therefore an important step toward re-establishing equilibrium.

From a strength point of view, if any muscle is habitually held at the fixed, shortened length, as the lower erector spinae are in a lumbar lock, they do not necessarily function well when asked to change length *eccentrically*[G] and *concentrically*[G]. The muscles may be strong in a limited range but behave as if functionally weak once asked to work outside this range. They may even forget how to release – which they should at end-range spinal flexion.[10] Releasing the lock allows the muscles to reset to a more neutral length at a lower baseline level of activation. This makes more of the microscopic cross-links within the muscle fibers available, which, in turn, creates greater strength potential.

Once you have released the lumbar lock, the next step is to integrate the change. Hot Toffee (see Chapter 8) and Superman (see Chapter 4) both offer a low-load opportunity for the deep abdominals, psoas, multifidus, and erector spinae to renegotiate their roles.

Posterior rib lock

In starting to address the lumbosacral lock, you will also have the opportunity to ease the *posterior rib lock*. This is another strong extension lock, associated with the trying hard, stand up straight, lots to do, have to be good enough, go-go-go! state of mind.

Serratus posterior inferior is one of the key characters involved in this lock (see Fig. 6.22). It acts on the back of the rib cage, drawing it down and toward the spine, compressing the joints of the lower thoracic/upper lumbar region into extension, and tilting the rib cage up at the front (see Fig. 6.23). As this spinal position reduces the potential for posterior expansion of the rib cage on inhalation, it can be associated with breathing dysfunction. The lungs are largest at the back and base of their structure, right about where the posterior rib lock occurs. If the rib lock blocks posterior expansion, it also robs you of efficient oxygen exchange. When such a large area for lung expansion is compromised, the body must seek another solution, often by redirecting breathing emphasis to the upper chest, or, alternatively, reducing abdominal postural tone to allow for more belly expansion. Attempting

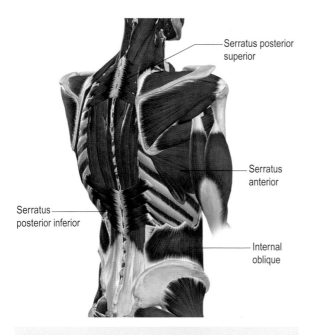

Serratus posterior
superior

Serratus
anterior

Serratus
posterior inferior

Internal
oblique

Figure 6.22

Serratus posterior inferior is positioned to pull down on the back of the rib cage

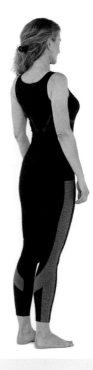

Figure 6.23

Posterior rib lock

to improve your breathing pattern can be frustrating when you are stuck in a posterior rib lock.

The posterior rib lock lifts the sternum and makes the posture look very erect, but, in fact, it creates a functional kink in your CLA that weakens the connection between your upper and lower body. Becoming aware of it is the best place to begin.

Movement exploration

The Giant Marble

Either sitting comfortably or standing with hips and knees softened, imagine that your rib cage has been placed over a giant marble, a smooth, lightly oiled globe that sits perfectly within the circular rings of your ribs. Place your hands on your rib cage, and experiment with rolling your rib cage all the way around the marble, feeling how this would invite it to adopt an undulating motion like the disk inside a gyroscope. Work out where your rib cage normally sits. Is it higher at the front and lower at the back, as if you have slid your rib cage over the back of the marble?

Slide your rib cage back to a position where it would be sitting straight over the marble. Allow it to slip over to the right side of the marble. Feel how this compresses one side and expands the other side of the rib cage like a concertina. Take a moment to breathe into the expanded space that has been created by your ribs mildly separating. Now slide your rib cage over the marble to the left, feeling how this reverses the expansion and compression. Feel how some ribs move together and others move apart, and breathe into the newly expanded space (see Fig. 6.24).

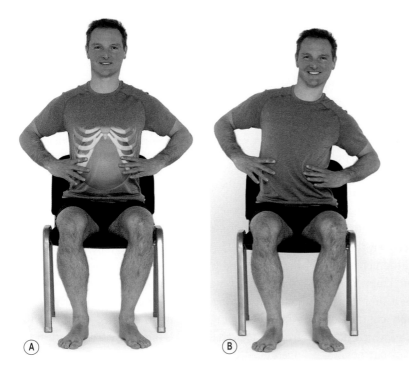

Figure 6.24

The Giant Marble. *A.* Start position; *B.* moving the rib cage around the giant marble

Slide the rib cage over the front of the marble and feel how this compresses the top of the abdomen and causes the lower belly to protrude. Then slide the rib cage over the back of the marble, feeling your spine compress and tighten into the posterior rib lock. Play with rolling your rib cage around the marble, pausing in different places to notice that when one area closes, the opposite side opens to allow you to breathe more deeply into it.

Come back to balance your rib cage centrally over the marble again. Having released some of the restrictions around your rib cage, this might not be where your rib cage normally sits. It may feel a little strange to experience the rib cage floating horizontally over your pelvis, rather than being fixed in place by the spinal muscles or abdomen.

Both the lumbosacral lock and the posterior rib lock are also commonly associated with the *anterior hip lock*. Whether in supine, prone, sitting or standing, the anterior hip locker will try to create a stable point of control by using hip flexors to fix the relationship between their femur, pelvis, and lumbar spine (see Fig. 6.25A). In standing and sitting, these people will have their hips slightly flexed, but their spine will compensate with increased extension to maintain an upright position (see Fig. 6.25B). In a supine heel slide along the floor, these are the people whose pelvis attempts to follow the thigh away from the body, pulling the pelvis into anterior tilt, which then draws the lumbar spine into extension. In sitting, the palpable bone at the front of the pelvis known as the anterior superior iliac spine (ASIS[G]) tilts down toward the femur, locking the relationship between the two bones. When asked to sit up straight, the pelvis and femur remain fixed, and the person compensates with the posterior rib lock to assume a more vertical posture. This is achieved through contraction of the upper fibers of the psoas muscle, which draw the upper lumbar vertebrae forward, in partnership

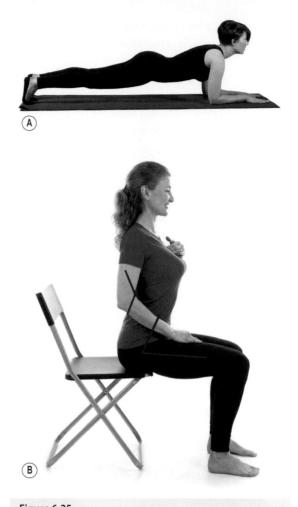

(A)

(B)

Figure 6.25

A. Upper, lumbosacral, and anterior hip locks demonstrated in the plank position. *B.* Posterior rib lock coupled with anterior hip lock. Trunk is pulled forward by hip flexors and compensates by upwardly rotating rib cage

with serratus posterior and the thoracolumbar erector spinae. The effect is like being cut in half at the waist: the upper and lower parts of the torso become disconnected. In standing, the effect is similar, with the pelvis appearing to be tilted downward at the front, while the rib cage appears to be tilted upward at the front. The overall effect is one of the front of the body opening.

Fortunately, everything that we have learned so far that addresses the lumbosacral lock is relevant for the posterior rib lock, as the spine needs to learn to relax out of extension. Now we can see that it is not just the erector spinae that can be caught in a narrow range of contraction. Serratus posterior and the hip flexors also need to reclaim their full range of motion.

To re-establish the active length of the hip flexors and interrupt the anterior hip lock, which, in turn, will reduce the lumbosacral and posterior rib lock, we are going to explore the Greyhound Heel Slide.

Movement exploration

Greyhound Heel Slide

The prerequisite for this technique is the sacral rock. The central resting place on the sacrum will be the point of reference for the person performing the movement, and the ability to feel a change of this position is going to play a major role in self-monitoring. If we don't do this first, we are reduced to abdominal setting again, and this commonly puts the pelvis into a shade too much posterior pelvic tilt for the hip to be able to move comfortably into extension.

With head supported on a rolled towel if necessary to relieve the upper lock, and knees bent, rest a moment, allowing your breath to find its own rhythm. Feel your body weight resting on the sacrum. Place the fingers of one hand on the front of the pelvis in line with your thigh. Place the fingers of your remaining hand on the top of your thigh (see Fig. 6.26). Feel the distance between your two hands. Now slowly and smoothly, move your thigh away from your pelvis by sliding your heel along the floor, feeling how your hands separate. We call this "opening the book." Notice how the back of your leg is lengthening, opening out behind the knee, and imagine that you are pressing your heel out into a piece of elastic that has been attached to your sitting bone (see Fig. 6.27). At the end of the movement, note that your weight is still supported on the same part of your sacrum and that your belly has sunk toward your spine in the Greyhound abdomen response.

If you have been an anterior hip locker, this will constitute a big change in the pattern of how you extend and flex your hip. The muscle length and activity around the entire hip–pelvis–spine region will be different, and so it is likely that some sensory input will be necessary to tell your brain how and where to bend once you have extended your leg. Find the crease of the hip (the line where your underwear might normally sit), which is where the hip should

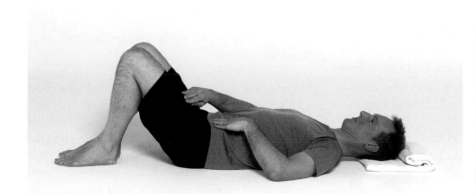

Figure 6.26

Greyhound Heel Slide start position

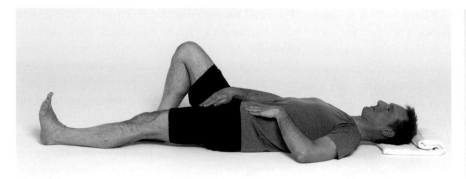

Figure 6.27

Opening the book into the lengthened position

bend. Tap it firmly with your fingers as you allow the imaginary elastic to draw your heel back toward you.

> Using the imagery of elastic between the hip and the heel helps to balance the effort between the hip flexor and the hamstrings.

Moving in this way persuades the hip flexors, which have been contracting with limited length change, to rediscover their eccentric and concentric action through range. By removing the habitual hip lock, deep, low-effort abdominal activity can flicker back into action, providing just enough support, but no more than is necessary.

Breathing: the universal key

If there is a single aspect that you could focus on to positively influence as many systems and areas of body function as you can, it would be breathing.

Unimpaired breathing is a whole-body affair. We have already discovered that the body accommodates the breath in multiple segments, and if it cannot do this, postural control is affected. The spinal curves themselves absorb each inhalation, flattening slightly at the cervical and lumbar lordoses as the trunk fills, before recoiling into their normal position with the out-breath. A stiffly held neck or a lumbar spine that is immobilized with bracing will therefore affect breathing mechanics as the body tries to find an alternative strategy to manage air pressure.

Movement exploration

Lie comfortably on your side with your head supported and your knees and hips bent enough for you to feel relaxed and balanced, but not so much that your spine flexes. In your mind's eye, see a gentle inwards curve at your neck and lumbar spine, even if you don't naturally have one (see Fig. 6.28).

Take a moment to let everything go (as much as is possible).

Starting from the point where your cervical spine joins your thoracic spine, visualize sending your in-breath to gently press out into this single vertebra from the inside, and then imagine it recoiling as you breathe out. This may feel difficult at first, and the first great breakthrough is actually noticing your own resistance. There's no need to force it – just keep thinking

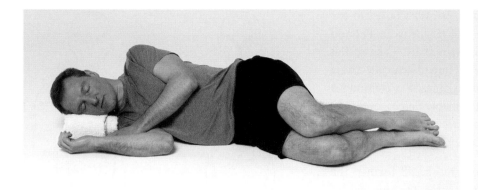

Figure 6.28

Support the head and relax in side lying to release the neck with the breath

of softening this area. When you are ready, move your focus up to the next vertebra and repeat the process, breathing the softness into one segment at a time until you reach the very top of your neck. Finally, listen to the sense of the head gently nodding on the in-breath, and releasing on the out-breath. You are restoring the expansion and recoil of the neck in response to your breath. This is ideal at any time, but especially for reminding the body to release an upper lock.

The diaphragm is one of the most interconnected organs in our body, anatomically, neurologically, emotionally, and functionally.[11] It is a surprisingly thin muscle that separates the thoracic and abdominal cavities, and at rest forms a domed shape with a concave undersurface. At its center is a thickened, white, non-contractile area called the central tendon, which – in addition to its role in breathing – also supports the heart. The diaphragm is connected via ligaments to the lungs, heart, liver, esophagus, and colon. There is even a link to the duodenum via the ligament of Treitz, which creates a connection between the duodenum and the spine via the diaphragm's spinal attachments (see Fig. 6.29).[12] The degree of connection between the diaphragm and its adjacent organs alerts us to its potential influence on their function and motion.[13–15]

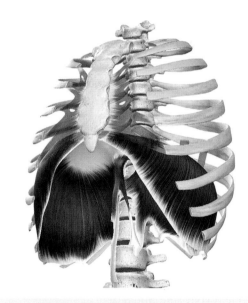

Figure 6.29

Diaphragm. Note the attachments on the spine

The anterior muscle fibers of the diaphragm reach forward to the xiphoid process to form its sternal attachment and then line the ribs with costal attachments connecting to the inferior six ribs. These costal fibers intersect with those of transversus abdominis, which attach to these same ribs from below.

From behind, the diaphragm is also secured to the vertebral bodies and disks, usually between T12 and L3, but occasionally as far down as L4. The two flat tendons that create this attachment are collectively called the crura. The diaphragm fascia is continuous with the medial arcuate ligament, which covers the psoas muscle, and the lateral arcuate ligament, which covers the quadratus lumborum.[12]

The anatomical connections reach still further: the fascia transversalis, spreading across the underside of the diaphragm and continuous with the diaphragm fascia, separates the inner surface of the tranversus abdominis from the membrane containing the abdominal cavity and arrives at the linea alba of rectus abdominis, thus connecting as far as the pubis.[16]

With such far-reaching connections, the potential for the diaphragm to influence multiple aspects of our posture is extensive.

Under pressure

Although we think of breathing primarily as a process of gas exchange, the role of breathing in postural control is one of pressure management. Imagine that your trunk is made up of a large rubber pressure chamber divided horizontally by the diaphragm into two cavities. The upper one is your thoracic cavity, and the lower one is your abdominal cavity.

In normal, quiet breathing, the contracting diaphragm descends, flattening out its dome shape. This increases the pressure in the abdominal cavity below it and reduces the pressure in the thoracic cavity, making space for air to enter to fill the vacuum. The intercostal muscles draw the ribs upward and outward, and the rib cage expands to create even greater space for a deeper breath.

The increased pressure on the abdominal cavity applies a subtle pressing action upon the abdominal

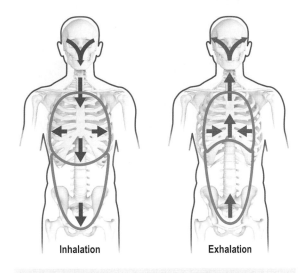

Inhalation   Exhalation

Figure 6.30

Inhalation increases pressure in the thoracic cavity causing it to expand, which in turn presses down upon the abdominal cavity

contents, applying a massage-like effect to the organs and assisting in lymphatic drainage of the abdomen (see Fig. 6.30).[17]

> The diaphragm rhythmically mobilizes the abdominal organs.

To accommodate the increased downward pressure, the abdominal muscles allow a controlled expansion, and the muscles of the pelvic floor also mildly lengthen while still remaining active. This relationship between the diaphragm, the transversus abdominis, and the pelvic floor is therefore intimate and synchronized.[18] Between them, they regulate the intra-abdominal pressure, which is a normal stabilizing action for the spine,[6] much like having a supportive balloon inflated from the inside running up the front of your vertebrae.

When pressure is managed effectively, it contributes to stability.

Pressure is beneficial when things are working well, but, if not, it can lead to mischief. Hernias, prolapses, reflux, incontinence, sexual dysfunction, pelvic pain and back pain are all associated with pressure management problems between the thoracic and abdominal cavities. Pressure problems fall into two categories: where tension is blocking the expansion needed to accommodate pressure due to tension, and where pressure is being allowed to escape too freely, like opening a valve.

Just for a moment imagine holding in your hands a partially inflated balloon. If you squeeze one end, the air escapes to the other end. If you squeeze that end, once again the air is pushed away. Your body performs the same trick – if you block expansion in one area, the pressure will seek a less restricted route.

Once you grasp this concept, you can relax about specific patterns and just ask yourself where the air is going.

To take a simple example, in the case of the posterior rib lock, the air cannot inflate the rib cage at the back, so it is redirected forward and up instead. Your client may look like an upper chest breather, but, in fact, to change the situation, the back must make itself more available for expansion.

Child's pose offers a nice opportunity to discover expansion into the back and softening of the posterior rib lock with breathing (see Fig. 6.31).

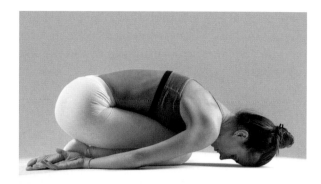

Figure 6.31

Breathing into the back with Child's Pose

One of the increasingly common breathing dysfunctions that I am encountering in clients with low back pain involves a misunderstanding about "belly breathing." As they breathe in, they skip past their rib cage and excessively inflate their abdomens, in the mistaken belief that this represents healthy diaphragmatic breathing. In reality, these distended bellies mean that intra-abdominal pressure is escaping out through the front of the body like a puncture in a balloon. The stabilizing effect of the intra-abdominal pressure is compromised.

In normal function, the abdomen expands proportionately to the rib cage, a gradual, coordinated motion that radiates throughout the trunk while retaining the elasticity of the abdominal wall. It is important, therefore, to help these people to rediscover rib cage expansion, embrace the whole breath, and find balance and coordination in the system.

Conversely, if the abdomen is consciously held in, as so many low back pain patients are taught to do, the normal abdominal expansion is blocked, and the air is pushed either into the upper chest or into excessive lateral expansion with disproportionate intercostal muscle activity. Alternatively, it may be pushed into the pelvic floor, which is unable to withstand the pressure, often causing distressing symptoms like incontinence.

The emotional diaphragm

Holistic movement practitioners have long appreciated the benefits of breath work for general health. Increasingly, the links between emotion and breathing (and therefore diaphragm function) are being identified in the research, emphasizing just how intimate this relationship is. Emotion can affect the position and function of the diaphragm, altering its biomechanics and elasticity as well as its effect upon its fascial and neurological connections.[19] Spinal stability and pressure-related problems are often amplified by stress for sound physiological reasons.

Fortunately, it is a two-way relationship in that breath retraining can positively influence our emotional state.[20,21] It seems that working with the breath, that most fundamental of physiological processes, is powerful medicine.

Base notes

The pelvic floor is a frequently misunderstood part of this system. The sling of pelvic floor muscles creates connections from the pubis anteriorly back to the sacrum and coccyx (see Fig. 6.32).[22] If you were a dog, some of these would be your tail-wagging muscles, but they have evolved to support the pelvic organs now that we are upright. Via fascial connections, the pelvic floor also has a relationship to the deep hip rotators that stabilize the femoral head.[23] If pelvic floor function is compromised and the coordination between the diaphragm and the pelvic floor becomes impaired, the resulting biomechanical disturbance of the lumbopelvic–hip complex can lead to low back,

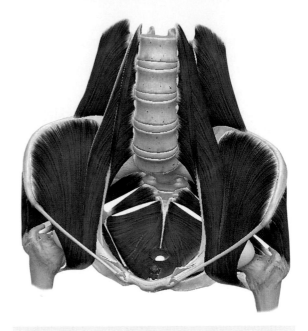

Figure 6.32

View of the pelvic floor from above

hip, and pelvic pain,[24] sacroiliac joint dysfunction, and even sexual dysfunction in both men and women.[25,26] Chronic pelvic floor muscle dysfunction can provoke postural adaptation in an attempt to alleviate the stress on these structures.

A normal pelvic floor maintains a baseline low-level hum of activity (a tonic level of tonus). Its muscles lengthen slightly on an in-breath as they accommodate the extra pressure, and – like a trampoline – are able to recoil afterwards.

Symptoms of incontinence or other pelvic dysfunction tend to automatically trigger a diagnosis of a hypotonic or weak pelvic floor, and treatment frequently emphasizes strength and endurance training for these muscles. In women where this condition has been associated with child birth, the hormonal changes associated with menopause, aging, or obesity,[27] it is certainly true that they will benefit from pelvic floor strengthening regimens.

This is not just a consideration in women, however: in men, symptoms of a weak or hypotonic pelvic floor (e.g., incontinence, erectile dysfunction, and premature ejaculation) have been associated with age-related change in the collagen and muscle fibers of the pelvic floor[28] as well as with pelvic surgery, such as prostatectomy.[29] These men will also benefit from a program to address pelvic floor weakness.[30] In terms of pressure management, the hypotonic pelvic floor loses pressure through the floor of the abdominal cavity, and, as a result, can contribute to low back pain by compromising the stabilizing mechanism of intra-abdominal pressure. The body's search for an alternative solution leads to other compensatory postural control strategies – which takes us back to the locking behaviors discussed earlier in this chapter.

While the underactive pelvic floor is old news, the overactive pelvic floor is presenting with increasing prevalence in both men and women. It can be caused by many factors, including stress, social discomfort, behaviors of delaying urination or defecation,[31] and compromised trunk stability. The result is an unyielding pelvic floor that can neither lengthen to modulate intra-abdominal pressure nor contract reflexively to manage impact (or even just a cough or sneeze). Remember: a muscle can only contract as quickly and effectively as it can release. You can't contract what is already contracted.

A chronically over-contracted pelvic floor loses its elastic quality. Instead of a responsive trampoline that supports the pelvic contents by finely regulating its tensions, it becomes an iron door slammed shut in an attempt to withstand an intolerable load. The distressing symptoms of incontinence, especially in higher load activities like running, jumping, and weight lifting, become an increasing problem as anxiety further increases the tension in the struggling

pelvic floor. In this case, conventional pelvic floor strengthening programs may not only be ineffective, but might actually exacerbate the problem.

> In the case of the overactive pelvic floor, it is important first to acknowledge that allowing the pelvic floor to relax is normal and healthy.

Incontinence in athletic women is widespread and, surprisingly, more common than it is in sedentary women.[32] It is often assumed that the pelvic floors of athletic women are not strong enough to withstand their sport, which leads back to the simplistic reaction of more strengthening, and potentially more tightening. However, if we understand that the pelvic floors of these women are under pressure, we can instead look at balancing their systems to alleviate it.

The diaphragm, for example, works in the same feedforward way that our pelvic floor and transversus abdominis do to prepare for movement.[6,33] It has dual roles – respiration and postural control – and it adjusts its function between them depending upon your activity.[34] If postural stability is being challenged, the diaphragm responds by increasing its stabilizing contribution, which, in turn, reduces its respiratory movement. Breath holding is therefore understandably common when postural control is challenged; but it does affect pressure management between the thoracic cavity and abdominal cavities. This ultimately imposes higher and more prolonged pressures on the pelvic floor. Rather than fighting the pressure, greater awareness of breath management is fundamental to healthy pelvic floor function.

> There is a circular relationship between posture, trunk stability, breathing, and pelvic floor function.

Mechanically, adequate shock absorption in the joints of the legs can reduce impact force in the pelvic floor. It is, then, perhaps not so surprising to learn that an inability to absorb shock sufficiently through the foot has been linked to symptoms of urinary incontinence.[35] The same principle can be applied to the knee and hip, being large joints that can alleviate the amount of downward force that the central body must bear. Working on springy, coordinated legs becomes a part of preserving or regaining urinary continence in the athletic woman. This is the principle of force sharing again, isn't it?

Movement exploration

To connect the normal in-breath to the pelvic floor, lie comfortably with knees bent and feet on the floor with your head supported on the folded towel if necessary to neutralize the upper lock. Alternatively, you can use relaxed sitting – sometimes one position is easier than the other to make a connection. Supported sitting can be even better: sitting on a chair with a fitness ball on the thighs right up against the front of the body, allowing the arms to rest on it, eases the postural stress and provides sensory input. As you start to slowly draw in a normal breath, visualize a long balloon progressively inflating through the center of your body all the way into your pelvic floor. Imagine the pelvic floor as an elastic membrane, and as your long balloon contacts it, it stretches to accommodate that gentle pressure, and then recoils again as your air slips away.

After repeating this a few times, shift your awareness to think about allowing the air to expand the area between your sitting bones, imagining them spreading gently away from one another, and then returning on the out-breath. Now think of your little tailbone, your coccyx, expanding backward away from your pubic bone, and let it return to settle again. Some directions will be easier, others more tricky. Find what

works for you, and then experiment as you explore the options.

This technique is all about rediscovering the normal stretch and recoil functionality of the pelvic floor. If yours tends to be overactive, this will initially be tough – you are accustomed to getting your feedback from a high level of muscle tension. Learning to release this tension will feel uncertain, but in doing so you will begin to re-establish the neural coordination between the diaphragm and the pelvic floor.

> If it is relevant to your clients to include pelvic floor strengthening, make sure that you balance it with this coordination exercise – the timing relationship is important for weak pelvic floors as well!

Real life study

My client was a young male professional squash player who had struggled with persistent patellar tendon problems. This wasn't surprising: he found it difficult to drop his center of gravity and told me that he had never been able to squat. As a very quick, multi-directional sport, squash requires constant change of direction, and to control momentum effectively, you need to be able to drop your center of gravity quickly. If you can't do this, the stress amplifies in the knees instead of being shared with the large hip joints.

An upper chest breather with a hyperlordotic posture, he was an intense, earnest young man who applied a great deal of pressure to himself. His squat demonstration took him quickly into a "tail tucked under" pelvic position, which often indicates a short pelvic floor. He only managed to achieve a third of his potential range of motion.

I asked him to feel where his coccyx was and to imagine it as a little tail. Allowing him to support himself through his outstretched arms on a firm vertical bar, I invited him to begin his squat, pausing at the point where his tail wanted to tuck under like an unhappy dog. Here he practiced "breathing his tailbone outwards," like a happy dog. After a few breaths, he was able to deepen the squat, repeating the process several times. To his great surprise, he ended up in a full squat and felt quite comfortable there. He was both delighted and bemused. The knee problems diminished rapidly once he learned to integrate his new ability to smoothly drop his center of gravity while playing. The pelvic floor was the key.

> From head to tail, breathing pattern and posture stand united.

People can become very anxious about whether they are breathing correctly. The truth is that there are many correct ways to breathe: it depends on what you are doing and the position your body is in. If you curl forward, for example, you limit the capacity for anterior expansion in the chest, but make the back very available. If you bend your trunk to the left, it compresses the left side of the rib cage but invites rib expansion on the right. The point is to have many options, not just one.

For this reason, we are going to practice breath moving, which is an activity of exploring different possibilities. Everyone is different – what is easy for some is difficult for others. However, we are going to work toward dislodging a single fixed habit and establishing a coordinated, more versatile breathing pattern.

Movement exploration

Breath moving

Breath moving can be performed in supine lying or in relaxed sitting. When lying down, remember to support the head with the folded towel to neutralize the upper lock, and bend the hips and knees, placing the feet flat on the floor to remove tension from the hips and spine.

We are going to take up the imagery of balloons once again, but this time we will use them to direct the breath to different areas. We are going to use calm, natural breaths rather than deep breathing; this is because we want to normalize the experience of breathing adaptability, rather than making it into a specific special exercise.

Begin by placing a hand over your sternum, and create the image of a round balloon resting within your chest under your hand. As you breathe in, fill this balloon, allowing the chest to expand from front to back. You will feel the sternum lift a little, and then, ideally, it should subside back down again. However, if you have a tendency toward posterior rib lock, or if your life is busy or stressful, you might find that your sternum is unwilling to return to the start position again. Deal with this gently – you need to allow the muscles that are stuck in a protective contraction to relax, and for the sternum to feel as though it is softening (see Fig. 6.33).

> Sternal softening is often the key to releasing the posterior rib lock.

Move your hand to the junction where your ribs come together at the bottom of your rib cage. Again, see a round balloon resting within your body under your hand. Following your normal in-breath, allow this

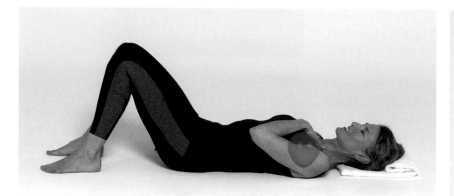

Figure 6.33

Inflating a balloon between your hand and your spine: sternum-level

balloon to expand within you, and notice how your body becomes deeper from front to back. This also helps to relax the back muscles, thus allowing the vertebrae to be mobilized gently to introduce a more elastic possibility to the spine (see Fig. 6.34).

Sliding your hands around to the sides of the rib cage, notice how (courtesy of your imaginary balloon) the lower chest can expand to fill the space under your hands here as well. In fact, it can expand in all directions, as you will find if you place your hands on different parts of your rib cage. No matter where you put your hands, you can expand your balloon between them. You might have noticed that some directions are less mobile than others, and this is a great discovery. It highlights where your greatest benefit is to

be gained, as you learn to soften and allow the air to move your body in this stiffer area.

Moving down the body, the balloon will now sit within your abdomen. To make sure that you don't just open the pressure valve by simply switching off the abdomen to blow it up, you are going to see how slowly you can inflate that balloon. It will still inflate within the body from front to back, so include your lower spine in your awareness (see Fig. 6.35). As you breathe out, let the air slip away easily and without any muscular effort.

Finally, you are going to replace your round balloon with a long one. On your in-breath, expand this balloon lengthwise all the way down through

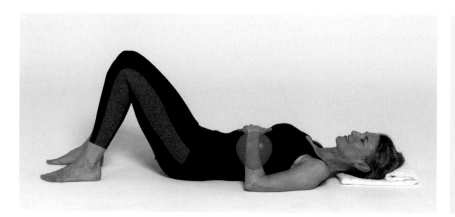

Figure 6.34

Inflating a balloon between your hand and your spine: diaphragm-level

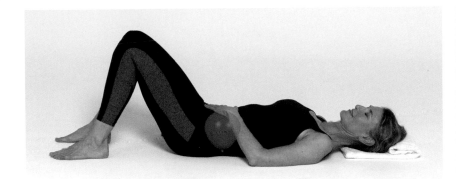

Figure 6.35

Inflating a balloon between your hand and your spine: abdomen-level

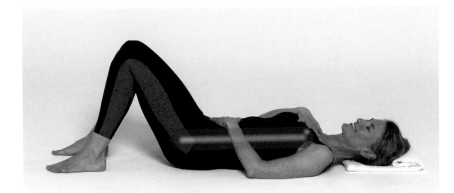

Figure 6.36

Inflating the long party balloon all the way through your body to gently press into your pelvic floor

your body and imagine it pressing gently on the pelvic floor to stretch it a little. As you breathe out, imagine the balloon subsiding to allow the pelvic floor to recoil (see Fig. 6.36). Let your whole body breathe each breath with no particular emphasis on the chest or belly.

It is powerful to know that improvements in so many postural presentations can be achieved through taking the time and care to support someone in finding a better way to breathe.

Power points

- Habitual fixing strategies, or locks, compromise our spinal posture.

- The common locks are often interrelated because they have biomechanical, structural, and functional relationships.

- Locks are often caused by muscle tension. Introducing tasks that invite muscle relaxation in those areas allows the spine to decompress.

- Unlocking areas of fixed tension can allow automatic postural muscle responses to emerge.

- Breathing is a powerful key to healthy global posture.

When I dared to stop holding my spine and start nourishing it with movement, the sense of fragility and brittle woodenness that I had carried since my teens began to dissolve into the glad, green welcome of a united body ...

Fear and misunderstandings have contributed to a persistent perception that the human body is flawed in its construction, and that degeneration will be hastened through repetition of certain harmful movements. It is not a great leap from here to an impression that, to avoid threat, we should limit certain motions. Nowhere is this more emphasized than in the spine.

Is this truly the case? A back injury frequently leads to avoidance of movements that are perceived as inherently risky, but avoiding spinal flexion or extension for the rest of life after injury is neither realistic nor necessary. The body knows how to heal when we set up the conditions that nurture and support it, and reclaiming these movements with confidence restores both body and brain. As with any other part of the body, the principles of force sharing apply in the spine, and this can guide our practice to ensure that our movement is sustainable and healthy.

Fundamental factors

The lessons that we have already learned so far about force management, physics, and fascia provide the guidelines for thinking about spines. When you observe or practice a movement, consider these factors:

1. Is the mobility demand shared? (Each link in the kinetic chain participates, preventing excessive movement stress in one specific area.)

2. Is the load demand shared? (Load applied to the body is spread across the kinetic chain, rather than being focused on one specific area.)

3. Is the spine supported throughout its range of motion by myofascial connections across the whole body?

4. Is the movement initiated from the most suitable area for load bearing and force creation? (The substantial anatomy of the legs and pelvis, for example, is more suited to generate force than the more intricately constructed spine.)

We are therefore very interested in the way that a person chooses to use themselves, especially if they have experienced an injury. The question you will ask yourself is this: *why is this painful structure under pressure?*

Using the four points above, we can consider the person's movement as a whole. There is no better medicine than robust, confident natural movement, and, as a movement teacher, you can help people to relieve the stress on an injured structure by balancing the forces throughout the kinetic chain.

This function-based approach to considering injury is a learning process, but with practice and the aid of the few tips that follow, you will soon start to recognize the pressure points in a movement and learn how to work toward smoothing out the demands upon the kinetic chain.

Strength in mobility

In Chapter 5 we introduced the CLA, a biomechanical concept that helps us to identify how force is acting on the body and how effectively we manage those forces. When we aren't managing forces effectively, a kink in the CLA points to where we are diverting or storing them.

Visualized as a firm but flexible line through the center of the body, the CLA is straight and secure when efficient rotation is required, and of course for zone stacking tasks. However, if you move your spine into side bending, extension, or flexion, an intact CLA is achieved when each segment contributes to the movement demand without being stressed beyond the limit of its structural capacity. When this is achieved, you will see a fairly evenly distributed motion throughout the spine. This shape is what transforms a relatively flimsy structure into a functionally strong one. In studies using dissected spines, applied pressures of only 80–100 N cause the spine to give way. Yet the spine in a living body withstands

1000 N just to stand upright.[1] It can manage even higher loads when we lift. It seems impossible, yet this is the magic of the living body: it transcends its structure with functional solutions. In this case it is physics.

The concept involved is called "follower load." It means that although the spine is under pressure, as long as the surface of each vertebra is positioned for optimal load transfer with respect to the next, it is able to tolerate far greater loads, even when it is bending in different directions. If this is tricky to imagine, think of your spine as a stack of children's wooden building blocks – when you apply a certain amount of compression to the stack, it becomes more rather than less stable. If you change the angle of pressure slightly, you can even start to bend the stack, and it continues to tolerate the pressure (see Fig. 7.1). Of course, there is a limit to how far you can bend a stack of detached blocks before it collapses: this is where our body differs, as it uses a sophisticated coordination of trunk muscles to maintain the relationship between each vertebra in the stack.[2] To achieve this, we need a sense

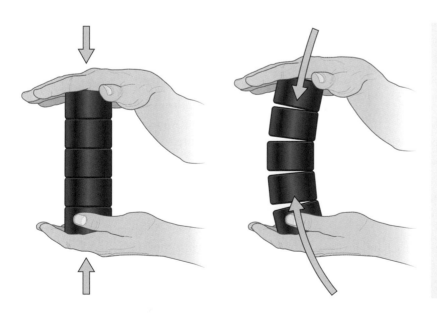

Figure 7.1

Follower load. Compression can actually increase the stability of the structure, as long as each segment is optimally positioned for load transfer. In the human body, muscle coordination and fascial support increases this capability

both of where forces are acting on our body and of our own spinal shape.

The demand of a movement or load on the body will run like water through the spine to find where the motion can most easily be exploited. If one area is stiff, an adjacent area may be more accommodating and thus experience more of the movement demand. This area of amplified movement at a specific spinal level can appear as an angle rather than a curve, or even a deep crease in the soft tissues that lie over it. It is like a speed bump in the road, interrupting the coordination and connection through the movement and attracting greater loading (see Fig. 7.2).[3]

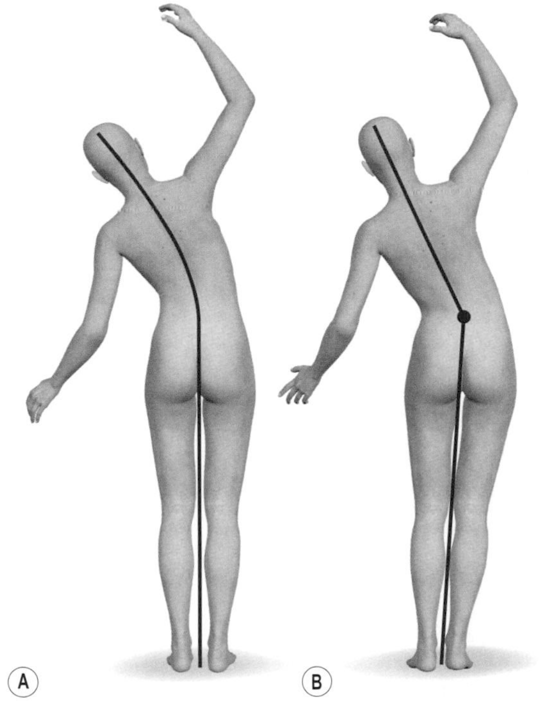

In the case of Fig. 7.2B, the body has compensated for the lack of spinal mobility by shifting the pelvis sideways. As a movement teacher, you might address this by emphasizing, first, awareness of the pelvic position over the feet, and then, second, the opening of the ribs on the upper side to facilitate the missing part of the curve.

Looking more globally, if our hips have restricted mobility, the lumbar spine attempts to compensate in order to offer greater range when our functional activity requires it. The movement demand is then amplified in the lower back instead of being distributed evenly across the kinetic chain. If hip flexion is insufficient, the spine flexes more to increase the range of motion (see Fig. 7.3). With restricted hip extension, the lumbar spine deepens its curve (see Fig. 7.4).

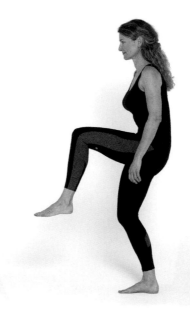

Figure 7.2

A. Look for a smooth spinal arc that indicates an intact central longitudinal axis. *B.* When you see an area of straightness, you will usually spot an area of increased bend nearby

Figure 7.3

The spine will often increase its flexion to accommodate restricted hip flexion

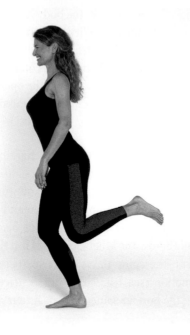

Figure 7.4

The spine will often increase its extension to accommodate restricted hip extension

The amplification of spinal movement to get around the hip mobility problem causes us to compromise the CLA. Although this is a great example of our body trying to solve a functional problem, unfortunately, it is often interpreted as evidence of insufficient core stability.

Movement exploration

In standing, place your hands around one side of your pelvis and start swinging that leg backward and forward under your hip as though you are kicking a ball (see Figs. 7.5 and 7.6). In a hip with adequate mobility, the pelvis should stay level as the leg moves. If you feel your pelvis tilting forward and backward in response to your leg motion, see what happens if you attempt to keep it level. If you are able to do this but find that you can no longer swing your leg, your problem is not with your abdominal muscles – they are clearly able to do their job in managing your pelvis. In this situation, either your hip mobility is restricted or the

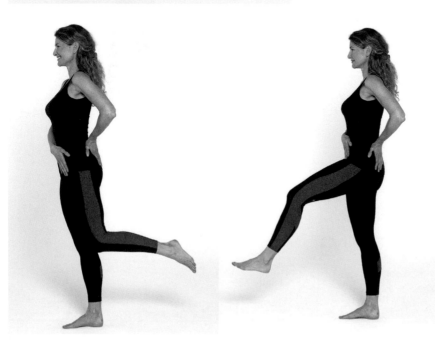

Figures 7.5/7.6

Maintaining the pelvic position as the leg swings into extension

Maintaining the pelvic position as the leg swings into flexion hip muscles are unable to lengthen quickly enough, causing the spine to respond instead. The result is a compromised CLA; it is not an abdominal muscle problem. First, ensure that you have the hip mobility and flexibility to perform the movement, and then practice letting the leg learn to relax as much as possible, so it can swing from the hip rather than the spine.

These CLA collapses put the trunk into a position of disadvantage when it comes to effective force production and ease of movement. But this does not in any way mean that our spines should not move in these directions – it is a question of what is appropriate for the task.

Fretting about flexion

Much anxiety has been generated about flexion and disk health. Disks in dissected segments of a spine (usually that of a pig or sheep) have been subjected to multiple repetitions of isolated movements to see how many of these can be performed before structural failure ensues.[4-6] Based on the findings that many cycles of repeated flexion, flexion/rotation, and flexion/extension eventually disrupt the disk, there has been a proliferation of training practices advocating restriction and even prevention of such movements with various bracing techniques.

While the isolated structural research provides helpful background knowledge, the spine in a living person works as part of an integrated system, and the loads that each segment experiences are dependent upon how the body as a whole performs the task. Flexion, for example, is a normal movement. Most of us use some as we roll out of bed in the morning. We use it to get the milk out of the fridge. We use it again to make sure that we don't dribble toothpaste down our shirts as we clean our teeth; and yet again to get into and out of our cars. Our grandparents may spend hours every week in their gardens, flexed over

their vegetables or flower beds. A child, transfixed by a butterfly, squats with their torso curled over their legs to watch it. Our biology has not made a mistake. We are human. We flex.

However, in our contemporary relatively sedentary society, we are not necessarily adequately conditioned to flex *well*. If this creates a force-sharing problem, stress can be amplified in a vulnerable area. It is therefore imperative that today's movement teacher looks beyond whatever repertoire or traditional sequences of movements they have been taught, regardless of their history and purported lineage, to identify the reality that modern bodies present.

Returning to our four points for sustainable movement, let us consider mobility. We ask ourselves: does each segment in the movement chain contribute adequately? To answer that question, we need to consider not just the movement within the spine itself but also the movement relationship between the pelvis and the lumbar spine, and the pelvis on the hip.[7,8]

So, in a natural standing forward bend, what do you notice? The lumbar spine begins the motion, and it continues to lead the movement until the pelvis engages and rotates forward over the hips. The flexion curve should proceed smoothly through the thoracic spine, ending finally with the head dropping toward the floor to release the cervical lordosis (see Fig. 7.7).

The proportion of spine to hip motion can vary, depending upon the flexibility characteristics of the individual. Those with very flexible hamstrings will emphasize the pelvic rotation component, while those with tight posterior legs are more likely to utilize more spinal motion.[9]

What else might you observe? Perhaps instead of the smooth curve throughout the whole spine, there is an excessive amount of thoracic flexion, which appears

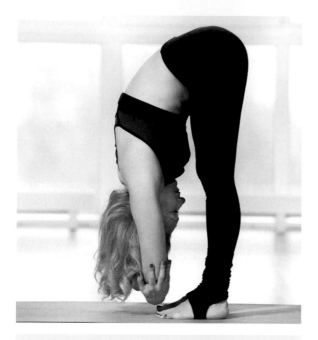

Figure 7.7

Even contribution of body parts through the flexion movement

as an accentuated angle in the mid back. This might be seen, for example, in a woman with osteoporosis whose spine has started to compress into its region of greatest stress.

Following the points for sustainable movement, exercises that emphasize thoracic flexion, particularly loaded flexion, will not be suitable choices in this case. Curl-ups (crunches) and Pilates Hundreds will apply significant compressive force into thoracic flexion, increasing the pressure on this lady's already compromised thoracic vertebrae. Strengthening of her spinal extensors will help to support her posture against gravity, but as flexion is an inevitable feature of everyday life, low load experiences can be used to help balance the flexion motion throughout the kinetic chain. Instead of fearing movement, she needs movement nutrition.

The Caterpillar technique, which is equally useful to improve awareness in a person with low back pain, teaches us to differentiate the flexion movement between our hip and pelvis, and pelvis from lumbar spine.

Movement exploration

Caterpillar technique

Curling from the bottom up

First, we are going to learn to move the hip independently. Take up a side-lying position with your head supported.

Starting with both hips and knees bent for support, place your uppermost hand on your sacrum, with fingers toward your tailbone (see Fig. 7.8). Stretch out your uppermost leg, leading from the toes until your body is aligned like an arrow with your hip straight (see Fig. 7.9).

Now slide this foot back in, drawing the knee toward the body so that your hip bends. Notice what happens under your hand. Does your sacrum move? It may act as though it is attached to the back of your knee with a piece of string, following your knee by gliding downward as the leg slides back to the flexed start position (i.e., the brain has forgotten how to differentiate between hip bending and spinal bending). If it does this, think of leaving the sacrum behind as your knee draws in (see Fig. 7.10). There is no need to actively resist the sacral motion, nor to attempt to stabilize the trunk in preparation. We are training the brain to work out how to effortlessly move one part on another. Practice a few more movements, and as your knee starts to move independently of your sacrum, you will notice the feeling of a hinge joint at your hip.

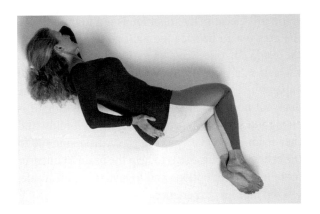

Figure 7.8

Caterpillar start position

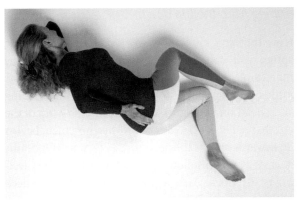

Figure 7.10

The sacrum remains quiet when the hip can move freely

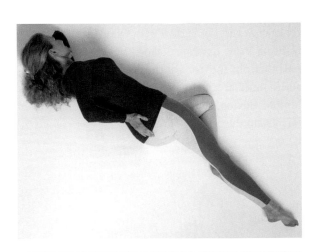

Figure 7.9

Sliding the leg straight

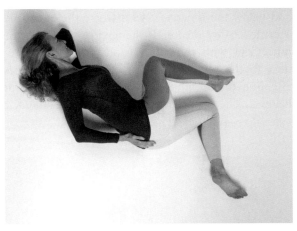

Figure 7.11

Allowing the pelvis to move on the lumbar spine

Now we can learn to differentiate the pelvis from the lumbar spine. This time as you draw your knee up toward you, allow your sacrum to follow the moving leg (see Fig. 7.11). Feel the sacrum under your hand gliding down and tucking under you, leading your lumbar spine into a comfortable flexion curve. There is no need to actively create a pelvic tilt: just imagine that a piece of string is attaching the sacrum to the

back of the knee, and let the pelvis be drawn into the movement.

Pause in the flexed position and breathe into the lumbar spine, experiencing a sense of expansion and elasticity between each vertebra. Then stretch out through the uppermost leg until your body is fully lengthened into a straight line.

Curling from the top down

Now that you know how to flex below the thoracic spine, you can further develop the movement by increasing awareness and mobility above it. Unfold the lordosis in your cervical spine by first gently nodding your head on your neck to release the very top of the curve (see Fig. 7.12). Notice how this movement begins an inwards curl as the head rotates forward. Once this is easy, you can follow that curl a little further, feeling how it opens each segment at the back of the neck without effort. When this feels comfortable, combine it with the leg motion from the first part of the Caterpillar to encourage lumbar flexion (see Fig. 7.13).

In the example of the woman with osteoporosis, this gentle process introduces the sense of motion above and below the thoracic region where she habitually accentuates her flexion. If she obviously initiates the movement with thoracic flexion, draw her awareness to the sensation of this before directing her attention to the motion possibility either above or below it. There is no need to cue to keep the thoracic spine still, because the intention is not to immobilize the area but to balance the total motion throughout the spine. In side lying, there is very little load, so she can safely explore the experience of folding and expanding the body without effort. She learns that she does not need to fight into flexion or extension; it is enough to sense each part of her spine as it folds, and then to lengthen like a piece of elastic from one end to the other. Our purpose is to help the brain to uncover more movement options and to give the spine a safe, relaxed mobility experience.

Thoracic dominant flexion is just as prevalent in a younger population. It is sometimes associated with persistent slouching; however, it can also be seen in otherwise very fit individuals who, through heavy training, have developed short, tight upper abdominals that pin the front of the rib cage down, or overactive lumbar erector spinae muscles that prevent lumbar flexion, thus amplifying the flexion demand farther up the spine.

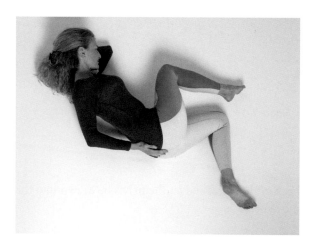

Figure 7.12

Gently nodding the head on the upper cervical spine to begin a reversal of the spinal curve

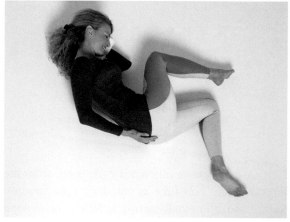

Figure 7.13

Curling from top down and bottom up

By modifying your cueing, you can use familiar exercises to help these people to balance their mobility through learning to differentiate at the spine, pelvis, and hip. A cat tilt is frequently used to encourage spinal mobility; however, cueing for a rich upward arch of the spine will provoke those with a thoracic flexion preference to press strongly through their shoulders into their already flexed thoracic spines, without substantially involving their lumbar spine. It is simply how their brain is wired at this point – they flex where it is easy to flex. If we shift the focus to initiating the movement from the tailbone, the lumbopelvic area becomes engaged, mobilizing the spine from the base upward and awakening the movement relationship between hip, pelvis, and spine. In a class situation, this creates an opportunity for the participants to discover the difference in their movement response between the two cues, using comparison to expand their body understanding and awareness.

Perhaps you have noticed that it is difficult for the person to open their lumbar spine as they bend. You might see excessive bending in the mid back instead, or an unwillingness to release the lumbar lordosis. This person is one who needs a little more sense of moving the pelvis relative to the spine.

Movement exploration

String of Pearls Bridge

This is not a new concept, but one that is often misunderstood. Its purpose is both to unlock the relationship between the pelvis and lumbar spine and to allow the lower back to experience relaxed flexion. We are therefore not aiming to work in a "neutral spine" position as is the case in a conventional bridging exercise. String of Pearls deepens the flexion experience that was covered in Chapter 6 (see Sacral rocks) and makes a connection between the posterior hip muscles and pelvic motion.

Begin with your sacral rock, remembering to support your head on a folded towel to ease any tension in the back of your neck (see Fig. 7.14). Feel the connection all the way to the tip of your tail as you roll over your sacrum, and then, using as little abdominal effort as you can, reverse the rock up to the top of your sacrum. At this point, become aware of the surfaces of your feet on the floor, and slightly deepen your connection through them as you continue to roll up to the top of your pelvis (and maybe beyond it into your lowest

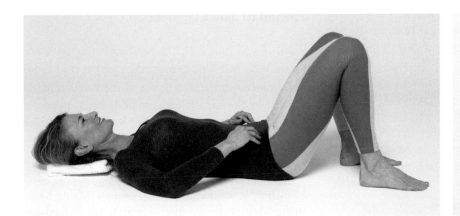

Figure 7.14

String of Pearls start position

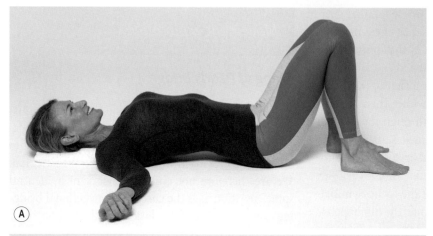

(A)

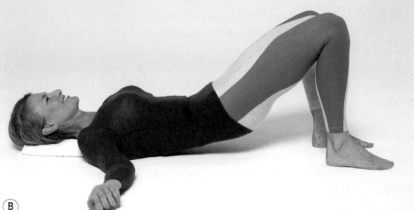

(B)

Figure 7.15

A. Rolling over the sacrum to its tip to release the spine and free the motion. *B*. Rolling back to the top of the sacrum and continuing the motion, progressively turning the pelvis by connecting with the feet to trigger the hip muscles

vertebrae), as if your pelvis is a wheel that you are winding thread onto. You will find that you do not move far from the floor – this is a release of the spine, not a lift (see Fig. 7.15).

Check that your abdominal wall is still relaxed, as if falling back toward your spine. Place a finger over your upper abdominals and sink your body away from it. Move your finger gradually down the middle of your belly, sinking under each point until you find yourself back on the floor in the starting position.

The hip to pelvis connection

What if you notice that a person's pelvis does not rotate over their hips to carry the trunk forward into standing flexion? If movement of the pelvis is being resisted by the hamstrings, the body needs to find a solution. This may result in the lumbar spine over-bending to compensate; alternatively, this link can be skipped over and the restriction will manifest again as excessive flexion in the thoracic spine (see Fig. 7.16). Most people would simply work on stretching hamstrings, but as we are discovering, targeting isolated

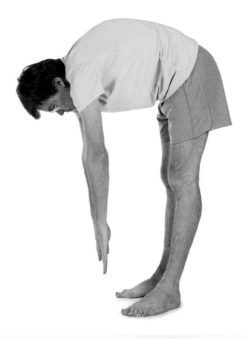

Figure 7.16

Tight hamstrings prevent the pelvis from rotating forward, so the flexion motion is pushed farther up the spine

muscles doesn't necessarily provide a complete solution as far as the brain is concerned. To make this an integrated intervention, address those hamstrings by awakening the pelvis–femur relationship. This provides vastly more information for the nervous system by introducing a new movement possibility.

Trunk tilt

The pelvis-on-femur relationship is an awareness gap for many people, and they are frequently frustrated with their lack of forward bending. This trunk tilt task is an awareness builder that provides a foundation for many different exercises that you may use in your classes or programs; it is equally relevant for yoga, Pilates, or gym work.

With your client either sitting on stacked blocks on the floor, or on a chair with their feet on the floor, guide them to sense when they are sitting directly on top of their sitting bones (i.e., neither in front nor behind them). Invite them to place one hand comfortably on their sacrum and the other on the front of their abdomen with fingers spread wide from pubic bone to ribs. Ask your client to identify the points of skin contact under their little finger and the thumb. These two points should remain the same distance apart for this first stage of the movement (see Fig. 7.17).

Ask them to think of gently pressing out through a point on the top of their head and to maintain this impulse throughout the movement. Now invite them to tilt their pelvis and trunk forward as a unit over an imaginary hinge joint in the hips (see Fig. 7.18). As they move, direct their attention to the sacrum: has it moved smoothly forward with the trunk or have they left it behind? If it has been left behind, what has happened to the two contact points under the other hand? They will have moved toward each other because the spine will have flexed instead of the pelvis moving over the hips (see Fig. 7.19). This is a great discovery! Knowing what you habitually do opens the way to another possibility. Repeat the movement with attention to what happens under either the front or back hand to uncover the solution.

If the sacrum has moved nicely forward, draw your client's attention to their sitting bones: they will notice that they have rolled over the front of them. As they come back to the start position and the sacrum returns to a more

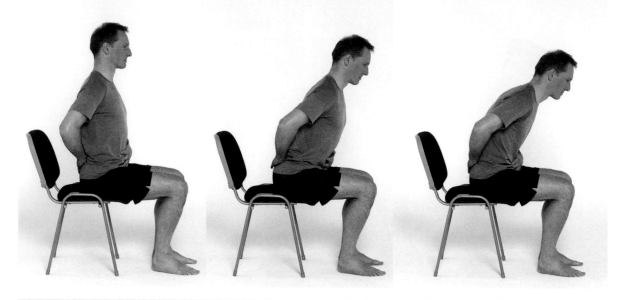

Figures 7.17/7.18 /7.19

Trunk tilt start position

The pelvis carries the trunk over the flexing hips

The sacrum is left behind, collapsing the trunk

vertical orientation, they will feel that they are once more on top of the sitting bones. Once the client has made this connection, they will start to realize that the pelvis carries the trunk easily in and out of a trunk tilt.

When your client is able to move the pelvis over the hip, you can introduce hamstrings. In the same start position, slide the left foot forward on the floor. Repeat the tilt, feeling the sacrum glide forward under the hand. Pause at the limit of hamstring stretch and breathe into the lengthening at the back of the thigh. Return and repeat the motion with the right foot forward (see Fig. 7.20).

Once this motion can be performed, there is a final learning step. To integrate the rest of

the flexion movement, your client needs to move into the trunk tilt (with a hand still on the sacrum), and once they reach the limit of pelvic motion, they can allow the rest of the trunk to fold forward to complete the flexion motion. This can be done over one or both legs (see Fig. 7.21).

The key point here is that the pelvis needs to learn to carry the spine. If practicing a forward fold of the trunk over straight legs on the floor, unload the hamstrings by providing a supportive block to raise the hips, and permit a little knee bending if necessary. The focus will be on rolling the pelvis up onto the sitting bones, and, if possible, a little farther over them to engage the relationship between the hamstrings, pelvis, and spine. We are teaching the brain to permit

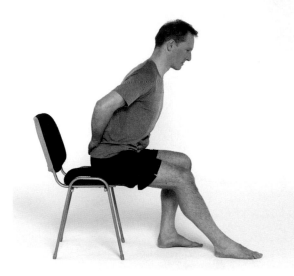

Figure 7.20

Introducing the hamstrings

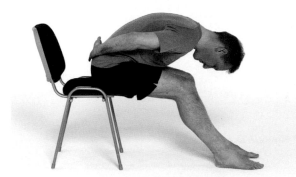

Figure 7.21

Completing the integrated flexion motion

motion of the pelvis on the leg, thereby encouraging a new neuromuscular response from the hamstrings.

Can you see the process? Look at the whole movement. Notice areas of greater or lesser mobility, *including the pelvis and hips.* Help the person's nervous system to learn new motion relationships while gaining mobility in the quieter links in the chain. Modify your cues, or select tasks that reintroduce these lost possibilities to the system.

Avoiding pitfalls and making a comeback

There are four main factors that contribute to flexion-related problems in an exercise setting.

1. Lumbar flexion appearing as a coping strategy because the person lacks the awareness, mobility, strength, or control of the spine or hips to achieve the appropriate position (see Figs. 7.22 and 7.23).

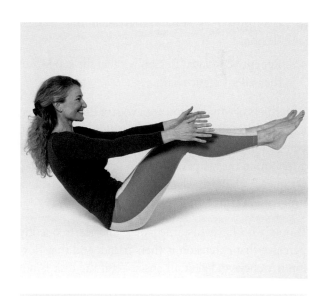

Figure 7.22

Lumbar flexion as a coping strategy when the load demand is too high

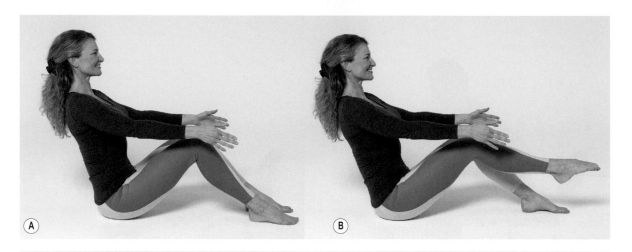

Figure 7.23

Reducing the load to establish lumbopelvic awareness and foundation control

2. Insufficient eccentric control and strength from the back and hip extensor muscles of the posterior chain.

3. Inadequately gradual progression into loaded flexion.

4. Repetitive isolated flexion without the support of the wider kinetic chain.

Regardless of whether you are a yoga or Pilates teacher, a personal trainer, or a rehabilitation professional, you can manage these factors as long as you: (1) pay attention to the shapes and form that you are seeing, (2) modify the task when necessary, and (3) create a progression plan.

People who have sustained disk injuries frequently perceive that extension is their friend, and that flexion is to be avoided at all costs. Yet if the disk is not exposed to some degree of flexion stress once it has moved beyond the initial phase of its healing process, it will remain vulnerable to the inevitable flexion that normal life involves. Of course, the "functional frozen" will strive to avoid these moments, but only

at the cost of never recovering normal movement. Physiologically and psychologically, restoring confidence in flexion is important.

Once the acute pain phase has passed, the person can be familiarized with lumbar flexion within their own control and self-selected range of motion. The tailbone-led cat tilts on all fours and the Caterpillar movement in side lying offer an active control element through a range of motion between flexion and extension. Actively rather than passively moving in each direction, with an aim of ease rather than range, reduces the chance of over-stretching the area initially. Once confidence is gained, and the person is more accustomed to flexing the spine, gentle passive movements can be introduced – such as drawing the knees toward the chest in supine within a pain-free range, or rocking the pelvis back toward the heels in quadruped, before gradually working toward Child's Pose. These positions offer a low-load, non-threatening experience of spinal flexion that can be progressed within the tolerance of the individual.

Coming back from a flexion based injury isn't just about the spine. Restoring the squat motion will reintegrate the legs to ensure that they contribute to sharing overall mobility and load bearing. Similarly, ensuring that the person has a foundation level of posterior chain connection and strength through the back extensors, glutei and hamstrings will develop support for standing flexion.

By ensuring that the person restores their flexion in addition to their other rehabilitation activities, you can help them to avoid joining the ranks of the functional frozen, and reclaim their normal movement.

> Flexion itself is not to be feared. We should ensure, however, that our clients are adequately prepared for it, that we understand their restrictions, and that we are prepared to modify our exercise choices to systematically progress them.

Rotation reservations

Misunderstandings about normal biomechanics have given rise to an emphasis on anti-rotation exercises for low back injury prevention. This is critical to address, because without rotation, our movement is profoundly compromised.

The relatively vertical orientation of the joints between each *lumbar* vertebra means that there is only a very small amount of rotation available at each level. But, having said that, rotation through the spine arises from the aggregate of multiple levels, each making their contribution. Each joint adds its small amount of range to the next, and so on up the spine. The *thoracic* spine's joints allow more sliding between their adjacent surfaces (and therefore more rotation), and the cervical spine, with its much flatter joint surfaces, allows the most of all (see Fig. 7.24).

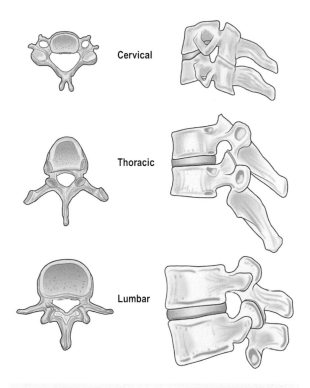

Cervical

Thoracic

Lumbar

Figure 7.24

The different shape and orientation of the joints between each vertebra in the cervical, thoracic, and lumbar spine determines how much rotation is available

The hips are also an important contributor because the range of their ball-in-socket rotation will influence the ability of the pelvis to turn over that hip when standing. This allows the pelvis to carry the lumbar spine around with it, reducing the rotational demand upon the spine itself. The problem comes when one area in this chain is compromised, increasing the demand on the remaining joints, which is sometimes beyond what they are structurally capable of offering. For example, a lack of hip mobility is strongly linked to lower back pain.[10,11] If the functional task requires more total body rotation, and the hip is restricted, the lumbar spine is asked to use the extent of its rotation as the next link in the chain. Once it reaches its limit, the brain looks for a new solution, and with no more potential available in the transverse plane, it looks for another plane to absorb the movement. This is frequently the sagittal plane, leading the body into lumbar extension. At this point, when the lumbar facet joints are pushed into combined extension/rotation, they are under high stress, which makes them vulnerable to potential injury.

Conversely, if the lumbar spine is beginning in extension, rotation range is limited.[12] Having so little motion to offer in the first place, it doesn't take much to push it beyond its limits. This is what has triggered the impression that rotation is harmful and must be prevented.

> Remember: to rotate effectively, we need an axis to rotate around.

Let's consider this calmly. The lumbar spine stress is a signifier that something needs to be addressed in the kinetic chain. This area, rather than being primarily weak, is often the victim of a workload inequality. Immobilizing it with setting of the core therefore only serves to remove even more mobility from the kinetic chain. To address the problem, we must reduce the pressure being applied, which involves optimizing the rest of the kinetic chain. In the case of the lumbar spine, make sure that you have relaxed the lumbar lock to reduce any excessive extension, and then turn your attention to mobility of the hips below and the thoracic spine above.

Movement exploration

Total Body Rotation gives us the opportunity to encourage rotation in the lower body in order to relieve spinal stress.

Begin by standing in a relaxed posture with feet hip width apart, allowing the feet to place themselves on the ground as they fall naturally. Feel how your feet rest upon the ground. Do you feel the pressure more under the outsides or insides of your feet, or do you feel that you are bearing the weight across your whole sole?

Draw yourself up with a helium balloon, and turn your body to the left to a comfortable limit. Note how far you go, and don't attempt to push further. Reverse your turn, following your eyes and head as you turn your body to the right. Again, note how far you rotate (see Fig. 7.25).

This time as you turn, notice what happens under your feet. As you turn right, you might notice that the pressure under your feet follows, taking you onto

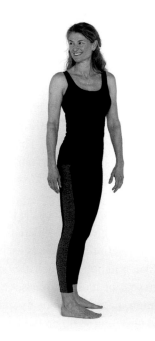

Figure 7.25

Turning to test rotational availability

the outside of your right foot, and the inside of your left foot. This would be ideal, but you may find that yours do the opposite. If this is the case, the next part of the exercise will help to reboot the natural movement.

Pausing with your body in relaxed right rotation, place your right hand on your right thigh. Smoothly and easily move the pressure under your right foot from the outer border toward the inner border without forcing the motion beyond what is comfortably available (see Fig. 7.26). Take your time, and feel every millimeter of the movement across your sole as it transitions toward the ball of your foot and the inside of your heel. As you begin to reverse the movement, feel how your thigh turns as it follows the foot. Repeat the movement, slowly back and forth, feeling the thigh (and therefore the hip) responding to the foot pressure. You are starting a conversation between your foot and your hip.

Once you have explored several of these movements, pause with your weight toward the outer border of your right foot. We are going to address the left hip now.

Place your left hand on your left thigh and let any tension in your leg melt away. With your body still turned to the right, you are most likely to be feeling more pressure on the inside of the left foot (see Fig. 7.27). Again, taking care not to force the movement, pay attention to what it is like to shift the pressure from the inner border of the left foot across the sole toward the outer margin of your foot, allowing the whole leg to relax and follow. If it feels blocked, simply pause, take a breath, exhale, and continue if more range becomes easily available. If not, reverse the foot pressure back toward the inner border again. Repeat this several times. Return to the start position. Recheck the right turn, and notice the pressures under your feet following along. You might find it easier to turn to the left now.

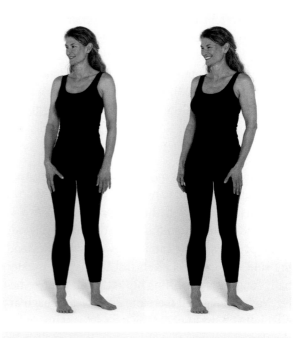

Figures 7.26/7.27

Feeling the right thigh turning in response to changing foot pressure

Feeling the left thigh turning in response to changing foot pressure

Repeat the process to the left.

Finally, retest your turning in each direction. Most people find that they turn further and more easily. This is because their first turn frequently only involves the spine. After Total Body Rotation, the feet, legs, hips, and pelvis are reminded to be involved, balancing the movement throughout the kinetic chain.

This process addresses rotational restrictions in your hips, and relaxes any tension you may be holding. If you are accustomed to standing with your weight on the outer part of your sole, now relax and allow the feet to rest their whole surface on the ground.

People also fear rotation when it appears unexpectedly. If you are performing a simple quadruped exercise like Superman, for example, the pelvis and spine can appear to rotate when one leg is extended out behind (see Fig. 7.28). The rotation is simply a signifier to tell you that the person is not moving the leg in the sagittal plane. Now you can set about identifying the reason.

The rotation is the symptom, so trying to restrain it with abdominal bracing is not addressing the real issue. Instead, note whether the problem is provoked on the side of the extending leg or the supporting side. If the pelvis is being carried upward on the extending side, the cause is often that the person is externally rotating at the lifting hip as they straighten their leg. Your cueing will therefore focus on an imaginary laser light on the kneecap tracing a straight line out on the floor to ensure that the person is using their hip extensors more effectively (see Fig. 7.29).

Alternatively, it may be that the pelvis is dropping on the extending side (see Fig. 7.30). If the lateral pelvic

muscles on the supporting side do not maintain a consistent length when the opposite leg is withdrawn, the pelvis will drop, and the hip may even move outside the support knee. In this case, you will direct the

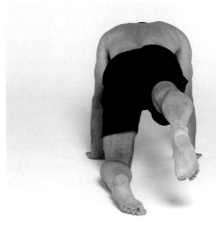

Figure 7.29

Imagining the laser light on the knee as the leg extends

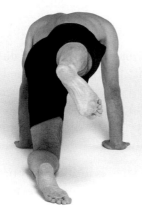

Figure 7.28

Trunk rotation caused by externally rotating the lifting leg in Superman

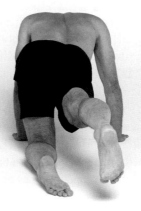

Figure 7.30

Trunk rotation caused by loss of control on the supporting side

person's focus toward stacking their hip over their knee in order to maintain the rotational relationship between the hip and pelvis. To achieve this, the person will unconsciously recruit a wider array of muscles in the pelvis and trunk in a low-level coordinated pattern, rather than using a high-effort conscious contraction. The emphasis is movement control, rather than anti-movement bracing.

Instead of viewing rotation as a pathological uncontrolled movement, look for what it is telling you. If rotation is not what you want to see in the task, ask yourself what it is that you do want? If the transverse plane is not appropriate, which plane should the person be moving in?

> Place your emphasis on restoring what you do want, rather than battling against what you don't.

Sacroiliac stress

Although the sacroiliac joints (SIJs) are perceived as vulnerable, structurally they are exceptionally stable, and in fact become more stable as we age. Over time, the bony surface between the sacrum and the adjacent ilium gradually develops a series of grooves and ridges that slot into one another like interlacing fingers, creating greater stability and an increased surface area for force transmission. Think of the SIJ as the marriage of an old couple who have rubbed along together their whole lives, each changing the other little by little to create an inseparable partnership. This is called *form closure*.

The SIJs are further supported by a broad network of ligaments, extensive myofascial connections, and additional compressive reinforcement from muscles that cross the joint, such as Gmax. This active compression is called *force closure*.

Despite this extensive support, anyone struggling with sacroiliac pain will tell you that the joint feels insecure and vulnerable. Force closure problems involve the balance of muscle activity around the pelvis and can be improved by addressing the activation of muscles such as Gmax,[13] but relative mobility also plays a part. If the adjacent body areas above or below are restricted, stress can be amplified at the SIJ. Limitation in thoracic or hip rotation can create SIJ stress in rotational stretches, so it is important to incorporate mobility work in these areas before performing movements like spinal twists.[14,15]

The body needs rotation for ease and effectiveness of functional movement. Rather than avoiding rotation with anti-movement cues, you can teach the system to work in a cooperative and integrated way.

If rotation is restricted or even painful, here's a checklist to help you solve the problem:

1. Does the person have a CLA? Rotating on an extended spine will increase spinal stress, so release out the lumbar and posterior rib locks, and encourage lengthening throughout the whole spine all the way to the top of the head (even in lying down positions like spinal twists).

2. Are they losing their CLA because the loading of the exercise is simply too high? Consider simple modifications like reducing the lever or increasing the base of support.

3. Have you ensured that the areas above and below are contributing their share of the mobility? When the lumbar spine is being put under pressure, increase mobility in the thoracic spine and hips to improve their contribution to overall rotation.

4. If rotation should not be a feature in the pose or exercise, do you need to communicate a clearer image of the direction of movement?

5. If unwanted motion is appearing, do you need to convey an image of solid grounding in the supporting body part, e.g. the legs and pelvis, which will allow the spine to expand and spiral with freedom and ease?

Extension anxieties

This natural motion has caused perhaps the greatest confusion for movement professionals, especially when considering back-bending movements, such as those involved in dance and yoga.

Somehow, we have become trapped between one side of the industry that is working to prevent back extension in the belief that it is harmful and another seeking increasingly extravagant back bending. The first thing we need to establish is that extending the spine is not in itself dangerous. As with rotation, problems arise when the extension impulse is amplified in one area instead of being shared throughout the spine, or when it appears inappropriately. When an area is stiff, the force will be directed to a more mobile site in the chain, as it was in the ballet dancer example in Chapter 4.

The challenge as a teacher is to note whether the extension is evenly distributed through the spine. As you tune your eye, you will begin to see the spine in terms of regions of excessive motion and regions of immobility. Figure 7.31 shows a fairly even distribution of motion throughout the spine. Notice how, in Figure 7.32, there is a lack of a spinal extension curve in either the thoracic or lumbar region. There is a visible "hinge" rather than a curve where the extension motion is amplified at the neck and the thoracolumbar junction. In Figure 7.33 there is very little extension available in the spine, leaving the very lowest of the lumbar vertebrae to bear the greatest load. Improving mobility and awareness in

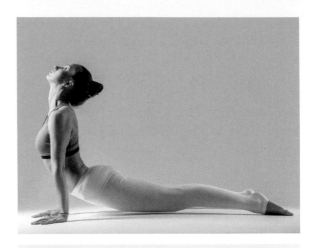

Figure 7.31

Reasonably even motion throughout the spine

the thoracic spine in all planes will be a priority in both of these cases.

In standing extension poses, more of the kinetic chain is available and distribution of the weight over the feet can become a factor, so an even greater array of strategies can be seen.

In Figure 7.34 the upper body has shifted forward relative to the pelvis, so the hips have been unable to extend. This is common in the person whose normal postural habit is the posterior rib lock, as they will already have a slightly upwardly rotated rib cage. Their thoracolumbar region is extended before they even begin. If they are then cued with an upper-body focus – for example, lifting from the waist or shining the sternum up to the sky are commonly used – they shift their rib cage forward in an attempt to gain more motion in an area that has already used up its extension range. Cues that focus their attention on the upper body also amplify their disconnection from the lower body, and the pelvis and hips look as though they have been "left behind."

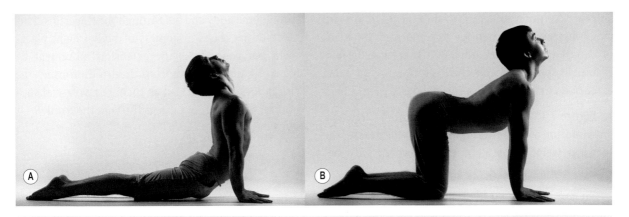

Figure 7.32

Extension accentuated at neck and thoracolumbar region

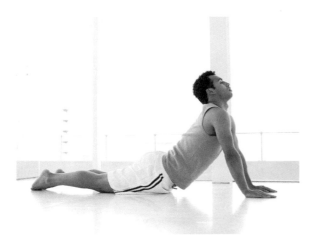

Figure 7.33

Extension accentuated at lower lumbar spine due to poor spinal mobility

If a cue does create the desired response, it does not necessarily mean that it is a bad cue. It could simply be that the person's individual structure and habits require a different focus.

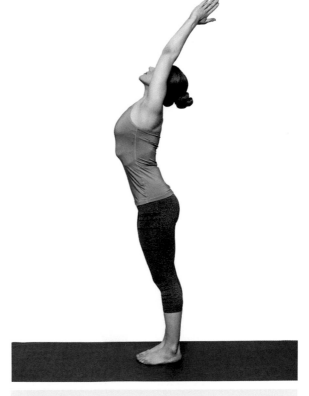

Figure 7.34

Extension focused on lower thoracic spine

Another common strategy is to shift the pelvis forward using increased hip extension to compensate for a lack of spinal extension. This amplifies the stress on the lower lumbar spine. Note that there is relatively little spinal extension curve above the lumbar spine (see Fig. 7.35).

In Figure 7.36 we can see a more balanced extension, with motion visible throughout the spine despite the forward weight shift. The hips, however, have not fully extended.

What are our cueing alternatives? Consider calling awareness to the feet. For those who are shifting their pelvis forward, cue for the weight to remain more central in the feet throughout the movement. If it looks as though the person is leaving their legs behind and performing the movement only from the rib cage, invite them to draw themselves up from the feet right through the body and out through the fingertips. This not only increases awareness of body-weight placement but coordinates the extension movement by including the hips and pelvis. It also diminishes the risk of localized overload as there is myofascial support all the way from the legs through the trunk.

> Focusing forces on any isolated body part, either through repetition or excessive loading, can create structural stress. Rather than avoiding the problematic movement direction, balance the mobility and load bearing throughout the entire chain. To do this, we need to think past the spine and into the hips and legs, which have a major influence on all spinal movements.

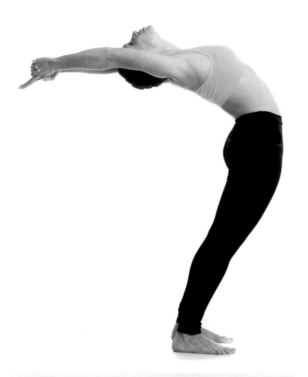

Figure 7.35

Extension focused on lower lumbar spine and hips

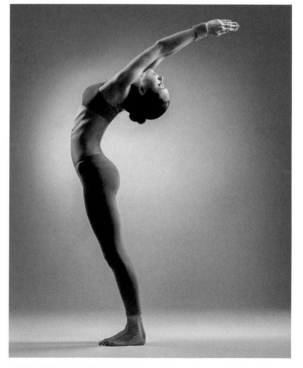

Figure 7.36

More balanced extension throughout the spine

Effect of active hip extension

As with flexion and rotation, looking for an area of increased extension motion in the kinetic chain helps you as a movement teacher to find the areas that are not pulling their weight. For example, in an active hip extension movement where the leg is lifted behind the body, the hip must first have sufficient extension range to perform the movement, and then it must have sufficient inner range gluteal strength to straighten the hip. If either of those criteria are missing, the person will do the only thing left to them in order to achieve a leg lift, and that is to work harder and further into lumbar extension. This is not a lack of core stability but another instance of the body offering an alternative solution to achieve the objective of raising the leg.

There are three elements that can provide stepping stones to more effective hip extension and that balance out the overall movement. The first is mobility. You ideally will have first introduced movements to open the front of the hips and lengthen the hip flexors to make the hip-extension range of motion available. The second element is learning to contract the gluteals into their shortened inner range. For some people this may be easier in a position like a bridge, where the load is more readily sensed at the hip. Finally, as we discussed in Chapter 4, the impulse of lengthening outwards from the pelvis down the leg will share the forces through the kinetic chain more effectively than thinking of lifting it upward.

Nourishing the spine

In these last two chapters we have looked at increasing awareness in specific areas of the spine, helping some areas to remember how to move so that others can experience less stress.

Now we need to integrate this potential into movement, so that each area learns to talk to the next in a fluent conversation. We are going to glide between flexion and extension as a continuum, imagining the delicious movement of fluid through the spine as it learns to open freely.

Movement exploration

Spinal elasticizer

Ideally, we want each part of the spine to participate in a conversation. If the spine is to work as a fully integrated functional structure, movement in any one part should trigger the other segments to respond in sequence.

Take up a position on a seat with an awareness of resting your weight through your sitting bones. Allow yourself to slowly roll off the back of your sitting bones so that your sacrum starts to draw your spine down, creating first lumbar and then thoracic flexion. Let your whole spine follow, until your head is released down toward your chest and your entire back line has opened (see Fig. 7.37).

Bring your awareness back to your sitting bones. Roll up and over them so that your pelvis starts to tip forward, and feel how the front of the body starts to progressively open as if you were a fern frond unfurling. Once you reach the top of the movement, your entire spine will have extended, ready to once again roll over the back of the sitting bones to begin the progressive opening of the back again (see Fig. 7.38).

Feel the difference between this and a traditional pelvic tilt, which changes lumbopelvic position but creates a motion block in the spine. Rather than thinking of a static posture, focus on how each body part can play more effectively with the structures above and below it.

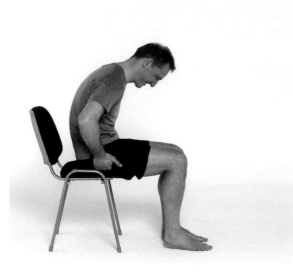

Figure 7.37

Spinal elasticizer opening the back of the body

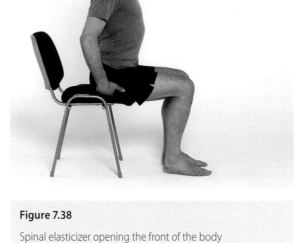

Figure 7.38

Spinal elasticizer opening the front of the body

In a class situation, the safe and enjoyable exploration of mobility can be found when we emphasize the journey. Instead of moving from position to position, pose to pose, exercise to exercise, we inhabit a continuous, joined up progression between points, which develops finer control, improves proprioception, and gives greater awareness of the motion itself.

It turns out that spinal control is not necessarily about keeping things still, but making sure that everything is playing its part as we move. When we introduce the limbs to the story, we have even more to explore when it comes to trunk control.

Power points

- Our spines are designed to move: we are not aiming to prevent their motion but to help them to move better.

- The CLA provides a simple reference point for assessing central body movement.

- We need to train our body to understand when the CLA's job is to be straight and when it should bend and curve.

- Kinks and collapses of the CLA into planes that don't support efficient movement may not necessarily be due to a primary loss of control. They may be the body's solution to a movement restriction somewhere in the kinetic chain.

- To ensure that this compensation effect is minimized, it is necessary to restore and maintain the mobility of the adjacent joints and muscles. For the entire spine, hip and shoulder mobility is key. For the lumbar spine and SIJs, thoracic mobility is profoundly important.

The willow which bends to the tempest, often escapes better than the oak which resists it.

Sir Walter Scott, *The Pirate*

With a clearer understanding of the array of different central body strategies that we have available for creating and managing forces, and an appreciation of the range of factors that can affect the posture of our central body, we can now put to rest some persistent misunderstandings regarding the core – or as we now know it, the central zone.

We all need to manage, withstand, and support the forces acting upon our central trunk. Some of these are externally applied, perhaps through lifting a load, being bumped in a crowd, or just controlling a dog on a leash. Other forces arise from the movement of our own limbs as they pull from their *proximal*[G] attachments. Imagine the force applied by the legs of a world-class sprinter to his central body with each powerful stride. It is not difficult to appreciate that we need central control, and the role of central stability in normal movement has been identified and supported in research from sports performance[1-3] to coordination in children.[4,5] However, unconvincing data on the effectiveness of stability training for low back pain has called into question the relevance of how we address it. It is not a surprising result: most of these studies have focused on programs that address certain key muscles to maintain a "neutral spine," but, as we discovered in Chapter 1, we need a wide variety of movement combinations and multiple integrated systems (including our psychological and emotional responses) to be globally stable in the context of functional movement.

Effortless control does not arise from the conscious activation of "deep stabilizing muscles," but from the body profoundly understanding where it is in space, where its body parts are relative to one another, and how to choose the best neuromuscular response for the task from a palette of many options.

To achieve this, we need to be able to feel how our spine is moving, which requires awareness. We need to sense its position, which requires proprioception. We need a variety of strategies, so we uncover and release the coping habits that restrict the spine's choices. We teach it to respond to the impulse to move and progress to being able to tolerate load, create torque, and transfer force. The process begins deep in the central nervous system and moves in layers out into the muscles.

So far, we have considered the reflexes that involve the vestibular system and help us to detect not only our body's orientation in space but the relationship of our head to our body. We have worked with our postural locks to create a relaxed but responsive foundation to work from. We have also started to develop awareness of relative movement between adjacent segments in the kinetic chain.

If we understand how to detect movement of one segment on the next, we must also learn the sense of how and when to keep them together.

Changing relationships

A great deal of stabilization training is devoted to preventing spinal motion in response to limb movement. In everyday low-load normal movements, this is creating an unnecessary battle. Rather than fighting against a movement, it is more often a case of learning clearer relationships between our body parts. The key is to understand how the brain perceives the movement task.

Simple movement tests can give you some insight into this. Every day, for example, we have to lift our arms to some degree, whether to put on a shirt or take a coffee cup off a shelf. How does the brain arrange our body to do this natural movement? To examine this, we can use a simple test, the Double Arm Raise, to observe a client's personal strategy.

Movement test

Double Arm Raise

In relaxed standing, ask your client to lift their arms naturally up toward the ceiling. By indicating the ceiling, you have provided a direction for the movement impulse. The interesting thing will be to see how their brain reads that impulse.

This is a movement that progresses up from the feet, through the central body and out through the fingertips. Ideally, you will see the arms stretch upward, drawing the body with it so that the center of gravity remains centered over the feet. The abdomen automatically draws inwards in response to the movement stimulus, and the pelvis remains level. The ribs spread a little as they follow the arms in a whole-body lengthening motion. The thoracic spine subtly extends, and the scapula continues the flow of movement impulse by rotating upward to create space

between the humeral head and the acromion (the bony arch that is the roof of the shoulder joint), thus protecting the sensitive structures on top of the shoulder from being squeezed as the arms are raised. It is a symphony of force management (see Fig. 8.1).

You may, however, observe a less harmonious picture. Instead of a nicely connected linear motion, the functional spinal locks may appear, which give the

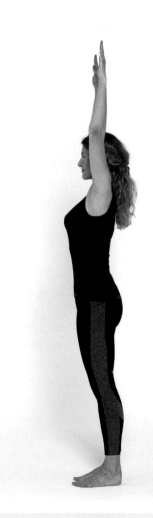

Figure 8.1

Double Arm Raise

impression of loss of central control in a number of different ways. For example:

1. a deepening of the lumbar curve with the pelvis tipping into anterior tilt (see Fig. 8.2A)

2. a deepening of the lumbar curve as the pelvis is drawn forward by the body weight sliding toward the front of the feet (see Fig. 8.2B)

3. the weight staying centered on the feet, but the rib cage rotating upward at the front as the posterior rib lock pins it down at the back (see Fig. 8.2C)

4. the abdomen becoming inactive, protruding passively (see Fig. 8.2D).

This is easy to fix, right? Usually people are instructed to set the abdominal wall in a static contraction, or consciously keep the front of the body closed by maintaining a consistent distance between the ribs and the pelvis. However, this is an anti-movement approach – by creating a new fixed point at the front, it simply replaces a posterior lock with an anterior one. Cues of this nature interfere with normal movement because they prevent the natural trunk lengthening that sets up the dynamic myofascial connection between the arms, trunk, and legs. Think of Olympic freestyle swimmers: they maintain their CLA like a straight arrow but allow the body to lengthen sleekly into the Greyhound shape as they reach for each stroke, so that their arms can access the power of the whole body.

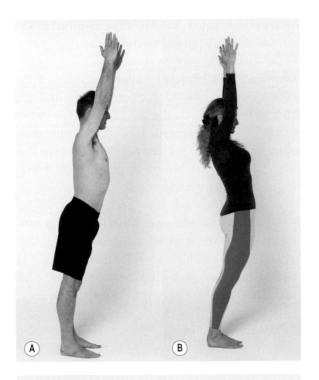

Figure 8.2

Double Arm Raise. *A.* Pelvis moving into anterior tilt. *B.* Pelvis sliding forward

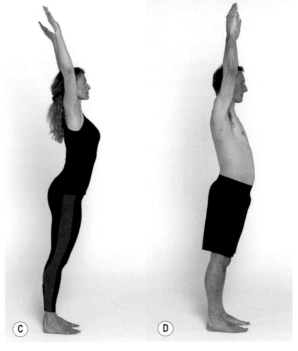

Figure 8.2

C. Weight centered on feet, rib cage drawn upward and a posterior rib lock. *D.* Passive, protruding abdomen

In elastic motion, lengthening through the body creates myofascial tension that connects each limb to the power potential of the whole body.

Consider the many tiny cogs in a traditional wrist-watch, where preventing one area from moving will affect all the others. Biomechanically, preventing movement with abdominal setting or consciously pinning the front of the rib cage down creates shoulder stress. When the lumbar spine is held statically, the body must compensate for the loss of motion elsewhere. Whether the increased demand on the thoracic spine can be accommodated depends on its mobility. The next cog is the scapula, which when forced to offer more motion, often expresses it in the form of either greater abduction (moving away from the spine) or elevation (moving upward). This alteration in the mechanics of the glenohumeral joint can then change the tensions and pressures on the soft tissues of the shoulder.

It is no great surprise that I meet so many people who have developed secondary shoulder pain some time after undertaking a core stability program for their lower back. So how do we address these functional spinal locks without pushing the problem elsewhere in the kinetic chain?

Consider how the brain is perceiving the Double Arm Raise movement. If you raise your hands in front of you to shoulder height, the overall sense of the arm movement is upward. However, once the hands move past shoulder height and continue, the movement can be sensed as a backward motion of the arms on the body. If the brain perceives that the movement impulse is in a backward direction, it naturally counterbalances itself by shifting the center of gravity forward. This takes the spine into extension.

If this is happening, there is no need to fight the motion. The brain needs to learn a new relationship between shoulder flexion, trunk lengthening, and dynamic balance. Begin with elbows bent and hands at shoulder height so that the fingertips move straight upward, drawing the body with it (see Fig. 8.3). You have simplified the task by removing the forward/backward dynamic. This enables the body to follow the arms more easily, learning how to lengthen without provoking the locks. To emphasize this learning, ask the person whether the front and the back of their body are a similar length when they reach up overhead. Let them compare their trunk shape between the original arm-lift movement and the modified movement, as comparison often makes change more obvious. They may notice that their normal habit in the arm lift is to shorten the back and lengthen the front of their trunks. Return to the modified movement so that they can feel the difference.

There may be other relationships to discover. If the pelvis is sliding forward, the weight glides into the front of the feet. Draw the client's awareness to this sensation. What happens if they maintain the pressure centrally in the feet instead? Can they draw that sense all the way up through the center of their body and up through their fingertips?

Perhaps there is an even easier cue: if the pelvis is moving forward as the arms lift, it is behaving as if they are tied together with strings at the front (see Fig. 8.4). Cutting that attachment will allow the pelvis to be left behind as the arms float away from it up to the sky.

If the spine looks like it is being caught in extension locks, have the person rest the back of their hand on their sacrum, and ask whether it stays relaxed in place as the other arm lifts or follows the arm up as if tied to it (see Fig. 8.5). What would happen if they just left their sacrum behind as the arm lifted? The imaginary piece of string between the sacrum and the

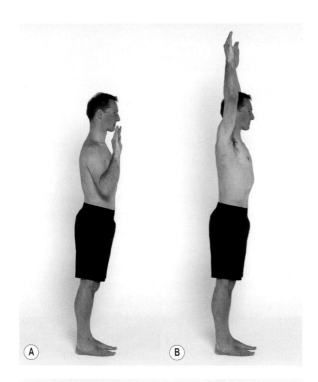

Figure 8.3

Changing the direction of the movement impulse.
A. Standing with hands at shoulder height. *B.* Stretching arms upward

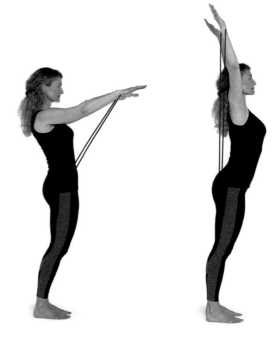

Figures 8.4/8.5

The sense of the pelvis being dragged forward by the arms

The sense of the sacrum being pulled upward by the arms

arm becomes a fine elastic thread that allows the arm to move away from the sacrum while still remaining connected.

When you leave your sacrum behind, notice that you remain connected to the ground and that the experience is one of the whole body lifting your arm from the feet upward, rather than just your shoulder muscles. Compare this sense with the conventional cue of holding the rib cage in place with the abdominals. When you set your abdominals, notice how your awareness shoots up to the shoulder: can you feel the restriction? Return to leaving your sacrum behind: can you feel the ease of arm lifting?

> The impulse of raising our arms begins in our feet.

If you compare these experiences for yourself, you may realize that it is not necessary to fight the extension response in the spine in such a low-load movement. Instead, we re-educate the system to understand the movement in a different way. The same principle can be applied for arm movements in any direction.

Extra credit: Remember the Greyhound Hand Slide in Chapter 6? When people are struggling to dissociate their arm from their trunk in standing, this simplified supportive position can be the key to unlocking the relationship.

> Sometimes the quickest route to dynamic stability is to understand how to leave something behind.

Limb integration

The Double Arm Raise illustrates that by promoting an elastic motion throughout the whole body, we can dissociate our limbs and move freely without sacrificing connection. This is frequently a light-bulb moment for many people who are struggling with hip, shoulder, and back problems, as they have often trained in a way that fixes one body part and forces disconnection from another.

Having worked out how to connect the upper limb to the trunk with Greyhound Hand Slide, and the leg to the trunk with Greyhound Heel Slide, we can progress to extending the link throughout the whole body by combining them.

Hot Toffee

Begin in the sacral support position and slide the hand away from the outward-pressing foot on the same side of the body. Let the sole of the foot slide along the floor until it naturally transitions onto the heel at the end of the movement. The sense of the movement is to allow the trunk to melt along the floor and let itself be gently stretched until it feels long and narrow in the middle, just like a warmed piece of toffee that has been pulled between your fingers (see Fig. 8.6). Notice how the abdomen falls into the Greyhound position. Once the movement reaches the end of the stretch, maintain the long and narrow feeling in the trunk as the arm and leg ping back in again. If that position of the trunk and sacrum is maintained, an efficient lumbopelvic stabilization pattern is triggered, and the hip and shoulder can move cleanly and easily.

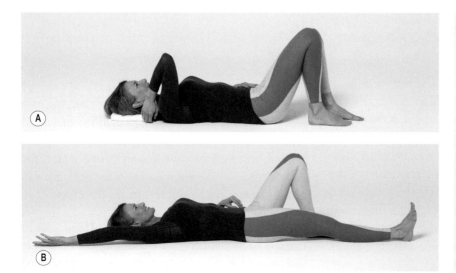

Figure 8.6

Connected lengthening

Hip freedom

We have learned already that to maintain the CLA, we need freedom of hip movement. Frequently, we see a spine being pulled into flexion, extension, or rotation because of restricted hip motion, and this is often addressed with various stretching and releasing techniques coupled with spinal stability training. This can be a circular, never-ending process if the activation pattern associated with hip movement habitually induces unnecessary tension. Restoring hip mobility is important, but it needs to be backed up with movement integration if it is to stick.

The concept of leaving something behind is familiar to us, having investigated the Greyhound Heel Slide in Chapter 6. This addressed the issue of the hip flexors struggling to actively lengthen, causing the femur, pelvis, and spine to move as a single unit. As the leg slides along the floor, the pelvis rolls anteriorly as if stuck to the femur, pulling the spine into extension. The primary problem could be a posturally over-involved psoas pulling on the spine itself or with rectus femoris or iliacus pulling directly on the ilium – but the movement result is the same in each case. Muscles that have learned to contract at a fixed length need to remember how to change length both eccentrically and concentrically. It is a problem of dissociation.

> Think of the movement rather than just the muscles. The movement shows the outcome to be changed. Releasing the muscles will not have a lasting effect unless the brain is given an alternative way to use them.

Learning to leave the pelvis behind while moving the femur away helps the brain to understand how to dissociate at the hip. This reveals that it requires a relatively low level of trunk muscle activation to support the hip extension/flexion movement at this level of load. When we use no more than is actually needed, our efficiency improves, giving us greater potential to pursue higher level activities.

We can use the same technique to balance the hip adductors and reduce the feeling of tight congestion in the hips.

Movement exploration

Hip Opener

Lie on your back with your head supported by the folded towel if necessary. With your knees bent and feet on the floor, use your sacral rock to find the balanced sacral support position. Take a moment to relax your breathing, letting any tension in your chest or abdomen subside. This is your reference point: you will simply rest on this sacral connection to the floor.

Place your left hand on the front of your abdomen just inside the ilium, the pelvic bone. This is your anchor point. Slide your right fingertips down the inside of your right thigh in the direction of your knee, to the point at which your elbow is nearly straight. Visualize a connecting line between your two hands (see Fig. 8.7).

Where your left hand is, imagine a small fisherman with a fishing rod standing on a rock. He has cast his line, and the hook has attached to the inside of your right thigh, exactly at the point you are touching. He is now going to let the line run out smoothly so that your right knee can move away from him, opening your hip (see Fig. 8.8). Enjoy that sensation of space in the hip, and then let your little fisherman reel your knee back in again.

If the fisherman initially wants to follow the leg, remember that you are aiming to move your right hand away from your left hand, creating space between them. You don't need a lot of strength or flexibility: your brain needs to understand that it can leave the pelvis behind and move the thigh by releasing the

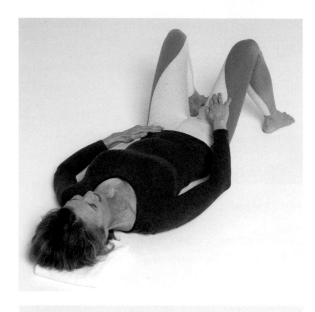

Figure 8.7

Hip Opener start position

tension in your inner thigh muscles. In doing so, the hip adductors remember that they can actively lengthen and shorten, rather than being caught contracting in a fixed part of their range.

Sometimes we need to offer the brain a different way of thinking about the idea of hip opening. Move your fingertips from the inside to the outside of your thigh. You may find that your brain responds to the idea of moving positively into your fingertips to open your hip (see Figs. 8.9 and 8.10). Select whichever option makes the movement feel easiest.

This is another example of clearing up a functional blur, as we first encountered in Chapter 2. If it is difficult to open the hip, the brain is considering the pelvis and thigh as a single moving unit. We want it to understand that it has two distinct body parts, which gives us more movement options and greater hip mobility.

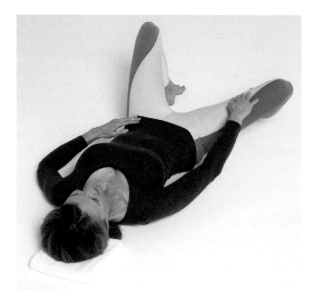

Figure 8.8

Open hip position

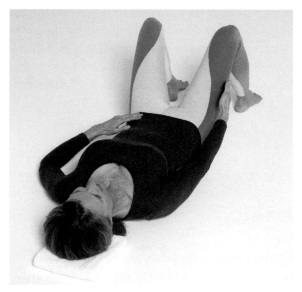

Figure 8.9

Hand placement on outside of the thigh

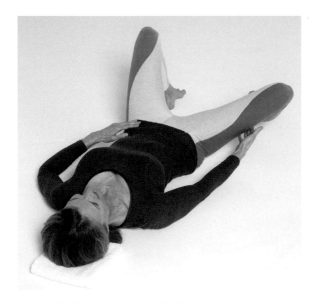

Figure 8.10

Moving positively into your hand to allow the hip to open

If we don't understand this, we start to fight for control, using far more trunk muscle activity than is necessary to keep our pelvis in place. When body parts are moving together, think of clarifying the functional blur rather than fighting an unwanted motion with increased tension in the system.

In the Hip Opener, we focused on the trunk and pelvis resting peacefully on the floor throughout the movement. Without us realizing, the brain has calculated how much muscle activity is necessary to stabilize them in a far more subtle muscle pattern than the one that we can cognitively generate. Anything more would be wasted effort and will increase the sense of restriction that we are aiming to relieve.

Extra credit: If you have made this connection, why not combine the Greyhound Hand Slide with the Hip Opener on the opposite side? Remember to let your body rest centrally on your sacral support, and

to allow your abdominal wall to fall naturally back to your spine in response to the movement impulse. Sense the diagonal movement of the myofascial connections between your upper and lower body as your body opens and then returns to the start position.

> To develop quality movement, use the solution that achieves the freest movement for the least effort.

Focus on the movement, not the muscle

At this point, it should be becoming evident that the art of teaching movement depends on an ability to direct a person's intention for the best effect. This means that focusing on activation of specific muscles may not be the route to better movement.

Many people struggle with the perception of hip tightness, for example, or experience pain at the front of the hip or groin. This feels like an imbalance of the anterior myofascial chain, a battle between the hip flexors and abdominals. However, we need to look further. When flexing the hip, there needs to be a pivot point within the joint around which the motion takes place for the movement to be mechanically efficient. This stable axis of motion within the hip joint is maintained by the small, deep muscles that secure the head of femur snugly in its socket, like a hand holding a tennis ball (see Fig. 8.11). If the muscle action around the hip joint becomes unbalanced, however, the mechanics of the joint can become compromised.

This problem can be created either inside or outside the hip. Internally, it can happen when the pull exerted by the hip flexors at the front of the hip is not balanced by the counter-pull of the muscles acting on the femoral head to stabilize it deep inside the hip joint (see Fig. 8.12). Alternatively, the axis can be lost due

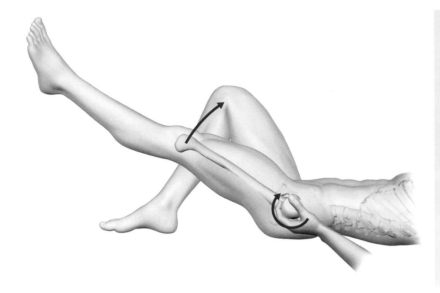

Figure 8.11

The deep rotators of the hip hold the femoral head securely in the socket to create a secure axis for motion

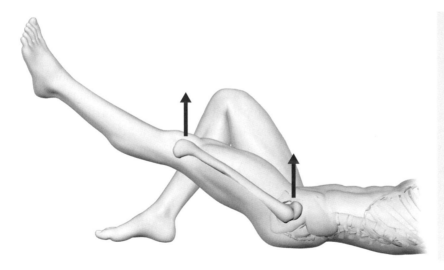

Figure 8.12

Dysfunction in the deep hip muscles can lead to a loss of the secure axis, allowing the hip flexors to exert an anterior dragging force on the head of femur as the hip flexes

to a larger external strategy, like hitching the hip with quadratus lumborum while trying to lift the knee (see Fig. 8.13).

In either case, the secure pivot point for the motion is lost, and movement efficiency is compromised. When we lose efficiency, we must increase muscle effort to get the job done. In this case, the common compensation is to increase the amount of hip flexor activity necessary to lift the leg. When this happens, active hip flexion usually creates a sense of congestion in the front of the hip, and, in some cases, anterior hip and groin pain. Attempting consciously to reduce the overactivity in the hip flexors while still flexing the hip creates a conflict of intention, and it is quite difficult to do. Consciously increasing gluteal activation

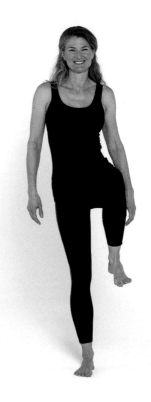

Figure 8.13

The deep axis of motion is lost if the pelvis hitches upward as the hip flexes

Movement exploration

Lifting from the back of the leg

Lie on your back with one knee straight and the other bent with the foot on the floor. If necessary, alleviate your upper lock with a folded towel, and find your sacral support point.

You are going to be raising your straight leg from the floor, but you will use two different cues for comparison. First, bend your ankle, bringing your toes toward you (see Fig. 8.14). Feel how this immediately provokes a sense of shortening through the front of the leg. Focusing on the front of the body – from the abdomen down through the quadriceps to the foot – lift the leg (see Fig. 8.15). Sense where the effort is experienced. This cue often creates a sense of heaviness in the leg and a feeling of load in the front of the hip as more stress is applied to the already irritable hip flexors.

Let's take the movement again, beginning with both knees bent and feet flat on the floor. This time, run your mind down the back of your leg as it straightens – think of stretching a piece of elastic all the way down and under the sole of the foot. Although the ankle moves into dorsiflexion at the end of the leg straightening action, the tensions are more balanced between front and back of the leg, and the muscles around the hip joint relax.

to counterbalance the activity at the front of the hip only increases superficial tension around the entire joint. Redirecting the movement intention, however, opens the door for the brain to recalibrate the muscle pattern.

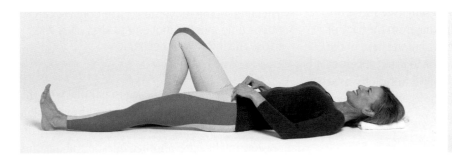

Figure 8.14

Start position for lifting from the back of the leg

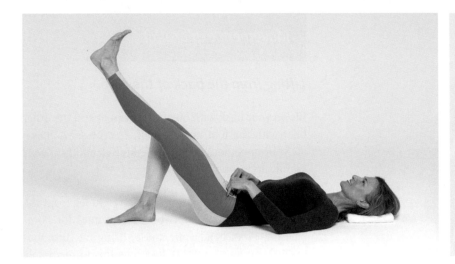

Figure 8.15

Tightening and shortening the anterior surface of the body

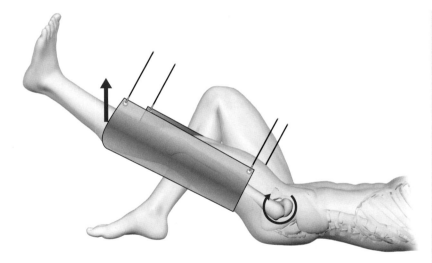

Figure 8.16

Lifting from the back of the leg

Feel what it is like to carry the leg upward as if it is being supported underneath by a sling (see Fig. 8.16). You have shifted your focus to lifting from the back of the leg. The leg still moves upward, but the head of the femur is encouraged to settle back and rotate nicely in its socket rather than being dragged anteriorly as it was before. The intention to lift the leg is transformed into the experience of carrying it.

By changing the movement intention, we can induce a cleaner hip movement that uses less effort and improved mechanics.

Here, we have been lifting the leg in parallel with the knee facing upward, requiring a neutral hip position with ankle dorsiflexion. But if you are involved in dance, you might have another question about this movement: what if I want to lift my leg with my toes pointed and hip in external rotation?

The principle is the same. Begin in the same position, with knees bent and feet flat on the floor. As you slide your leg out into extension and external rotation at the hip, let your toes lead the movement out until the leg is straight, and lift from the outside of the thigh (again as if it is in a sling) rather than squeezing with the inside of the thigh. There is far less hip compression, and the femoral head can sink nicely back to provide a cleaner motion.

How about seated positions?

The hip axis is once again the key to cleaner, more effortless hip flexion.

Movement exploration

Sit on the edge of a chair in balloon posture and your weight through both sitting bones. You are going to experiment with two cues.

The first is simply to lift one foot off the floor. This may cause you to take the pressure off one sitting bone, shortening that side of your body (see Fig. 8.17). If this happens, it causes you to lose the hip axis and increases tension around your waist and hip. (At the same time you will notice high activity in your quadratus lumborum and rectus femoris.)

The second cue is to settle both sitting bones onto the chair. They will both stay connected to that surface throughout the movement. While maintaining this connection, imagine a balloon attached to your patella. The balloon will lift the knee, which is at the end of the movement lever created by the femur. Placing the focus at the far end of the movement lever allows the hip to remain settled on the seat, securing the axis of motion and minimizing anterior hip tension (see Fig. 8.18).

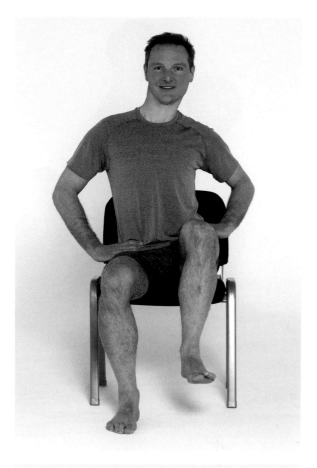

Figure 8.17

Hip hitching prevents efficient hip flexion

Changing the focus point can transform the movement outcome.

Knowing where we are

It seems contradictory to need to learn both dissociation and association of body parts: surely we must have at least one of these abilities?

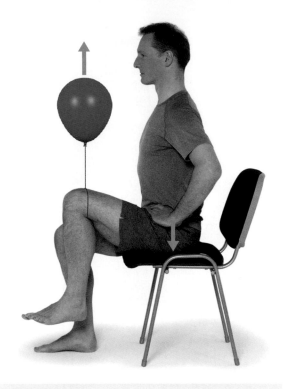

Figure 8.18

Connect the sitting bone into the surface beneath it, and maintain this connection while floating the knee upward

The functional transference of this is limited, however, if performed without awareness. It creates a dependence either upon high muscular noise or external feedback (e.g., from the floor) for the person to know where their body parts are relative to one another. Neither provide transferable solutions to the varying conditions of everyday life.

The quick boost of sensory input that comes from the slapping, rubbing, and shaking that we mentioned in Chapter 5 is a great start to let the brain know where various parts of the body are. You can then add more direct proprioceptive challenges.

When you work with proprioception, you are not so much teaching a person to maintain the position of their spine as to sense the *shape* of it. You can use simple images: is it an arrow or a banana? Even children are able to identify this within themselves, and they can move between these shapes with ease without any specific coaching on how to achieve them – or indeed any core stability training. It isn't strength but proprioception that enables them to sense their spinal shape.

In side bending, has the spine the graceful curve of a rainbow, or does it feel like it hits a kink in the road? If the spine is blocked in the frontal plane, the pelvis will react by displacing in the opposite direction. It looks as though the pelvis is unstable, yet it is simply acting as a counterbalance to the spine (see Fig. 8.19A).

Reaching up and out of the pelvis and tracing a smooth curve all the way through the body can help to iron out the kink. It is the quality of the shape through which you are moving that is important, not the range of motion. Interestingly, if you iron out a frontal plane kink, you will reconnect the spine and pelvis, making the entire chain more stable and controlled (see Fig. 8.19B).

It is not so. Those who hold themselves together with the high-tone suit of armor strategy, those whose postural control depends upon locks, and even those with low postural tone all struggle both to move their limbs and body segments freely and to demonstrate an efficient controlled connection between them. As we discussed in Chapter 5, in both high-and low-tone presentations, the problem is the same: they cannot adequately sense themselves.

This ability to sense the positional relationships between our body parts is called proprioception. The effect of diminished proprioception is frequently misinterpreted as poor control, and it is consequently addressed with stability or strength training.

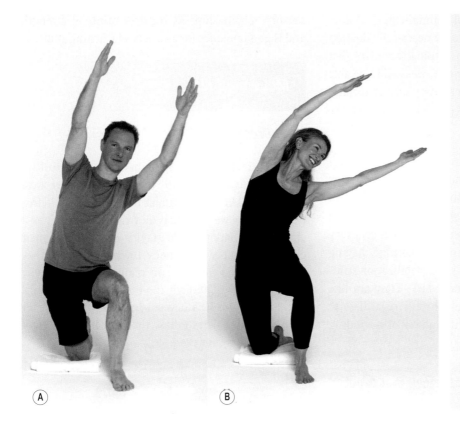

Figure 8.19

A. Reaching over flattens the spinal curve and displaces the pelvis. *B.* Reaching up and out of the pelvis into a graceful spinal curve

Making the grade

To carry ourselves with ease and efficiency, we need to be able to sense ourselves without the need to create sensory noise with excessive muscle contraction. This capability enables us to optimize our use of muscle activity so we don't waste energy and effort.

For example, if you stand upright with your hands on the wall at shoulder height, you need no more than a faint background hum of abdominal activity to maintain spinal posture, as gravity is falling straight through the body. If you then bend your elbows to tilt your body into a vertical press-up against the wall, gravity acts on the spine at a progressively greater angle. Your brain then needs to calculate how to gradually increase the amount of abdominal activity so it

can control the shape of your spine while maintaining your CLA. It grades up the muscle activity as you approach your maximum body tilt, grading it back down again as you press your body back to a vertical orientation. Your body performs this feat multiple times each day as you take it through the demands of normal life, from getting in and out of your car to pushing a supermarket trolley.

This ability is fundamental to our movement performance, yet many people lack trunk proprioception. Low back pain patients tend to demonstrate difficulty in consistently sensing where their spines are,[6,7] but conventional training programs often neglect this fine-tuned quality of proprioception. It is much easier to teach someone to preset or brace the abdominal wall to maintain a constant contraction throughout a movement. While this might maintain the CLA during the specific exercise, it doesn't necessarily develop the proprioception and deep automatic control that transfers to everyday life. For this, we need to be able to regulate our trunk muscle activity such that fluid, adaptable spinal movement is possible, using no more than is necessary.

It is not unusual for highly trained athletes to struggle with injury or performance problems when they have developed great strength, but have no sense of their body segment relationships without the extra feedback from high muscle tension. They meet every situation as if it was a high-load challenge, having trained themselves to use the same stabilization strategy regardless of the movement task. They are like Ferraris that are driven at full throttle regardless of whether they are on a straight highway or a winding mountain pass.

> A world-class racing driver knows that to get the best out of a powerful vehicle, it must be handled with finesse. We should do the same with our bodies.

Before proprioception in the trunk can be addressed, we need a sense of the body alignment that will be our reference point. The postural work of Chapters 5 and 6 establishes this foundation, which in relaxed standing requires minimal muscular effort. However, the effort level of the trunk muscles will vary according to the task and the angle at which gravity is falling on the body. The key will be to make it look easy regardless of what you are doing. How little muscle can you use to maintain the arrow shape of the spine, or to keep the length of the front and back of the trunk equal?

The following task is a sneaky low-load proprioceptive challenge, which I often use as a simple test of trunk awareness and control. Although it calls on deeper

sensory relationships, it requires minimal strength and is good practice for a variety of teaching skills.

Movement test

Wall Press

Have your client place their hands on the wall at shoulder height, and ensure that their body is vertical (see Fig. 8.20A). If they are able to find the CLA in this position, now we will see if they can maintain it as it changes its relationship to gravity. As they bend their elbows and move their body toward the wall, they should have no difficulty in maintaining this body relationship even though the body is tilted forward (see Fig. 8.20B). It is nevertheless very common for even trained athletes to lose the CLA in a variety of ways. They may, for example:

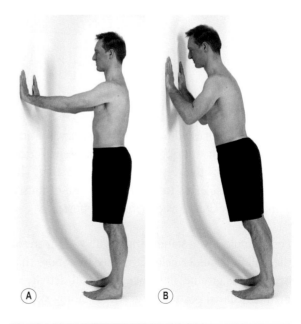

Figure 8.20

Wall Press. *A.* Start position with the body vertical. *B.* Finish position with the body tilted forward

- immediately move into upper lock, which inhibits their abdominal wall (see Fig. 8.21A)

- lead with their pelvis, pulling their spine into extension (see Fig. 8.21B)

- leave their pelvis behind, flexing at either the hips or back (see Fig. 8.21C)

- manage their CLA quite well on the way toward the wall, but leave their pelvis behind as they push their upper body back (see Fig. 8.21D)

The temptation is strong to teach presetting of the abdomen, isn't it? This might improve the CLA for this task, but it is a coping strategy that does not teach the features of deep control.

What are our options? If the starting posture is poor, and your cueing is not working, check that the arms and pelvis are not "tied together" when lifting into the start position (see Fig. 8.4). For a surprising number of people, this is the key.

Next, take care of the upper lock. This is the master lock because of its reflex effects, so it may be all that you need. Fold your middle fingers and thumb around the upper neck just below the skull, and apply a light upward impulse. Then, with your client's permission, rest your fingertips lightly on their abdomen, just below their belly button (see Fig. 8.22). With your hands in place, follow their movement toward the wall. If their abdominal muscles are grading properly, the abdomen will firm without protruding under your fingers as they approach the wall and gradually soften as they move away.

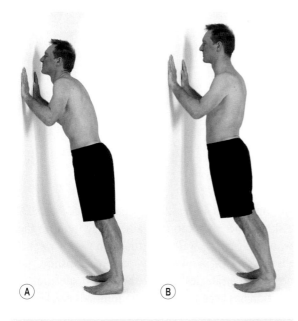

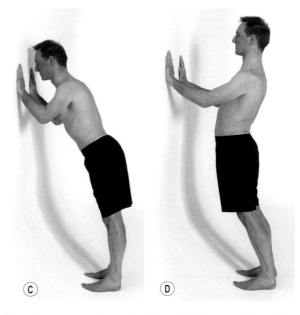

Figure 8.21

A. Compressing into upper lock. *B.* Leading with the pelvis. *C.* Leaving the pelvis behind as the body moves to the wall. *D.* Pressing out with the upper body and leaving the pelvis behind

Figure 8.21 Continued

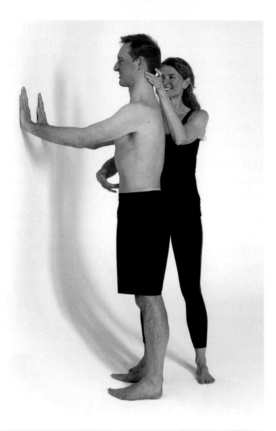

Figure 8.22

Releasing the upper lock and increasing awareness of the front of the body

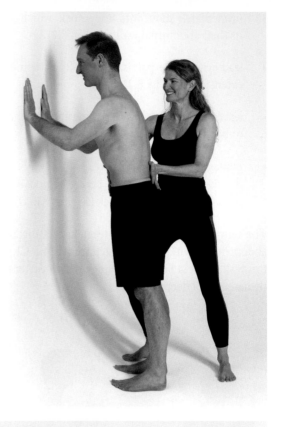

Figure 8.23

Spanning the breaking point

If you do feel the abdomen protruding or the pelvis sliding forward ahead of the upper trunk, call the person's awareness to any pressure they can feel as they lean on your fingertips with their abdomen. Are they aware that they are trying to get their stomach to the wall before the rest of their body? Or perhaps they are leaving their hips behind: can they notice that their chest is leading the movement?

If you place your hands on the front and back of their body, spanning their waist with your hands spread wide, you bring awareness to the "break point," where the upper and lower body separate (see Fig. 8.23). Ask whether they can find a new way to move their whole self to the wall, and their whole self away. In discovering their own body–part relationships, new activation strategies emerge, but as no specific contraction has been taught, the abdominals can learn to grade their activity appropriately.

Once the person can feel this, you can use one of the verbal cues (e.g., the balloons or arrows) to give them a sense of independent support.

If your client cannot perform a plank or press-up, check the Wall Press. If they can't manage to maintain their CLA at low load, it indicates that before strengthening can be of benefit, proprioception may be the missing link.

Once the proprioceptive awareness of relative body segments is established and the person can grade their muscle responses, then loading can be progressed. For example, you may choose to manipulate the load by changing the angle of gravity on the body. Depending upon the person's strength, you might choose a greater angle of gravity but shorten the lever (for example, a floor press-up from the knees), or a slightly more acute angle of gravity with a longer lever, like a knee drive from a bench (see Fig. 8.24). Once you have established proprioception, you have many choices to develop CLA control.

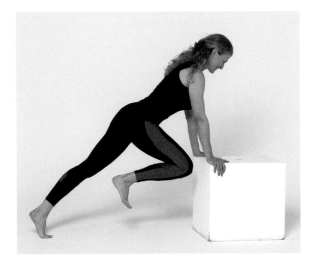

Figure 8.24

Knee drive. Progress the loading once the awareness is established

Inhabiting the whole movement

This issue of grading of muscle activation is seen in the limbs as well as the trunk. Someone may appear strong, but if they cannot detect lower levels of muscle activity, they contract much harder and faster than is necessary in order to be able to sense the action. It is a case of too much, too quickly. This works well to get the limb to end of range fast, but creates control problems when the joints must make coordinated *mid-range*^{G} angular changes. Walking is an example of this: for the knee to participate in our shock-absorbing system, it must be brilliantly coordinated to achieve the smooth, quick flexion and extension motions that create an accepting spring on every step. Too much tension in the quadriceps will compromise this tiny but important movement, increasing knee load and affecting the rest of the kinetic chain.

When you observe these people in motion, they seem to have a beginning and an end to their movement, but no sense of the journey between these two points. If their movement was represented by a children's join-the-dot picture game, it would look as though the pen had missed most of the dots instead of moving smoothly and continuously between them.

 Key cue: Can you join all the dots in your movement from beginning to end? Can you tell when you skip over some?

These people prefer to perform a task quickly, especially if it involves low load and greater control. If you ask them not to push so hard, they will not understand you – they are unaware of their own force. The key is to interrupt their output with a completely different stimulus: speed.

Chapter 8

Key cue: How slowly can you perform this movement? How slowly can you return to the starting position?

Lest you think that I am not in favor of strength training, nothing could be further from the truth. Strength increases potential. The problem at hand is inappropriate tension, which – as we have already seen – compromises movement in ways that limit power and eliminate grace. Brute force without finesse does not triumph in most pursuits.

With the deep neuromuscular connections in place, however, strength work can be progressed so that it enhances and elevates the power and control in our movements without sacrificing the fluency and grace.

Power points

- Our aim is to nurture more effective functional movement, but misunderstandings can transform stability into rigidity.

- Core strength without integration of proprioception, dissociation, and movement sense does not lead to deep adaptable control.

- Apparent loss of trunk control may have less to do with our ability to activate our abdominals than how the brain perceives the motion.

- Free movement of the shoulders and hips is necessary for trunk control. This requires that we balance the tensions in the myofascial chain rather than simply activating more abdominal muscle.

- "Leaving something behind" creates an anchor from which muscles can more easily lengthen.

- Proprioception can often be more effectively developed by cueing for the shape of the body rather than the position of the body.

- More is not necessarily better: for efficiency, we look for the cue that creates the best outcome for the least effort.

The higher your structure is to be, the deeper must be its foundations.

St Augustine

The evolutionary triumph of standing erect has opened physical horizons to us not available to any other creature. We may not be as strong, fast, or agile as other creatures, but we possess an incomparable versatility of movement, and an ability to adapt that movement to a multitude of environments, from water, to mountains, to snow.

Without a strong, stable, yet mobile lower body to carry our upper body, none of this would have been possible. However, despite its fundamental role, this secure, responsive lower-zone platform can be remarkably elusive in modern life. Many people yearn to move freely in their lower body but are trapped between the twin senses of weakness and tightness. From grumbling knees, painful feet, and obstinate Achilles tendons to grumpy groins and hamstrings, our bodies clearly communicate our issues with loading in our lower body. We shake our heads, blame gravity and the passage of time, and label it as "wear and tear."

Is this an inevitability, or is there an alternative to the merry-go-round?

Force fundamentals

As with the rest of the body, force sharing is key in maintaining healthy, versatile lower body movement. When we coordinate the motion in our ankles, knees, and hips, we distribute the load over a large surface area, reducing the pressure that any one joint must bear.

When one area moves less than the others, a negotiation has to happen throughout the rest of the body to work out how to accommodate it. Fortunately, we are masters of adaptation and can find many ways around a restriction, although some of these strategies are more robust and sustainable than others. If the strategy is efficient, it will be well tolerated by the body, but if it isn't, we can push pressure into structures that may not be well suited to bearing a high degree of repetitive loading. This can affect how the body manages forces, and in time can cause symptoms of complaint from those body structures. For example, if the hips cannot open out into lateral rotation adequately in a floor sitting position, the rotational stress is passed to the next link in the chain, the knee. The knee experiences the pain, but the hip is the culprit.

When we look at movement, we are perceiving this negotiation of force management – a dance of relative mobility, coordination, and control throughout the kinetic chain. Nevertheless, in many sectors of fitness and rehabilitation training, the focus for addressing injury and technical performance is heavily weighted toward strength training in one specific area.

The great glute swindle

When we talk about pelvic and lower limb function, it is the gluteals that seem to dominate the discussion. Just about any and every lower limb problem seems in some way to be attributed to "weak glutes," and glute strengthening has acquired the aura of a universal panacea. Yet, the gluteals are subject to as much mythology and faulty thinking as the core, and despite the effort invested in popular techniques for addressing them, many problems stubbornly persist.

When looking at the scientific literature on gluteals and rehabilitation, it doesn't take long to realize that the prevailing train of thought is overwhelmingly to identify which exercises create the most gluteal activation. The assumption is that more must be better. On the surface, this seems like a reasonable idea. Yet when we look at the gluteals in function, they are very rarely working at such maximal levels of activation, so there is more to this story than just strength if you are hoping to influence movement. In gait, for example, the actual activation levels of Gmax during walking is relatively low,[1] but this doesn't mean it is insignificant: the timing of that activation is key to its contribution in force management as we step onto that leg.

> Getting the right body part to the right place at the right time is critical for the glutes to fire.

In most of these research studies, the highest level of gluteal activation is recorded when the muscle is working bilaterally in its most shortened position. This has led to exercises that emphasize strong bilateral hip extension being recommended for virtually any lower limb complaint. The big squeeze feels good and can help to build potential, but it doesn't necessarily confer transference across the spectrum of normal functional movement. We rarely use a bilateral, maximal gluteal contraction in full hip extension in our daily lives.

We do, however, use submaximal levels of muscle activity through a wide range of different hip positions and hip muscle lengths, and often use quite high levels when the hip is bent, such as when lifting a heavy load from the floor. Strength is going to come in handy, but it needs to be trained in a variety of positions.[2]

Strength of course does not necessarily translate into power. The most physically strong individual is not necessarily the most powerful. Power has its foundation in strength but requires speed, coordination, and timing throughout the kinetic chain to actually unleash that potential. This is critical for gluteal activation. No matter how much we clench, squeeze, and thrust, it is our movement and postural strategies that will determine whether these hip muscles engage or disengage spontaneously in functional movement.

As has been emphasized in the previous chapters, the lower body muscle pattern will come through connection and intention, rather than conscious muscle activation. Focus on the direction of the movement impulse with all the smoothness, ease, and precision that you can muster. A clear intention and sensory awareness will allow you to make the most of your potential.

> Power and grace require efficiency. Tension costs energy and interferes with movement fluency. Aim to make it look easy to ensure that you are using the appropriate amount of muscle activity to perform the task.

Despite the obvious biomechanical advantages of the gluteals, we can easily use alternative options, such as our hamstrings or adductors, to get the job done.

Our aim is therefore not to simply strengthen a weak muscle but to set up the necessary conditions for the brain to make the most effective choice – in other words, one that produces a balanced, effective, coordinated response through the entire lower-zone unit.

Fit for function

A handy way for us to understand the gluteals' role in normal movement is to consider Functional Force Management, which is as relevant in the lower zone as it was in the central body. A few basic concepts can help us to appreciate the different demands that we might expect from our gluteal muscles.

First, we need to consider whether the lower body is working unilaterally or bilaterally. When we sit down in a chair, we are lowering ourselves through both legs, so it is a bilateral activity. When we climb the stairs, we alternate between one leg and the other. It is a unilateral activity for each leg. The reason we need to consider this is that they involve completely different neuromuscular patterns.

We must also think about whether the muscles are contracting while lengthening, or shortening. When they are controlling the speed and range of joint bending, lengthening like a fisherman letting out his line, they are contracting *eccentrically*. When contracting *concentrically*, the muscle is shortening, creating force while straightening the joints. When there is muscle work but no length change and therefore no joint movement, they are working *isometrically*^G.

Finally, the length of the muscle matters when it is contracting. When it is at its longest, for example, as the gluteals would be when sitting into a deep squat, it is said to be working in its *outer range*^G. At its shortest, for example, in a bridging exercise, it is called inner range. We are usually strongest in the middle of these two extremes.

If you are striving to become more flexible, just remember that a longer muscle isn't necessarily a stronger muscle: for every gain in flexibility, time needs to be taken to develop strength in the new range.

> Take a moment to reflect on your programs, and analyze the balance within them from this functional perspective.

Equipped with this knowledge, we can now appreciate the different functions that the lower zone must perform, and how this can help us to shape our programs. Functional Force Management in the lower zone is made up of the following.

1. **Vertical force management**, which is our ability to drop and raise our center of gravity smoothly, in balance, and at varying depths and speeds in the sagittal (flexion/extension) plane. This involves the hip and knee extensors contracting eccentrically, that is, working while lengthening as we lower our bodies, and then shortening as they work concentrically, to raise our body again. The more deeply we lower our body, the further the hip extensors work toward their outer range (i.e., where they are longest). The primary hip extensor is Gmax, working in partnership with the hamstrings and adductor magnus (see Fig. 9.1).

2. **Support**, which is the acceptance of weight through a single leg. This will also involve the gluteals, but in a neuromuscular pattern that involves a greater hip abductor contribution. Gmax is still involved, but gluteus medius (Gmed) and gluteus minimus, along with tensor fasciae latae, now become major players.[3] Effective support is very sensitive to posture and requires the balanced placement of the trunk over the foot to be most effective (see Fig. 9.2).

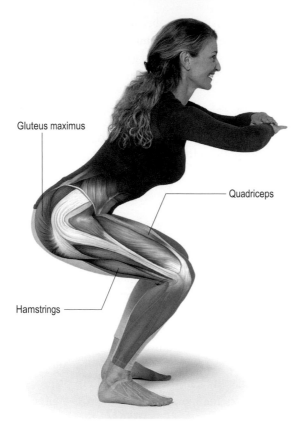

Figure 9.1

Gmax working eccentrically into outer range for vertical force management

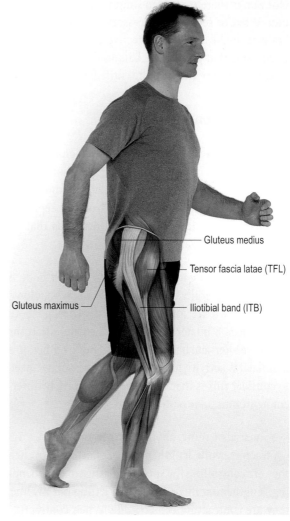

Figure 9.2

Accepting the weight onto a single leg for support

3. **Propulsion**, which is the impulse that overcomes inertia and moves the entire body through space for walking, running, and leaping. The hip extensors powerfully contract concentrically toward their *inner range* to create the dynamic propulsive movement of the body over the foot (see Fig. 9.3).

4. **Momentum control**, which we need to decelerate or change direction. To effectively control the momentum of our body movement, we redirect the energy of our initial direction of movement by pushing it downward into the springs of our leg joints, collecting it in our leg muscles, and releasing it in the new direction. This is one of the secrets of great movers: they keep the energy flowing by catching and reusing it like a form of rapid recycling, rather than blocking the motion and having to recreate more energy for the next movement (see Fig. 9.4).

5. **Balance**, which is the outcome of integrating sensory inputs and of the resulting adjustments and

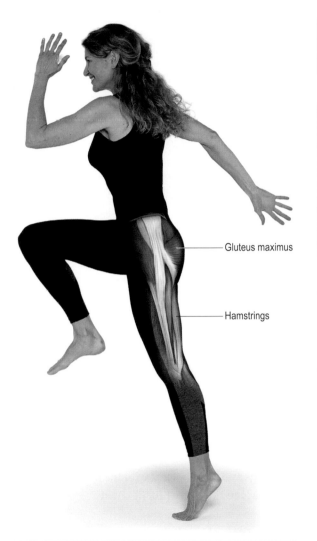

Gluteus maximus

Hamstrings

Figure 9.3

Hip extensors working concentrically for propulsion

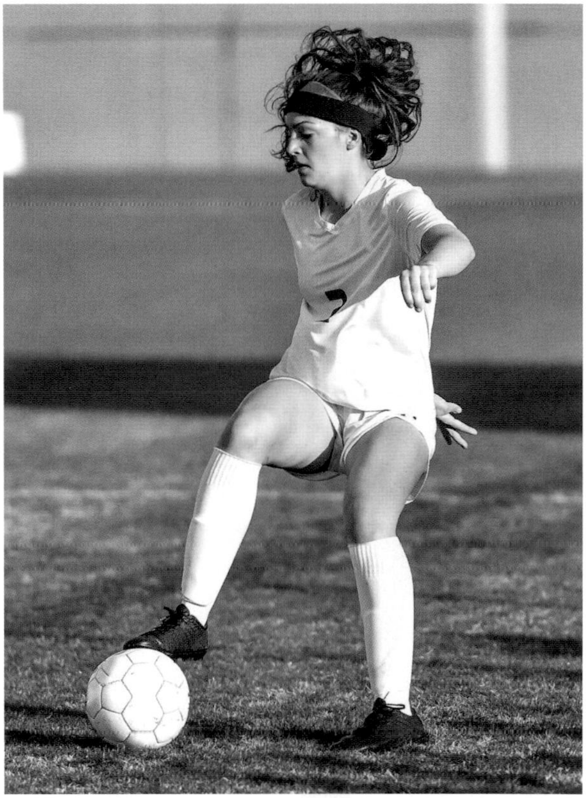

Figure 9.4

Capturing and redirecting forces in the lower body for momentum control

neuromuscular responses throughout our bodies. This is important not just for postural equilibrium but also for achieving an instantaneous sense of where load is being experienced in the body, in order to channel it optimally for force production and absorption (see Fig. 9.5).

6. **Projection**, which is the free, open chain motion of a leg on the pelvis – for example, when kicking a ball, or expressively moving the limb in dance. Here the movement impulse is sent, or "projected," from the pelvis in the direction of the foot. The gluteals are required to smoothly and sometimes rapidly shift their role between concentric and eccentric actions as the limb accelerates and decelerates throughout the movement (see Fig. 9.6).

Each of these force management conditions involves the gluteals, but with different requirements in terms of muscle length, speed, and type of contraction. In none of them is it helpful to clench or squeeze (which

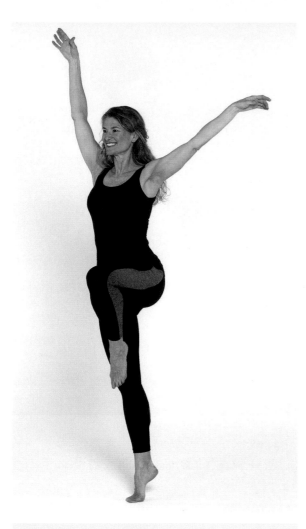

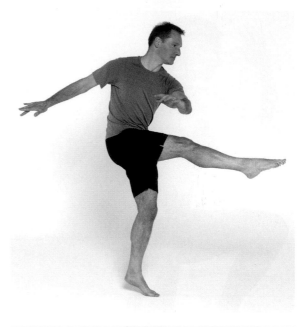

Figure 9.6

Projecting force from the body

Figure 9.5

Control of our center of gravity over our base of support

simply creates tension and resistance to motion). Anti-movement cues in the lower zone are no more helpful for normal function than they are in the central zone.

When taking into account all of these functional roles, it is not difficult to see why the bilateral, inner range, maximal concentric gluteal contraction only offers a limited solution for improving movement. Fortunately, we can use this knowledge to balance our programs and work not just with the muscles but with their place in the entire kinetic chain.

Start with the global picture

To encourage your brain to choose to use these gluteal muscles automatically in a wide range of activities, we must integrate the postural, anatomical, and movement relationships that invite them to participate. Many people spend a significant time strengthening their gluteals, but the performance and symptoms don't change. This is not so much an issue of weakness, but of accessibility and connection.

We need to look wider. Why are those glutes so disadvantaged?

Gravity matters

For the gluteals to function appropriately, it matters how we carry ourselves. If we think about the sheer cross-sectional area of the muscular family around the posterolateral pelvis, it is quite evident that it is designed for power and load bearing. However, in normal quiet standing, the gluteals are not highly active if the body posture is carried in balance. The energy investment in keeping large muscles contracting strongly while the body is at relative rest would be contradictory to our evolutionary drive for efficiency. Instead, they exhibit a low level of activity that fluctuates in response to the small movements we naturally make while we think we are standing still.[4] This fluctuation flickers between left and right to maintain our postural stability as we utilize a natural, very subtle side-to-side load/offload strategy for our hips.[5,6]

> It is time to let go of the longstanding myth that good posture involves tight glutes when standing relaxed and upright. This behavior does not reflect normal function, and in fact is associated with hip and low back pain.[7] Bilaterally contracting gluteals frequently indicate a lack of postural control or pelvic stability, which in turn impedes normal breathing mechanics and opens the door to a host of other biomechanical reactions.

The muscles of the pelvis and lower body are as responsive to the line of gravity as our central trunk. As we noted in Chapter 5, difficulties in sensing ourselves in relation to the fall of gravity through our bodies can cause us to carry our weight in front, behind, or to the side of that vertical line. Each time we do this, we compromise our opportunity to minimize muscle effort and joint stress as we strive to effectively bear the body through its wide array of functions.

We have already discovered that the trunk reacts to pelvic position, adapting the spinal shape and trunk muscle activity in response to anterior, posterior, or lateral pelvic tilt. We understand that "the pelvis carries the trunk." Conversely, the way in which we position our spine influences the muscle activity in our pelvis, so it is a two-way conversation.[8,9] The CLA has a profound effect on the automatic activation of our gluteals.

Extended relationships

Traditional postural cues have worked on sliding body parts horizontally backward or forward until they are positioned in a vertical stack. If we look at the body segments as a series of interlocking cogs, at the head, rib cage, and pelvis, we see different relationships emerge. The cogs will tend to alternate their direction of rotation, so when we turn one cog, those above or below will respond in the opposite direction when the spine is allowed to move in a normally integrated way (see Fig. 9.7).

The posterior rib lock that we discovered in Chapter 6 can be imagined as a cog that has been turned backward to lift the ribs at the front, and become stuck.

The head cog will counter-turn forward, dropping the chin unless the person overrides it by "keeping their head up." The pelvic cog below also turns forward, taking the person into an anterior pelvic tilt while the body weight drifts forward over the feet. The abdominal wall lengthens and the erector spinae and hip flexors become tight and active, as the person's choice for staying upright against gravity. This combination can influence gluteal activation.[10]

When we rotate that rib cog forward to drop the front of the rib cage, the pelvis and head will start to counter-turn backward. The body weight glides back toward the heels. It is important to know that this is a normal movement response; there is no need to resist or try to control it.

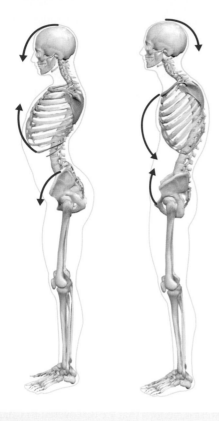

Figure 9.7

The interlocking cogs, each turning the next

Movement exploration

If you look straight ahead with your hands on your rib cage, practice rotating it forward and backward, feeling how the whole spine responds above and below if you don't restrict it. When each segment of the spine is talking fluently to the next, everything responds from the feet to the head. Notice the change in pressure under your feet. Then move your awareness down to your pelvis. If you don't feel a response, check whether there is something that you might let go to allow it. Perhaps move your hands to your pelvis, and turn this cog forward and backward instead. Notice how the rib and head cogs above it respond.

After that, allow your rib cage to float in the horizontal balanced position described in Chapter 6.

Sometimes the ribs sink at the front and become deeply stuck, compressing the ribs down onto the abdomen to produce the *anterior rib lock*. To feel this, put your thumbs onto your lower ribs and your fingers onto your upper abdominals; now drop your thumbs toward your fingers (see Fig. 9.8). Just like the posterior rib lock, this has a profound influence on gluteal function. The anterior rib lock can either be a passive collapse against gravity or an active over-tightening of the upper abdominal muscles, as seen in the slightly kyphotic posture that a male model adopts to delineate his abdominals for a swimwear shot.

A common response to this downward pinning of the ribs is to shift the hips forward. You can try this for yourself. Stand in a relaxed upright position with one hand on the bottom of your central rib cage, and the fingers of the other hand on the side of your hip, right over your greater trochanter (see Fig. 9.9A). Collapse your rib cage down at the front, and feel how the hip bone under your fingers glides forward (see Fig. 9.9B). The hips are driven into passive extension, the body weight falls into the heels, and the gluteals become inactive. No matter how great your glutes are, they will just hang off the back of your pelvis in this posture. This is a normal response, because with your weight already sitting heavily on your hyperextended hips, the hip extensors have no work to do.

> If the body weight is being carried in the heels, check for an anterior rib lock.

If you do feel your glutes squeeze in response to the anterior rib lock, you are using a compensated version of the movement. Those who are relaxed when they perform it take up a swayback posture as their pelvis

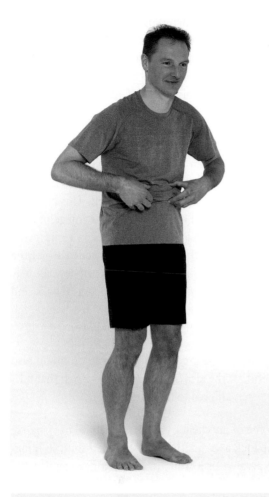

Figure 9.8

Feeling the anterior lock

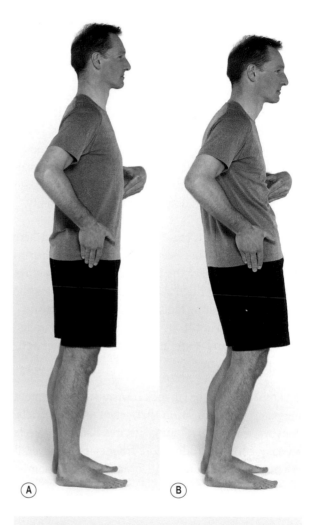

Ⓐ   Ⓑ

Figure 9.9

Hip alignment exploration. *A.* Start position. *B.* As ribs compress at the front, the hip glides forward

glides forward, increasing the extension in their lower spines. Those who compensate counteract the increase in lumbar extension with a mild posterior pelvic tilt, creating a flat back posture. Both are problematic because they prevent the state of relaxed readiness in the gluteals that we need for efficient functional movement.

To feel the uncompensated response, relax your legs and feet, switch off, and just deflate the front of your rib cage. Feel your pelvis drift forward. When you

reinflate yourself back to a normal upright position with your rib cage floating level, the pelvis will come back under you again. The hip is placed in an optimal position for the glutes to fire once you are ready to move.

Once you know to look for it, you will see this rib–hip relationship everywhere: the shortened front of the body with the hips pressed forward, and the associated flat buttocks. If this is your normal posture throughout the day, it won't matter how much glute work you do because they simply can't activate properly from this position.

This is an interesting posture as it is associated with such a breadth of communication possibilities. In the weights room at the gym, you will frequently spot the tensed upper abdominals of the *active* rib lock, calculated to project a readiness for action, nonchalant self-confidence, and don't-mess-with-me capability.

It is also seen in certain types of exercise class where participants may have been instructed to "fold the ribs down" to counteract the posterior rib lock. Its effect is frequently amplified with instructions to tuck the pelvis under or draw the pubic bone upward, creating a posterior pelvic tilt. In this setting, it is associated with control and containment, and creates an anti-movement posture.

The *passive* anterior rib lock transmits very different messages. It is a position that, when used positively, conveys a non-threatening impression, or projects an easy-going attitude. More frequently, however, it is a position associated with low self-esteem, submission, or feeling overwhelmed.

> When you spot an anterior rib lock, what is the message behind that posture? If you want to make change, this is often where you need to start.

Simple keys

As mentioned earlier, the passive anterior rib lock is usually an issue of being "switched off" and deflated, either due to underlying low tone or as a somatoemotional response. Accessing positive brain associations through imagery; increasing global body sensation with rubbing, slapping, and shaking; boosting the positive support reflex with the Listening Foot, and using buoyant cues like the colored helium balloon from Chapter 5 are all possible keys to play with.

Both passive and active anterior rib lockers can respond to direct opening cues. First, have them feel the area where their ribs connect to their abdomen at the front. Ask them to imagine filling this area with something that would invite it to open. This can have varied responses. For some people, the image of their rib cage as a paper lantern that has been compressed at the front gives them the insight needed to let the compacted area expand (see Fig. 9.10). They can play with shifting the compression from front to back and either side, before letting the lantern just hang, each level loosely dropping from the one above.

The giant marble imagery from Chapter 6 might also be useful, or the idea of the rib cage as a bell that falls silent when allowed to hang freely.

For some of my clients, it has been helpful to visualize the rib lock as a mouth that is clamped shut, so imagining a yawn or a smile in the area has enabled the release (usually a corresponding smile on their faces as well). Each person's associations are entirely their own. Where possible, it is often far more powerful for them to tap into their own neural data bank for the solution than to be cued.

Real life study

My client was a tough outdoorswoman, who had taken a blow through her pelvis six years previously having hit a rock while whitewater paddling. She had suffered with hip pain ever since, and despite diligent practice, was distressed at her inability to activate her gluteals despite having been told repeatedly

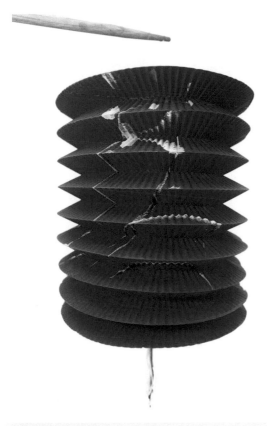

Figure 9.10

Imagine the rib cage as a paper lantern hanging freely

by healthcare professionals that this was the source of her problem.

She demonstrated a very strong active anterior rib lock, so her pelvis was sitting in posterior tilt with her hips pushed forward. This position would naturally cause her gluteals to be inactive. No matter what she did, she couldn't get a connection to the muscles. When I asked her what she could put in the space to open her rib lock, she was extremely surprised to find herself seeing a sunflower. Yet, when she imagined her big, wide-faced sunflower in place, the front of her rib cage released and floated back up, the hips slid back under her again, and, as she walked, the gluteals fired up just

fine. That sunflower turned out to be key in enabling her to return to walking up mountains with an active connection between her feet and her hip extensors.

> Carrying the body in balance under gravity puts the gluteals in a position to function.

Ball bearings

For long-term hip health and function, we ideally need to bear our body's weight in a way that spreads the load on the weight-bearing ball and socket joint surfaces of the hip. We don't all do this in exactly the same way; there is considerable variation in people's spine–pelvis–hip relationships as they solve the challenge of weight bearing. Preferably, their postural solution will center the femoral head (ball) of the hip in the acetabulum (socket), and the pelvis will apply a vertical force on top of this. This load is further dispersed by the formation of fine columns called trabeculae, which are arranged within the neck of femur itself to reduce stress upon the bone.

When a posterior rib lock moves the pelvis into anterior tilt, it shifts the body weight forward, and the line of gravity falls just in front of the central point for weight bearing in the hip. To gain a slightly greater surface area over the weight-bearing surface, the femurs will often rotate medially to compensate. The internal rotation can transmit this compensation all the way down to the foot, where it is eventually translated as increased postural pronation.

If the pelvis slides forward instead, owing to the influence of an anterior rib lock, the vertical load of our body falls slightly behind the hip, altering the pressures on our hip structures. The combined effect of this posture and the gluteal inhibition that

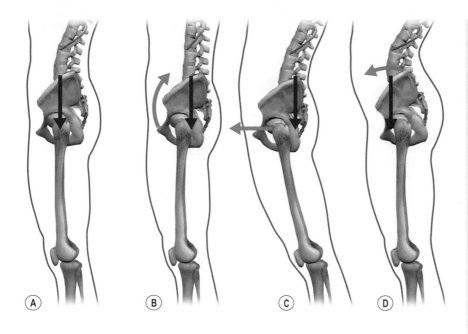

Figure 9.11

A. Neutral pelvic tilt: line of gravity is directed through the supportive architecture of the hip for even weight bearing over the femoral head. *B.* Posterior pelvic tilt: line of gravity falling posteriorly, amplifying the load on the back of the hip. *C.* Anterior rib lock/swayback: pelvis shifted forward, line of gravity falling behind the hip creating a forward push and increasing pressure on the anterior hip structures. *D.* Anterior pelvic tilt: gravity falling toward the front of the hip joint, shifting weight bearing anteriorly on the hip structures

is associated with it leaves the hip relatively unsupported while under greater stress (see Fig. 9.11).

The empty feeling that this creates can cause a person to actively tighten the gluteals to compensate. Sometimes this is an automatic adjustment made by the body to maintain force closure in the SIJs. Sometimes it is a trained response, which feels pleasing because it effectively locks the hips in the pelvis, making them feel strong and secure. Unfortunately, the sense of stability is bought at the price of effective movement and normal postural function. Remember that simply to breathe requires hip mobility.

> Imagine your pelvis as an umbrella over your hip, with your thigh as the shaft and your foot as the handle. Imagine gravity pouring down but flowing harmlessly off the umbrella, with your hip safe and dry within.

The centered hip

Whether we are weight bearing (closed chain) or moving our leg freely (open chain), the femoral head needs to be securely positioned in the acetabulum to create an axis for movement (see Chapter 8). Think of a pendulum swinging, or even the hands on your watch – they move relative to a fixed point. The hip, when functioning well, works in a similar fashion.

The smallest and deepest muscles of the hip have the role of creating this secure central point. If the trunk and pelvic posture puts them into a position where it is difficult for them to activate, the internal stability of the hip can be compromised and pain can develop. Gluteal strengthening exercises are often prescribed, but this often trains the superficial layers of the gluteal group instead of activating the inner layer at the root of the problem.

Think of the gluteals as a team with dual roles: some parts of the team act to stabilize the femoral head, while others move the femur. It is a coordinated partnership of muscles.

If considered in layers, the most superficial of these muscles are the powerful Gmax and the tensor fasciae latae, both of which increase supportive tension on the iliotibial band (ITB). The middle layer is made up of Gmed and piriformis, and most deeply in the hip is gluteus minumus, which has a direct attachment to the hip joint capsule itself and acts to stabilize the femoral head in the socket[11] along with rest of the so called "deep six," which includes gemellus superior, obturator internus, gemellus inferior, obturatur externus and quadratus femoris (see Fig. 9.12).

The route to balancing these relationships is through awareness and the management of gravity on the body.

> The cog-like interactions between our body segments can make attempts to alter pelvic positioning feel contrived and awkward if performed in isolation. Recognizing and addressing the spinal locks releases more movement potential for the pelvis, in order to explore the sense of gravity falling through the hips and feet.

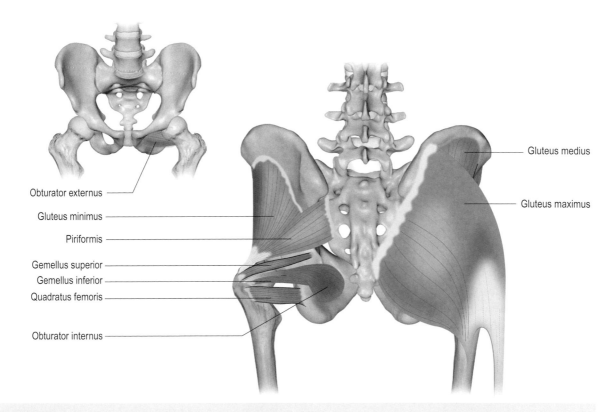

Obturator externus

Gluteus minimus

Piriformis

Gemellus superior
Gemellus inferior
Quadratus femoris

Obturator internus

Gluteus medius

Gluteus maximus

Figure 9.12

The muscle layers of the pelvis

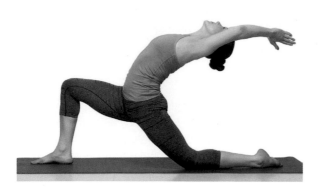

Figure 9.13

A centered hip, with motion shared throughout the spine

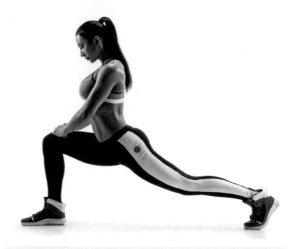

Figure 9.14

A centered hip, with hip stress avoided with slight knee flexion and forward tilt of the trunk

Considerations for deep hip extension poses

The issue of femoral head stability is of concern to yoga practitioners and anyone attempting to stretch out the sensation of tightness at the front of the hips.

In positions such as those shown in Figs. 9.13 and 9.14, healthy hip extension involves the femoral head remaining centered as the shaft of the femur eases back under it, like the hand on a wristwatch moving toward seven o'clock. The shaft of the femur and the bony point at the front of the pelvis, the ASIS, move gently apart.

If the femur does not release from the pelvis, it will drag it forward into anterior tilt. When there is no separation between the bones, there is no muscle lengthening and therefore no sensation of stretch, so people move further into the pose in a search for more sensation. If the pelvis–hip relationship isn't opening, the additional motion must come from elsewhere. The two most likely candidates are the lumbar spine sinking more deeply into extension, or the femoral head being driven forward (see Fig. 9.15). This is neither healthy nor effective for the hip.

To address this issue, we need to focus on what range is actually available in each person's body, rather than aiming for a more extravagant position.

Movement exploration

Relax and place your hands on the front and back of the body. Feel that shape, and see if you can adjust yourself so that the front and back of your central body feel to be a similar length (see Fig. 9.16). There is no need to "neutralize the pelvis" with your abdominals and glutes to begin with, as this will block your movement. Just notice whether the back of your body is curved in while the front is curved out, or vice versa, and nudge it back into balance. Now you will simply move your whole body through your hips as a single unit (see Fig. 9.17). Notice that your trunk is now tilted forward of the vertical but is still the same shape. Breathe and feel how your hips are allowing themselves to open, yet the back hip is not being forced forward in the joint.

It is useful to experience comparison to deepen your understanding, so, while in this position, bring

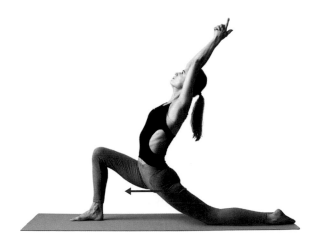

Figure 9.15

The head of femur being forced forward, compensating for poor motion in the spine itself

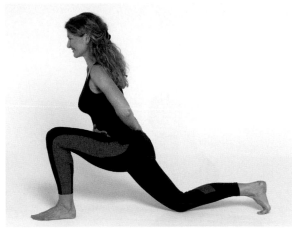

Figure 9.17

Carrying the whole body through the hips

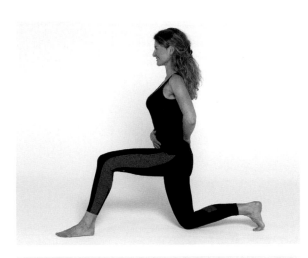

Figure 9.16

Finding a similar length on the front and back of the body

reduced. It feels more extravagant but is not effective. For many people with restricted hips, the centered approach will achieve a greater sensation of opening than the more exaggerated and stressful erect pose.

To progress using the centered hip method, maintain the hip and pelvis position and reach outwards with the fingertips before stretching upward into a smooth spinal arc, balancing the extension throughout the spine and facilitating a long, even lengthening through the front of the body from the supporting knee all the way through to the fingertips (see Fig. 9.18).

your trunk into a vertical position and let go of your pelvis, feeling what happens as you let your hip sag toward the floor. The front of the hip is put under more stress, but the sensation of stretch tends to be

It seems then that the hips are far more influenced by the wider body than is commonly recognized. Equipped with an appreciation of the functional interplay between seemingly separate body parts, we are now ready to explore the next step in the story of our relationship to gravity and the ground.

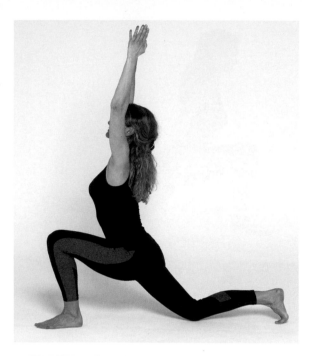

Figure 9.18

Completing the lengthening through the anterior chain

Power points

- The prevalent focus on gluteal strengthening does not necessarily translate into improved function.

- Our hip muscles perform many functional roles in different ranges and different lengths, and our movement training practices should reflect this.

- Strength training is not enough to bring the muscles on line: our global body carriage has a major influence.

- To manage forces within the hip itself, we must remember to place the pelvis directly over the hip, and to keep the centered hip in mind as we move.

Flying starts from the ground. The more grounded you are, the higher you fly.

J. R. Rim

Imagine watching a small monkey sitting on the slender branch of a tree. She decides to drop to the ground to investigate a nut, and you notice as she descends onto the scattered leaves that she absorbs the impact of her landing by folding the joints of her legs so quickly and smoothly that she seems almost weightless.

You look through the undergrowth and spy a small spotted wildcat poised to pounce upon its prey. You see that before it leaps, it first compresses its joints like preloading a spring, coiling in preparation for launching itself in a fluid ripple of gleaming fur. The sudden movement disturbs a giant heron nearby, who propels himself upward from spindly legs that have first pulled his body in toward his feet and then released him like a giant jack-in-the-box to catch the air in his wings.

From frogs to flamingos, we share this mechanism for absorbing force and energizing our movements. It is a movement that happens in the sagittal plane – the plane of flexion and extension in our joints – and it allows us to use ourselves elastically, to ground ourselves, and to manage loads effectively. This Functional Force Management feature is called *vertical force management.*[1]

Vertical force management is our negotiation between gravity and the ground reaction force. Every time we sit down or get up from a chair, absorb the shock of a step when we run, squat to pick up a load, or jump up high, we are managing vertical forces.

In essence, it is how effectively we lower and raise our center of gravity.

Vertical force management involves three main components:

1. unlocking the gateway between the lower and central zones

2. dropping and raising the center of gravity

3. absorbing shock.

In each of these categories, vertical force management will be most effective when the ankle, knee, and hip are timed and coordinated to contribute to the total movement. For example, even if the hip does not bend adequately, the same total force must still be managed, so more movement demand is pushed into the knees and ankles. If you happen to be stiff in your ankles or inflexible in your calves, that just leaves you with your knees to take the majority of the load. It isn't unusual for knees to become grumbly in these circumstances. To relieve the knees, working on more effective ankle and hip bending will be key, along with strengthening the movement into its new configuration. Force sharing is key in maintaining the health and performance of the legs and pelvis.

It's easy to see that this triple joint bending is so necessary that everyone should be able to manage it, yet that is far from the case. There's more to this story than meets the eye.

Opening the gate

We know that to create powerful whole-body movement, we need to transfer energy between the lower and upper zones. Many people never access the energy potential generated in their legs, because it gets bottled up in the hips and blocked from transferring into the trunk.

A small but mighty movement, the vertical hip release (VHR) is the key that unlocks the gateway between the lower and central zones.[2-4] It is responsible for energy generated in the powerful legs being transmitted smoothly upward via the hips to the trunk. From there, rotation of the trunk on the pelvis can transfer this force into the upper body. Whether you are performing a tennis serve, running a marathon, or throwing a ball (or even a punch), this transmission from lower to upper body is the mechanism that creates power. From boxers and dancers to squash players and runners, and to patients who have had joint replacements, low back pain, or knee problems, this is the one little movement that opens up a whole range of new possibilities for my clients (see Fig. 10.1).

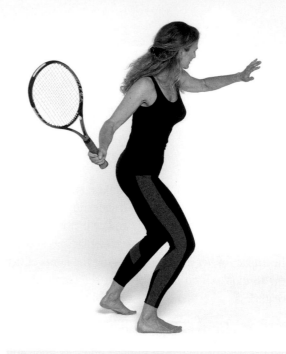

Figure 10.1

Opening the hip gate for forces to flow from the legs up into the body for a tennis shot

Movement exploration

Vertical Hip Release

To perform the VHR, stand and feel your weight settling evenly over the soles of your feet. A string lightly suspends you from the top of your head. Place a hand on your sternum, and adjust it a little so that this long flat bone faces straight ahead in a vertical position. Rest your other hand on your sacrum, and imagine your tailbone pointing toward the ground (see Fig. 10.2).

Now imagine the string on your head being loosened, just enough for your hips and knees to bend a little with your feet flat, allowing your body to drop

without resistance. It is only a small downward movement to unlock the hips from the pelvis (see Fig. 10.3). As you think about dropping vertically, does the tip of your tail want to point forward or backward during the movement? When the bottom of the sacrum has been pulled forward, you have bent your knees more than your hips, emphasizing the pressure on the knees (see Fig. 10.4). When the bottom of your sacrum lifts up at the back, it biases the quadriceps to work more than the gluteals, so, again, the loading increases on the front of the legs (see Fig. 10.5).

Ideally, as the joints in your legs bend, your sacrum angle will not have changed, because the pelvis itself has not moved relative to the spine. You will still have a sense of your tailbone pointing toward the ground. Your entire central body will have simply dropped a little toward your feet, cleanly releasing the hips and

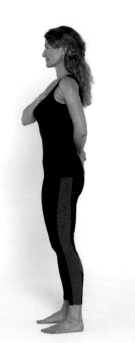
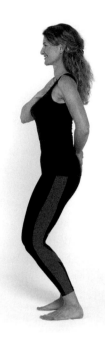
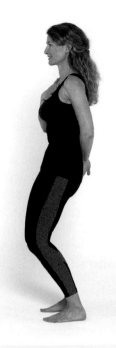
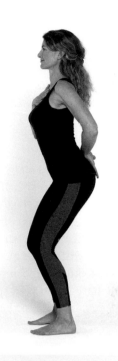

Figures 10.2/10.3

Vertical Hip Release start position

Vertical Hip Release finish position

Figures 10.4/10.5

Vertical Hip Release with sacrum pulled under and hips not flexing

Vertical Hip Release with sacrum lifting and lumbar spine extended

sharing the load more evenly throughout the lower body. The movement should be so free of tension that you can bounce easily in and out of it with very little effort.

It is such a small movement, this unlocking action, which makes it sound as if it should be easy. Yet for many people that is not the case, as it exposes deep habits. The VHR is not a mini squat: it is a completely different movement with its own unique purpose, yet people may try to use the same brain map as they do for their deeper squat. Some people take their hips backward, tipping their trunk slightly forward and blaming this on ankle inflexibility (it isn't, because the required range of motion is so small). Alternatively, they forget to bend the hips at all, moving mainly at the knees, which tips their trunk backward.

Notice that I have not once mentioned squeezing, clenching, or even being aware of any particular muscles. This is a small, effortless movement key that opens the gateway for force transfer. It requires a balanced, low level of muscle activity at the hip and knee; if you actively think about your glutes, it tends to interfere with the bending of your hip. The VHR is about letting go of tension and creating more freedom to move. Get this right, and a whole lot of other things are going to fall into place, because once the hip learns to move, the entire leg learns with it.

Movement exploration

Elastic Pulses

Let your breath and your muscle tension go and now fall into the VHR motion, bouncing rhythmically and easily like a weight on the end of an elastic band attached to the top of your head. Once your body is in balance with your trunk vertical, it should cost you very little energy to let yourself bounce. Feel the ankles, knees, and hips all moving softly in unison. You have found your springs.

In movement classes, the VHR increases the effectiveness of so many standing exercises. It allows the placement of the body in balance over each foot in t'ai chi or dance. It allows ease of rotation as we move the shoulders relative to the pelvis in turning movements. It allows us to relax our backs and drop into our supportive hips, igniting the triple joint partnership in our legs that is so necessary to efficiently produce power. It improves our ability to quickly regain balance, and to do so with reduced tension.

Once the VHR is integrated into a coordinated pattern, it becomes a shock-absorbing spring component in gait. It also prepares the body for quick movement in any direction by carrying the body in balance over the three major leg joints as they flex to prepare the muscles for action. This ability to easily maintain a vertical trunk supports better balance, even at walking speed, so it is relevant to people of all ages. It is so critical for effective movement that you would think that everyone uses it, but this is not the case, and, in fact, modern training techniques and old postural habits make it alarmingly rare.

Small but so significant, the VHR can be the key to improved force management throughout the body.

The jack-in-the-box

Being able to raise and lower our center of gravity is fundamental to normal human function. Stripped back to its essence, in the normal movement environment, we need to be able to drop our center of gravity smoothly, cleanly, and in balance – adjusting our vertical position in space as easily as an elevator in a high-rise building. We need to do that to sit in a chair, lift a low box, land from a jump, or change direction at speed. That should be simple, right?

It turns out that this is not the case, and that is not only a functional problem but a source of low self-esteem for many people. The way that we think about the squatting motion, which is so fundamental to ease in everyday tasks, has become stuck in the context of barbells in the gym environment and subject to many complications, rules, and misunderstandings. The natural management of our own body weight as we move it up and down is nevertheless within reach if we let go of some of the myths and work progressively to reveal each body's potential.

The movement intention for a natural squat is an up/down motion, rather than a backward/forward one. Think of yourself as a jack-in-the-box being pushed down into its box. If you push your hips too far out behind you, you won't fit in the box. If you push your knees forward instead, you will have the same problem. If instead you think about a giant hand pressing gently on your head, your trunk, hips, knees, and ankles fold into a zigzag as you sink down, fitting neatly into the center of the box. Although your joints appear to move forward or backward, the movement *intention* is downward (see Fig. 10.6).

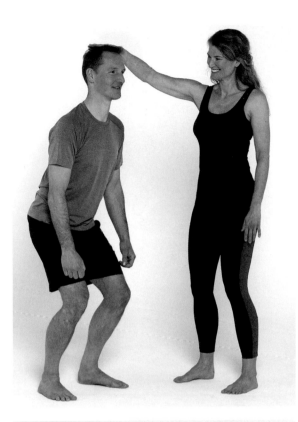

Figure 10.6

The "jack in the box": folding the body segments

This is the direction that makes us most effective in the sagittal plane, where our lower body is most powerful. It is the direction of shock absorption and agility, as it allows us to efficiently recycle the downward energy by storing it as we flex our hips, knees, and ankles, and then releasing it like the jack-in-the-box as our joints extend to propel us forward, sideways, or upward. A centered balance point also reduces body stress – equalizing the motion between our hips and knees means they share the load as we lower our body.

If this seems impossible, there are a several keys that can help to open the movement.

Lose the tension

One key is starting posture. People often approach this movement in a state of tension, and three areas are predominant.

The first area to work on is the head and neck. Releasing the upper lock allows the head to hover in balance directly over the body. This can immediately restore a little more freedom at the hips and knees.

The second is the hip. If you begin with the hips locked forward and with tense gluteals, it is difficult for the brain to determine how to initiate the movement of dissociating the hip from the pelvis. To avoid this problem, feel the entire surface of your feet expanding on the floor to access the foot–hip communication, then imagine creating a little space between your sitting bones to let the pelvis settle onto the hips. This unlocks the hips and opens movement potential. It also reminds you to let go of excessive tension in your pelvic floor.

The third is the upper back. Before you begin the movement, relax your upper body and allow your sternum to sit vertically, as if it is focusing a beam of light straight ahead. The initial angle of the sternum drives what happens throughout the kinetic chain, right from the beginning of the movement. There is interpersonal variation in how the kinetic chain responds, but here are some common examples.

A downward-tilting sternum caused by an anterior rib lock (collapsing the front of the body) will often initiate a spinal flexion response, blocking the hips from bending as the motion progresses (see Fig. 10.7). However, a downward-tilted sternum caused by a forward tilt of the trunk will have the opposite effect, pushing the hips backward.

An upward tilting sternum, as you would see in a posterior rib lock, can also have two effects. In some people it pulls the anterior surface of the body tight and

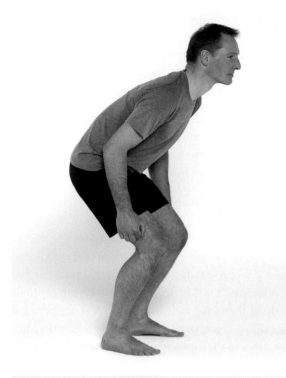

Figure 10.7

Squatting with the sternum downward at the start of the movement leads the spine into flexion

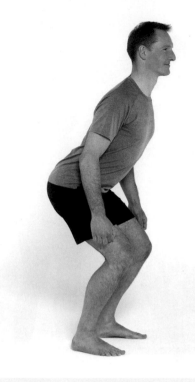

Figure 10.8

Squatting with sternum facing upward at the start of the movement leads the spine into extension

prevents them from bending their hips. More commonly, it triggers increased spinal extension as the movement begins, which pushes the pelvis backward (see Fig. 10.8), thereby increasing the pressure on the knees and biasing loading toward the hamstrings and erector spinae.

Roll your rib cage around the giant marble a few times to remove any tension, and allow your sternum to hang vertically. With a relaxed starting posture, we can further explore the natural squat.

Rotate to go straight

Understanding how to access the control and strength from your legs most easily, and being able to make

small adaptations in response to a changing balance point, takes you a long way toward mastering the vertical.

In Chapter 5 we encountered the positive support response, the neurological link between the soles of the feet on the ground and the effective antigravity action of our leg and hip muscles. Our natural knee biomechanics integrate with this neurological response to ensure that we are able to effectively transfer and support load throughout the kinetic chain as we lower our center of gravity – to squat or sit down, for example.

We often think of the knee joint as a simple hinge, but our body is much more sophisticated than that. As our knees flex into the squatting motion, the condyles of the femur roll backward on the tibia, creating

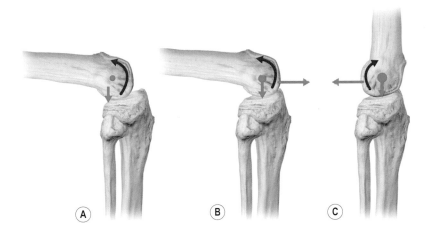

(A) (B) (C)

Figure 10.9

Biomechanics of knee flexion and extension. *A.* As the knee moves into flexion in a standing position, the femur begins to roll backward on the tibia, but this shifts the center of pressure backward. *B.* To counteract this, the femoral condyles glide forward as they roll backward. *C.* As the knee straightens into extension, this action reverses – the femur rolls anteriorly and glides posteriorly

the bend. However, if they continued to do this as knee flexes further, the center of pressure between the two bones would move too far back to safely and effectively support the load (see Fig. 10.9A). To counteract this, the femoral condyles also glide forward relative to the tibia, keeping the pressure between the two joint surfaces more central (see Fig. 10.9B). As we straighten the knee, this action is reversed (see Fig. 10.9C).[5]

This is not the end of the knee-bending story, however. Our menisci – the cartilage rings that sit on top of our tibiae – are wonderful solutions for distributing pressure, decreasing friction, and increasing knee stability by effectively cupping the femoral condyles. However, they are not the same size: the medial meniscus is larger than the lateral (see Fig. 10.10). With the lateral meniscus being smaller, the lateral femoral condyle will have a shorter distance to glide forward before it starts to stress the outer margin of its meniscus. The farther you bend your knee the more pressure will be applied to that meniscus. Repetitively stressing it in this way is a potential source of knee pain.

However, the body is so much smarter than that. We can keep each femoral condyle relatively centered on its meniscus if we introduce rotation between the

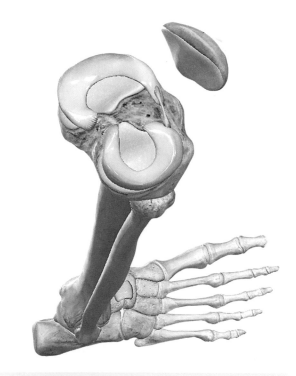

Figure 10.10

Looking down upon the menisci of the right leg. Note how much larger the medial meniscus is compared to the lateral meniscus

tibia and the femur as we bend our knee. As the knee moves into flexion, the femur rotates laterally (externally rotates) and the tibia rotates medially (internally rotates) relative to each other. This allows the smaller lateral meniscus to maintain its relationship with the lateral femoral condyle as it glides forward. As we straighten the knee, there is a reversal, with the femur moving toward internal rotation and the tibia moving toward external rotation. In each case, the femur can continue to glide without over-stressing the menisci, as the relative rotation between the tibia and the femur keeps the meniscal cups under the femoral condyles. It is an incredibly clever bit of engineering.

However, if your weight is falling predominantly on either the outer or inner border of the foot, this can be compromised. If your weight is directed into the inner border of the feet as you squat, your femurs are being drawn into internal rotation, preventing them from externally rotating as the knee bends.

If you tend to weight bear mostly on the outsides of your feet, it is likely that you are one of the many people who hold their hips in external rotation. This is increasingly the case: it is common for people to be taught to draw their pubic bones upward to achieve a "neutral" pelvic position, or to actively squeeze their glutes as a postural cue, which frequently shifts the hips in front of the vertical line of gravity and externally rotates them.

Movement exploration

Try it for yourself: simply put one hand on your pubic bone and the other on your sacrum, and draw the pelvis up at the front into a posterior pelvic tilt. Can you feel how it shifts the weight bearing to the outsides of your feet?

If your femurs are already externally rotated before you begin, they have nowhere to go once you begin to squat, because you have already used up your femoral rotation. When the knee joint can't bend properly, owing to this barrier to normal mechanics, or where the rotation availability between the tibia and femur is lacking, both the hips and the knees have to find another solution. Some people bend in their spines when they can't bend in their legs. Others push the hips backward, shifting their weight into their heels and even further onto the outsides of the feet. These movements are not dysfunctions: the brain is attempting to alleviate potential knee stress by offering alternative strategies to solve the problem. However, they are not sustainable solutions for effective functional movement, as they do not lead to effective vertical force management and frequently divert the pressure onto other body structures.

How, then, do we deal with this?

Although it seems counterintuitive, restoring rotational mobility in the hip and at the tibiofemoral joint in the knee can help the performance of the natural squat. Our eye tells us that it is a sagittal plane motion, but it is the small, subtle transverse plane movements that ease the joints and smooth the movement.

If you are finding yourself standing on the outer borders of your feet, or have rolled heavily into flattened arches, we need to make sure that your hips and knees are able to perform the normal rotational motion necessary to squat in the sagittal plane. You already know how to address these two components!

The Listening Foot (see Chapter 5) helps to restore the tibiofemoral rotation at the knee necessary for a natural squat, and also places your whole foot on the floor to more effectively press back up.

The Total Body Rotation technique (see Chapter 7) addresses the rotational mobility of the hip, and starts a conversation between the hip and foot. It also helps you to become aware of any tension you may be holding in your hip muscles. If you are accustomed to standing with your weight on the outer part of your sole in your normal posture, practice some Total Body Rotation and reassess, allowing the feet to rest their whole surface on the ground.

Having prepared the hips and knees, the next consideration is the balance point.

Striking a balance

If your natural habit is to move your weight backward as you squat, you will end up with your weight in your heels. Your body then activates the muscles at the front of your ankles to stop you from falling backward. The stiffening caused by this strong contraction makes the ankles feel restricted, and also creates a belief that the barrier is the stiff ankles, because this is where the strongest sensation is experienced. Far more frequently, it is how you manage your balance that unlocks the movement.

A little external support can help to reveal that we have choices in where our balance point is during the movement. To assist someone to experience this, stand in front of them and take their hands. Invite them to release their feet wide on the floor, and to become aware of the entire surface area under their soles coming into equal balance. Release them from their squatting associations by asking them instead to simply sit down toward the floor. As you may recall (see Chapter 2, Changing the game), this is an opportunity for exploration. If they slide their weight into their heels, pause, and invite them to bring their weight forward onto their whole foot again. They often don't believe that they can, but as soon as they do, they are rewarded with a greater range of motion. The process can then be repeated.

Once someone has started to appreciate that they have choices, you may want to draw their attention to any excessive rolling inwards or outwards on the feet, encouraging them to find the centered sense under their soles. Experiment with pressing up from the centered feet, and compare again from the overly pronated or supinated position, feeling the difference in muscle connection throughout the legs.

If a client becomes stuck and their spine flexes early in the motion, they may find it useful to breathe into their pelvic floor, "releasing their tail" as did my client in Chapter 6.

There's no need to overload anyone's thinking brain with details about their body angle at this point in the learning. It is enough to learn how to sense and control the balance point to begin with. We don't need to entangle them with corrections or constrain them with control cues; they simply need some time and support to work out in their own way how to allow their body to descend in balance. When we relieve them of their customary struggle, they can release their habitual tension, which in turn makes more mobility available.

To stand from this position, ask the person to find the position over their feet from which they can effectively press out. The positioning of the body over the feet for powerful, propulsive leg extension is an important sensory discovery. When they press from centered feet, they can follow the upward impulse all the way as if drawn up lightly by a string.

> Whether ascending in the vertical means launching into a jump, lifting a box, or rising from a chair, the principle of pressing through centered feet is the same

The natural squat is a witness to people's histories of injury, movement habits, and beliefs. It is an unfolding process for those to whom it does not come easily, so encourage exploration.

Three tips for easier natural squatting:

1. balance point
2. rotation at the tibia and at the hip
3. pelvic floor elasticity (see Chapter 6).

Clarity of action

Taking a look at the anatomy of the largest of the gluteal group, Gmax, you can see the line of its attachment across the upper rim of the posterior ilium (see Fig. 9.12). It also arises from the sacrum itself, so it crosses the SIJ on its way toward its insertion. Gmax also has slips of attachment at the coccyx. The fibers descend diagonally to extensive sites of attachment, with some slightly more vertically orientated to insert onto the gluteal tuberosity of the femur, and others reaching more laterally to insert into the fasciae latae of the ITB. This is important, because it gives Gmax two actions – that of extension of the hip, and that of external rotation of the hip. When training, it is important to know which of these actions you are addressing. Most people don't think about it: they just try to get the biggest contraction sensation – the most satisfying inner-range squeeze they can – in the belief that this will cross over into better function.

This frequently leads to an imbalance between the extension and the external rotation actions of the gluteals. You can recognize these people: every time they attempt to move their hip actively into extension, their thigh turns outwards. In a supine bridge position, their knees move apart as their pelvis lifts from the floor. In quadruped, they cannot extend the leg without lifting the pelvis upward on that side.

They stand with their knees pointing outwards. Their shoes tend to be worn down on the outer borders, and when they walk, they turn their feet outward as they push off.

> Cuing to maintain space between the sitting bones throughout the movement will help the soles of the feet to maintain contact with the floor, and encourage a clearer hip extension action.

When squatting, sometimes these people create high stress in their knees by trying to keep their feet pointing straight ahead, while their femurs are being pulled into external rotation with conscious gluteal squeezing. This creates a twist in the knee joint before they even begin to squat, and blocks the natural tibiofemoral rotation that we need for normal knee function.

> To relieve rotational stress at the knee, first warm up with Total Body Rotation (see Chapter 7) to relax the hips out of excessive external rotation, which will in turn allow the soles of the feet to make better contact with the floor. Then throughout the squat motion, maintain a broad sense of pressure centrally under the feet.

Sometimes the issue is the actual anatomy of the hip joints. There is immense interpersonal variation in the orientation of our hip sockets and our body proportions, and this will dictate the angle at which we can bend our hips most deeply. When rotational stress is being experienced at the knee in squatting, the solution may simply be allowing the feet to point slightly outward, so that the femur and tibia can follow the same track throughout the movement.

Tibia tilting

You might commonly hear that the tibia should be vertical in a squat. The genesis of the vertical tibia myth is understandable. If your squat is knee dominant and with a delayed or reduced contribution from the hips, your knee will slide forward, tilting your tibia forward as it goes. You end up with your knees moving past your toes, instead of your whole body moving downward.

To control the forward knee slide in a squat, people are often instructed to keep the tibia vertical, but to do this they must shift their hips backward. This of course shifts the balance point back as well. As we now know, this isn't functionally helpful, as it doesn't allow the center of gravity to efficiently drop in order to prepare the leg muscles for force production. This is not the natural squat, the adaptable key movement that enables us to move easily and elastically in any direction.

Dropping the center of gravity means sitting down in the jack-in-the-box action, and this creates a zigzag of alternating angles in the tibia, femur, and trunk. The angle of your tibia is just telling you what your hips are doing. If the knee is moving forward of the foot, tilting the tibia more, your hips need to "bend and descend" more to bring the movement into balance. You need to sit down into your squat with your weight spread evenly across your soles.

The downward impulse is the key to sharing the forces between the hip and the knee in asymmetrically loaded positions like a lunge or Warrior pose. Excessive tibia tilting in this case is an indicator that you are not allowing your hip to descend effectively (see Fig. 10.11), so the movement impulse is forward rather than downward. In the lunge, sink your fingers into the crease at the front of the hip and cup your buttock with your hand to encourage you to sit down into it. When you find the downward direction, your tibia will remain more upright. In a Warrior pose, you may need to create more space with a wider stance, which will allow the sense of the body settling downward onto the hip, rather than driving forward into the knee (see Fig. 10.12).

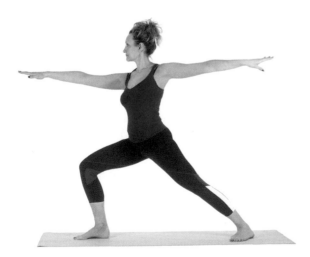

Figure 10.11
Increasing knee stress by leaning into the front knee

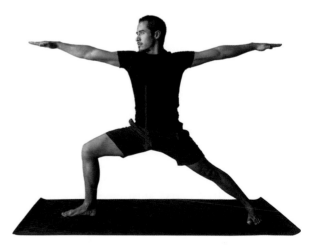

Figure 10.12
Sharing the load between hip and knee

To relieve stress on the front of the knee, ensure that weight is being accepted down into the hip.

Just letting go

The term "squat" conjures up a picture of the gym context for many people, and as soon as they start thinking about it, they block themselves with excessive tension. It's not all about moving heavy weights, so now is the time to free the term from the gym and reclaim it as a natural, fluent, utterly human motion. It's just getting near the ground. It's time to let ourselves go there.

Change the emphasis by sliding a dowel rod under someone's glutes and inviting them to press it toward the floor. It gives the brain a positive direction to move into, releasing it from the struggle for control that is blocking the movement. This can have surprising results. An awareness dawns on people: despite thinking that they were initially aiming to move downward, they were in fact resisting the motion with their own tension, like using the accelerator and the brake at the same time. When we release the brake, they realize that gravity is actually their friend in this movement.

Let gravity do the work.

But let's go further. Forget squatting – just softly drop. Issue an invitation to your body to drop through your hips as if your muscles have turned to water. If you over-balance, your brain will register it and start making adjustments. A different combination of muscles flickers into play. That's perfect. You might find that you automatically widen your stance a little. That's

fine. Just connect with the soles of your feet, let the tension go, and allow your system to find the way down.

This has been incredibly helpful for many people, especially those who control their vertical motion with excessive quadriceps tension. It relieves pressure at the front of the knee, and in agility sports, for example, squash, the resultant balancing of leg tension has a direct performance impact on speed in and out of the lunge. Releasing the handbrake issues an invitation to elasticity.

Inner springs

Now that you have found your "elevator," having learned to drop and raise your center of gravity, it is time to teach the muscles how to be elastic in the movement. This means balancing the tensions in your leg muscles, as well as teaching them to coordinate their contractions not only with one another but also within themselves.

First, we will keep the movement simple, and focus on the muscles.

Elastic pulses

To achieve springiness, the leg muscles must switch between eccentric and concentric contractions rapidly, a coordinated action that we need for power and shock absorption. It also means that the muscles must learn to release excessive tension, so this exercise will be performed with the intention of making it as easy as possible.

As you descend into your natural squat, imagine that you are passing different "floors" in your elevator. Stop a little way into the range and pulse the movement, bouncing lightly up and down a few times, before continuing with the downward motion to the next floor. Three floors will mean that you have worked at three depths and muscle lengths, giving you lots of opportunity for neuromuscular learning. As you ascend, stop to pulse again at three floors.

It is easy to throw the emphasis into the quads with this task, as the hips are often not accustomed to the speed of bend in these small ranges. Focusing on bouncing into the "sitting down" motion helps to facilitate the hips, and thereby the gluteals, to learn their roles.

Superfrogs

It is a wonderful feeling to unleash a sense of power from our legs. Once we have learned how to bend our joints in proportion and timing, we win the ability to access the explosive straightening that propels us.

This can be both easy and fun. Take up the frog position, with your hips and knees bent and fingertips on the floor (see Fig. 10.13). You do not need to have your heels on the floor. Imagine a stretched bungee cord attached to the top of your head, straining with tension and just waiting for you to let go of the floor. Now let it ping you up to the sky as you leap from the floor like a supercharged frog (see Fig. 10.14).

Does that sound silly? Not nearly serious enough? It's time to let go and feel your animal self. Using this technique, I get to see people who had no idea how to use themselves suddenly encountering power from their legs. They benefit not only from the leap but also from the rapid coordination of their joints as they return to frog position again. I see experiments with head position – clients learn that looking down just uses their calves and knees, whereas looking ahead gives them hips. I see moments of clarity as they learn that the propulsion comes from the feet, not from the shoulders. I see faces flush and smiles emerge.

And that's the best result of all.

Grounding

We cannot leave this discussion without considering the concept of grounding. This term is used widely, yet it is so poorly understood in practice. We know

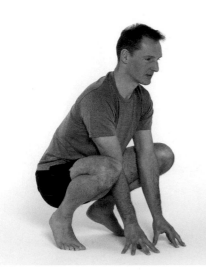
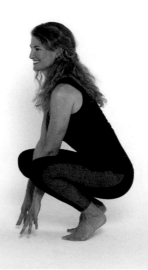

Figure 10.13

Superfrogs: coiling at the start

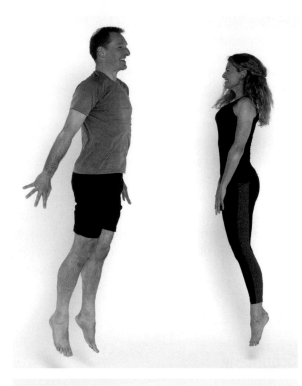

Figure 10.14

Superfrogs: releasing lower body energy

You have already practiced your Listening Foot, so it knows how to adapt its surface to the ground. You do not need to push down or try to be heavy. This only makes you a passive load, and to be grounded is to be vibrantly self-supporting. Simply be aware of the surfaces of your feet meeting the surface of the ground like two sheets of paper resting on each other.

Move into VHR, and feel how dropping your center of gravity in balance is key to your communication with the ground. From here your aikido, t'ai chi, dance, or yoga can flourish. If you cannot drop vertically without pushing your pelvis forward or backward, however, you will not be grounded (see Fig. 10.15).

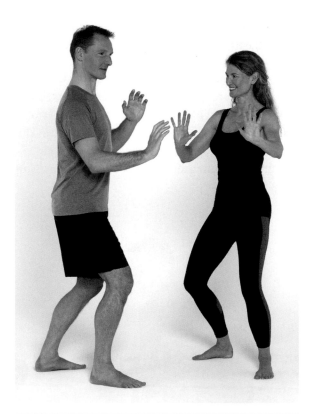

Figure 10.15

Allowing yourself to settle onto the ground while vibrantly self-supporting

what it looks like when someone appears well-grounded, but it is not always so easy to achieve.

The fundamentals for being beautifully grounded are now within your grasp. First, to feel the feet on the ground, think back to the zones that we learned about in Chapter 4. Visualize the three cylinders stacked on one another. Let your upper zone settle onto your central zone, imagining a soft click as they connect. Feel how that sinks your feet farther into the ground.

Check your sternum with your hand. If its face is tilted upward or downward, simply shine it forward. Feel how changing the sternal position changes the sense of connection through the feet.

Finally, it is not necessary to think "down" to be grounded. The key is to experience the sense of vertical suspension in your posture that we have been exploring through the past few chapters, and to allow your weight to settle onto the ground through that central line. For example, a ballet dancer can still be grounded while *en pointe*, as this ethereal position is actually an outward expansion between the toes and the head, a simultaneous impulse that travels down to the foot as it stretches up through the body.

From here on, we shall seek and find the sense of being grounded.

Power points

- Our ability to drop our center of gravity involves much more than our glutes. Our spinal posture, hip posture, and balance point all substantially influence our movement ability.

- The small movements make the big movements easier.

- Finding the hips relieves pressure from the knees.

- The tangle of instructions and associations with squatting can be set aside to allow us to find a natural way to drop and raise ourselves, smoothly and in balance.

- This skill opens up our potential for powerful leg movement and agility, as well as managing our everyday tasks with ease.

Gravity is a habit that is hard to shake off.

Terry Pratchett, *Small Gods*

Our bipedal nature has gifted us many movement options, and we can choose to walk, run, skip, leap, and dance as we exploit our ability to alternate between one leg and the other.

This means we have to be masters of accepting and managing weight on each leg independently, a Functional Force Management feature that in JEMS we call *support*. Support is the buoyant carriage of our pelvis over each foot as it contacts the ground – a sense of secure connection throughout our whole leg as we manage the challenge of receiving and propelling our body weight.

Once again we find ourselves negotiating between the vertical press of gravity and the upward push of ground reaction force, but this time it is through a single leg. The most direct line of force will be the most efficient for our body structures. If you imagine a cascade of water flowing down from your pelvis through one leg, it will fall straight into your foot. If you move your knee in or out, you create a kink in that flow – a diversion that increases the distance that the water must travel – and this produces a pressure point at the apex of the bend. Forces work much the same way in our legs.

To achieve support, however, requires us to meet a new challenge. If we lift one foot off the floor, we need to somehow prop our pelvis up with only one strut. We need an additional neuromuscular solution.

Feet first

To negotiate with gravity, we first need that "up" impulse from the ground: the communication from the soles of our feet that triggers the reflexive anti-gravity response in the legs and pelvis in response to weight bearing.

This communication from the feet blends with vestibular and visual processing to stimulate global postural control responses, among them the activation of the gluteals.[1] This link is so important that a past ankle injury can change your hip extension pattern by delaying gluteal activation on both sides of the body, even after the original injury has resolved.[2]

The natural response of a well-functioning foot is to calibrate its activity according to the level of postural control demand you are experiencing.[3] When standing on one leg, you will see and feel fluctuating muscle activity within the foot. It should not become functionally rigid with a fixed high level of muscle activation: a rigid foot is unable to make the finely tuned adjustments necessary for us to maintain our balance on a single leg. A foot that is not listening to the ground is not talking to you either.

Fortunately, we already have the Listening Foot (see Chapter 5) under our belt, to help place the sole on the ground, increase sensory discrimination, and reduce foot tension such that this accurate information is made available. This is an essential start if you want to achieve natural, automatic hip control with appropriate gluteal engagement.

> A significant key to accessing hip control is a responsive, connected foot. A spiky ball massage under the foot to awaken the sole, and the Listening Foot exercise to encourage tibiofemoral rotation are simple but effective keys to facilitating support.

Pelvic partners

Unsurprisingly, there are many muscles involved in stabilizing the pelvis over the foot.

Gluteus medius (Gmed) arises from the upper, outer surface of the ilium and inserts into a strong tendon on the outer surface of the greater tuberosity, giving it ideal leverage as an abductor and rotator of the hip. When we stand on that leg, its action places the level pelvis over the thigh, assisted by its partnership with quadratus lumborum on the opposite side (see Fig. 11.1).

When it is not functioning well, Gmed allows the pelvis to either slip sideways over the stance foot, or to drop on the opposite side, pulling the CLA into a side bend (see Fig. 11.2). This is known as the Trendelenberg sign, and it shifts the muscle activity emphasis from the gluteal muscles to the hamstrings, adductor longus, and vastus lateralis of the outer quadriceps (see Fig. 11.3).[4] It places the femur into relative adduction, which increases the tension down the outside of the

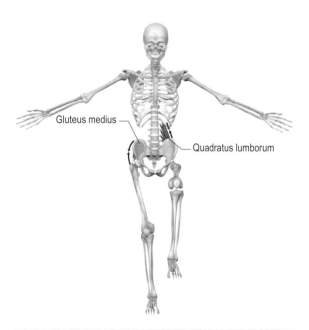

Figure 11.1

Quadratus lumborum and gluteus medius working in partnership to maintain pelvic position over the standing leg

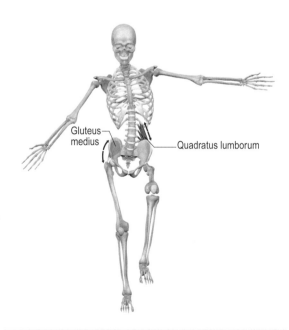

Figure 11.2

Gluteus medius and quadratus lumborum lengthen, and the iliotibial band is placed under tension. Adductor longus and lateral quadriceps increase their activity

hip and thigh. This can particularly stress the lateral hip and may be associated with symptoms like "snapping hip" and trochanteric bursitis, a painful inflammation of the small sac of fluid that lubricates and cushions the interface between the prominent bone on the outside of the hip (the greater trochanter) and its overlying soft tissues.[5] This adducted position of the femur also stresses the ITB, which must bear increased load in a stretched position. This chronic heavy tension can provoke symptoms at its insertion at the lateral knee, a common runner's complaint.

Meanwhile, the quadratus lumborum attempts to counteract the downward pull of the pelvis. If overworked in a lengthened position, it can start to feel tight and irritable, when in fact it is chronically overactive. When this happens, direct treatment for the muscle yields only short-term relief.

Our brain knows that we need to carry our weight effectively over the leg, and, as always, there is more than one solution if we lack strength in our pelvic partners. Instead of adopting the dropped pelvis option (see Fig. 11.3), it sometimes chooses instead to throw the trunk even further over the stance leg. This raises the opposite side of the pelvis, and brings the hip back underneath us. This is a compensated Trendelenberg sign (see Fig. 11.4).

Gmed tends to attract the most attention when considering single leg stance, while Gmax's significant role is often overlooked. With its lateral insertion into the tensor fasciae latae, Gmax helps to steady the pelvis on the femur, firming up that strong fascial band down the outside of the leg to support both the hip and the knee. As an external rotator, Gmax can also prevent excessive internal rotation at the hip as

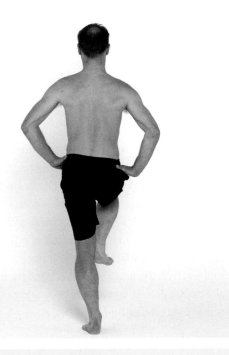

Figure 11.3

Trendelenberg sign

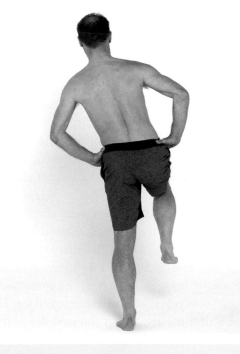

Figure 11.4

Compensated Trendelenberg sign

we place our weight on the leg. This prevents us from rolling into excessive pronation at the foot and ankle.

By all means, build gluteal strength using the many common exercises available, but resist the urge to cue people to squeeze their glutes when standing on one leg. This may feel pleasantly strong but has little to do with normal dynamic function. Instead, when moving into single leg stance, call the attention to centering the pressure under the stance foot, and then stack each body segment vertically over it (see Chapter 5). If you feel that a little more active sense of the hip muscles is needed, cue to gently press the floor away through the foot. If we work with body placement instead of muscle squeeze, the brain can find the low-level muscle partnerships that it needs without sacrificing joint mobility and dynamic balance.

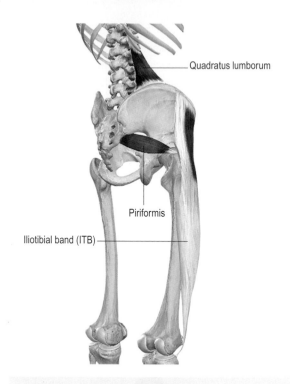

Figure 11.5

Piriformis and tensor fascia latae

We have other possibilities to turn to when Gmed and Gmax are not providing adequate control of the pelvis–femur relationship. Piriformis, for example, can have an abducting role at specific angles. Tensor fasciae latae is also an abductor of the hip, stabilizing the pelvis over the hip in weight bearing. Its supportive action continues all the way down the outside of the leg to the lateral knee via the ITB (see Fig. 11.5). Although both of these muscles offer abductor functions, they can nonetheless become very irritable if asked to take a consistently more significant role than they are designed for. The ITB and piriformis are two of the most frequently foam-rolled and pummeled structures in the lower body, but both are more likely to be victims of an unbalanced muscle synergy than a primary cause of dysfunction.

More distant relatives

Many muscles are involved in the myofascial web that maintains the balance of stabilizing tension in the pelvis known as tensegrity^G. The brain calibrates the fluctuating pulls of one muscle against another as they change their roles during movement, making lightning-fast computations to balance the tensions across and throughout the pelvis. If one muscle group is underactive, the brain will search for alternatives to make up the deficit, sometimes provoking other muscles into overactivity and discomfort.

Gmax is well connected into a fascial network that incorporates an extensive web of pelvic ligaments, merging into the fascia wrapping the erector spinae and multifidus, and proceeding farther up into the thoracolumbar fascia. As discussed in Chapter 4, latissimus dorsi also inserts into the thoracolumbar fascia, creating a diagonal relationship called the posterior oblique myofascial sling between Gmax on the one side and latissimus dorsi on the other thereby anatomically and functionally connecting the pelvis to the shoulder. From below, the hamstrings can also contribute to pelvic stability, providing tension through the sacrotuberous ligament, which blends with the dense pelvic ligaments. If Gmax is not performing, the latissimus dorsi, hamstrings, and erector spinae can all be called upon to make up the difference (see Figure 4.12).

If we look at the internal stability of the pelvis, the SIJs benefit from the balanced action of a number of muscles including the pelvic floor, deep abdominals, and hip muscles. Muscles that span the SIJ contract to pull the surfaces of the joint together, creating the force closure stabilizing mechanism. As mentioned in Chapter 7, this reinforces the structural form closure of the joint surfaces and the strong ligaments that bind them. Gmax and the much misunderstood piriformis both cross the SIJ, and as such can support it through force closure.

If one muscle is not playing its part in the dance of SIJ force closure, another will pick up extra responsibility to maintain the integrity of the pelvis. For example, if Gmax is prevented from working appropriately, piriformis is once again a candidate for stepping up its contribution. Given that it is rather small in comparison to Gmax, this work inequality is likely to irritate it, creating soreness and tightness deep in the buttock. Rather than trying to beat it into submission with strong soft tissue releases and heavy stretches, start by appreciating its efforts to support the SIJ. It needs to be gently persuaded to relax and lengthen, and the key to alleviating its stress is to identify why it is having to behave in this way. Although piriformis can be affected pathologically by irritation coming

from the spine itself, the majority of cases have a significant functional component. This means that it arises from how a person is using themselves to stand on one leg.

Movement test

Support: a quick check

When any of these related muscles keep presenting as tight or painful, you can perform a quick and easy movement check to see whether there is a functional element behind it.

Ask your client to stand with their feet just a little narrower than hip width apart and arms held out to the sides without excessive tension. This arm position can

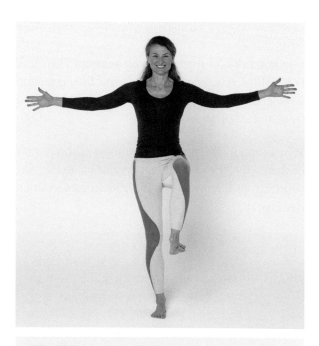

Figure 11.6

Standing Knee Raise

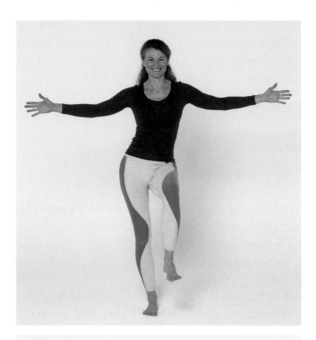

Figure 11.7

Loss of support: pelvis sliding sideways

help you to see changes in trunk position. Their task is simply to raise one knee. The arms should remain level, and the CLA should stay vertical, from both a front and side view (see Fig. 11.6).

When support is not secure, a number of things may happen. First, the stance hip may slide out to the side, which drops the pelvis into a Trendelenberg position (see Fig. 11.7).

Ask the person to place their hand on the outside of their hip, first to notice the sideways movement, and next to see if they can discover an alternative possibility. Sometimes, the problem is not gluteal weakness so much as the brain choosing one option habitually when others are available.

The pelvis can in fact react in any of the three planes. Imagine a car headlight on the front of each hip: they should stay straight and level. If you see the headlights turn toward the lifting knee, this is the pelvis losing control in the transverse (rotational) plane. Headlights tipping sideways suggests a frontal plane control issue. The headlights may even tilt down toward the floor, pulling the spine into extension, which is a sign that the body is trying to use the sagittal plane to manage the situation.

Call the person's awareness to their headlights: this may be all the information that their brain needs to construct a different neuromuscular strategy.

Signs of support trouble might also be visible in the trunk. The body may tilt in the direction of the stance leg, and you will see that the arms will no longer be level. Alternatively, the person might access their latissumus dorsi to increase pelvic support via the posterior oblique myofascial sling. This will pull the arm down a little on the opposite side to the stance leg (see Fig. 11.8). It is also possible that they tip the trunk backward, or even fold it forward (see Fig. 11.9).

In these cases, the person needs help to find their CLA. Our postural visualizations can help here, with the balloon helping to create a sense of verticality, or the "long ear" imagery opening and lengthening the compressed side of body (see Chapter 5).

If you see any of these signs, the symptoms of tightness and irritability in related muscles are likely to be linked to an inadequate support response from the standing leg. Balance the time spent on symptomatic relief, such as through stretching and soft tissue

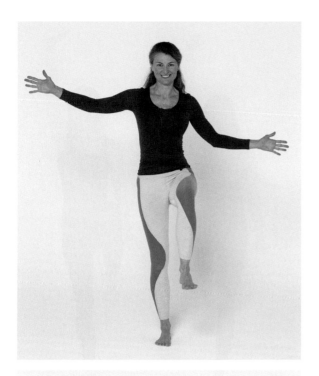

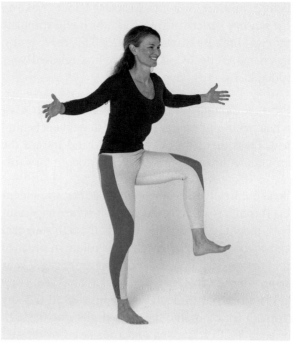

Figure 11.8

Arm dropping and trunk shortening on left as latissimus assists the pelvis on the right

Figure 11.9

Trunk folding

treatment, with that addressing the functional issues, starting with the Listening Foot and stacking of the body segments that we covered in Chapters 5 and 9.

To sum up, persistent tightening in muscles like latissimus dorsi, hamstrings, piriformis, quadratus lumborum, and erector spinae may indicate that they are being called upon to increase their role in stabilizing the pelvis. If issues showed up in the support quick check, stretching or releasing them may feel temporarily good but won't stop the problem from recurring.

If you have addressed the passive mobility in these muscles, ensure that you integrate this new potential with an activation task. This allows the brain to respond to

the change in myofascial tension and assimilate the new condition. Techniques like Heaven and Earth, below, are ideal for this purpose, bringing together the balance system, the pelvic stabilizers (as a coordinated group), the CLA, and myofascial connection through the whole body.

Movement exploration

Heaven and Earth

This move has its roots in Eastern movement traditions and introduces the body to a sense of dynamic expansion.

Before you start, do a little Listening Foot to wake up the sensory surface of your sole, which will stimulate the "up" impulse through your leg. This move is also much more effective if you have first released your spinal locks.

Press the palm of one hand toward the sky. Your wrist is bent with your fingers stretching straight out behind you. Press the palm of your other hand toward the ground, with your fingers stretched straight forward.

Press out firmly with both hands together, straightening through your elbows. If your elbows are hypermobile, imagine a straight line of light through your arm and follow this out through your palms in order to find that strong impulse. Once you have engaged your arms, choose a stance leg and stack yourself onto that ankle. Press out through your stance leg all the way through your foot into the ground, allowing the back of your leg to straighten and your pelvis to lift and place itself on your hip. Float the opposite knee up, and pause to feel the full lengthening through your body as you continue to press (see Fig. 11.10).

If you feel wobbly or insecure, you will sense a need to contract your body inwards, tightening the knee, hip, or belly, or shortening the side of the trunk. Compression is the position of insecurity, inefficiency, and defensiveness. Instead, dare to "go long to be strong." Hold the intention of this two-way press out through your foot and hands until your brain works out how to place your body in balance.

Maintain the arm position, but now swap legs, lifting the other knee. This engages a different neuromuscular pattern – a new combination to balance and integrate (see Fig. 11.11).

This is a task that my clients of all ages love, because it improves their balance, sense of connection, and stability very quickly, as well as feeling good. The active muscle work of pressing pulls on fascial tissue, which is itself being pulled taut by the movement, and this

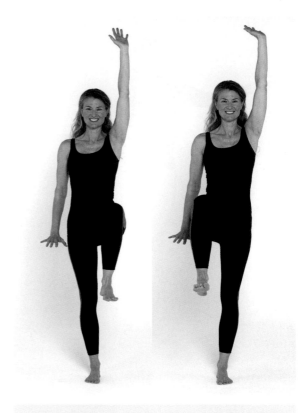

Figures 11.10/11.11

Heaven and Earth position 1

Heaven and Earth position 2

combination provides widespread proprioceptive feedback to improve the sense of where our body parts are with respect to one another. The movement addresses the synergies involved in single leg support, which involves the hip abductors and rotators accepting the load, allowing the compensating muscles (like hamstrings and latissimus) to ease their excessive tension.

If your client is struggling with Tree Pose or single leg balance, a little Heaven and Earth first may open up their possibilities.

Support in motion

Support isn't just for standing: we need it in many different hip angles and tasks.

Accepting a step

It is one thing to stand on a leg, but quite another to step onto it. You may have strong enough hip muscles, but if they don't switch on in time to actually use them as your foot contacts the ground, the result is the same as if you had weakness.

Let's look at what happens ideally. You take a step forward, with your pelvis carrying your body in balance as if you were carrying your trunk on a tray. Your body makes a rapid calculation and alerts the muscles at the hip and knee to prepare to trigger the positive support response. As your body weight begins to move onto your leg in what is called the preloading phase of gait, the hip and knee prepare with a soft sagittal plane springiness that will straighten into extension as your weight passes over the foot. The entire leg acts like a closed system filled firmly with air between the foot and the hip, allowing you to buoyantly contain the ground reaction force and gravity.

Now let's consider what often happens. You step forward, but your trunk tips forward, backward, or even sideways. This, as already described, affects the ability for the hip muscles to activate. The hip and knee don't make that small transitional movement between flexion and extension to prepare for the rapid application of body weight, so the force finds a different route. Instead of collecting and positively redirecting the force to help drive the next step, we let it slip upward past the hip, creating a Trendelenberg effect at the pelvis. Alternatively, it shoots sideways, and the hip protrudes laterally as we move onto the leg, meaning the closed system of support has sprung a leak.

We need to train the body to create the closed pressure system in each leg. To do this, we will use a technique called Hunting in the Forest. It was named when I developed a simple version of this with children to train their balance, stability, and postural control. Their task was to sneak up on an imaginary moose, but you are just going to investigate one leg in detail.

Movement exploration

Hunting in the Forest

Drop yourself into a VHR, so that the hips and knees are softly springy. First, we need to make sure that you can carry your trunk in balance, in order to set the pelvis up to support you. Place one hand on your chest and the other on your lower belly for feedback. Look straight ahead, and place the heel of one foot a little in front of you (see Fig. 11.12). Transition your weight onto the front foot, carrying your trunk in vertical balance. Your upper hand should sit directly over your lower hand throughout the whole movement (see Fig. 11.13).

Next, let's investigate what happens at the foot. Start in that softly springy posture, and place the heel a little in front of you again. Move your body forward onto that foot, noting any excessive tension and releasing it to feel your sole spread onto the ground. Pulse some pressure into your foot with a little springy hip and knee bending, adjusting yourself as necessary to connect with the sense of the whole foot on the ground. Step back again to the start position.

Now it is time to check the pelvis. Take up the start position, and fold your hands around one side of your pelvis, covering as much of it as possible by stretching your fingers apart. These hands will tell you whether your pelvis is secure on your leg as you stand on it or whether the ground reaction force pushes it up, back, or out to the side (see Fig. 11.14).

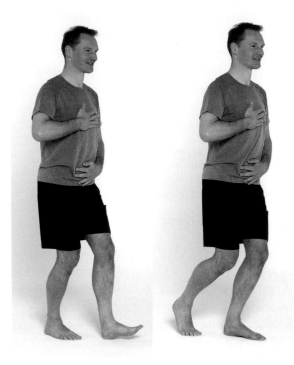

Figures 11.12/11.13

Hunting in the Forest start position

Hunting in the Forest finish position

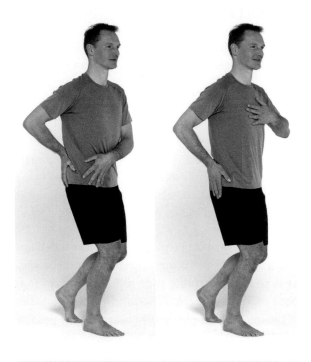

Figures 11.14/11.15

Pelvic hand placement

Focusing on the hip carrying the trunk forward onto the foot

Note what happens under your hands as you move your body onto the front foot. Does your pelvis stay level or push upward under your hands?

Start again, but this time focus on the hip and knee softening as you accept your body weight. By absorbing some of the early load in the sagittal plane as we fully commit our weight to the front foot, we reduce the demand on hip abductors as they activate to control the frontal plane. The hip extensors share responsibility for support with the hip abductors, allowing the pelvis to float serenely over the foot.

It turns out that the little VHR is the key to the gluteals firing as you step onto the leg. If you have already built strength with hip abductor exercises, this is the key to transitioning that potential into function – by integrating the timing and body carriage that will encourage them to fire.

Now place your palm on the side of your hip, fingers pointing downward. Notice, as you step forward onto the leg, whether the hip bone simply moves forward with you or deviates out to the side instead. If it pushes out into your hand, start again, this time focusing on it moving forward onto the foot. When my clients do this, they are making the movement intention clear to the brain, and they quickly notice a connection with their gluteals as they transition their weight onto the front foot (see Fig. 11.15).

I can't stress enough that it is the small movements that influence the big ones. Squeezing and clenching the gluteals is just trying to wallpaper over the real issues, which are self-carriage, force acceptance through a soft knee and hip, and a clear direction of motion. This combination of factors sets up the conditions for the glutes to respond to weight bearing.

Support in deep angles

If you are performing a lunge, or gliding into a yoga warrior pose, the loading experience is emphasized on the front leg, which should trigger a support response. There should be a balance of activity between the quadriceps, gluteals, adductors, and hamstrings to control the hip and knee in this sagittal plane movement. Those glutes should be cupping the back of the hip joint like a giant supportive hand in order to bring a stable buoyancy to the pose as you sink into hip and knee bending. When moving deeply into the pose, however, many people drop their pelvis into anterior tilt, pushing their sitting bones back, and driving their lower backs into extension (see Fig. 11.16). This disadvantages the glutes and shifts the majority of the hip load onto the hamstrings by placing pressure on the hamstring insertion. This is a common source of pain.

> When someone is struggling with hamstring insertion pain, check whether they are falling into anterior pelvic tilt as they descend into their pose.

Remember how our sternal position influences our hips? This is another key area of influence in both a warrior pose and lunge. Cues to "stay open" or "lift" in the chest can cause some people to overextend in the upper back. As they move into the pose, their sternum progressively tilts upward, leading the front of

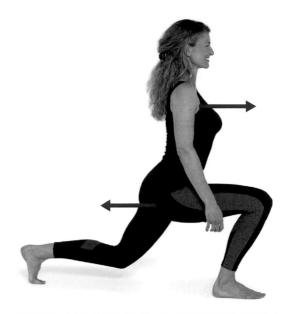

Figure 11.16

Collapsed lunge: the pelvis moves into anterior tilt, carrying the spine into extension and driving the hip backward

the body to lengthen and the back to shorten. Once again the hip slides behind the fall of gravity, and the pelvis no longer provides a level platform to carry the trunk. In these circumstances, the hamstrings must work harder to support the hip, and without the significant contribution of the glutes to share the effort, the quadriceps are also under greater load. This can make the pose more difficult for people struggling with anterior knee pain.

Movement exploration

To investigate this, place your feet in the start position for either a lunge or a Warrior pose. Place one hand on your sternum and the other on your lower belly. As you start to move, do your hands stay the same distance apart, or do they move away from each other? You may notice that your belly hand moves downward or your sternal hand moves upward.

Return to the start position to begin again. This time, maintain a consistent distance between your hands as you move into the pose. This keeps your pelvis aligned under your trunk, and directs your hip to move down into the supportive glutes. Can you notice the change in muscle work in the leg? When the hip is supporting you, the quadriceps and hamstrings do not have to work so hard because the load is shared between the hip and knee (see Fig. 11.17).

To allow your hip to support you, Gmax must be able to contract eccentrically deeply into its range to allow the bending. If it is weak in this position, your brain will find a solution to allow you to continue, and will alter your body position accordingly. It may evade the load by shifting the pelvis back or tilting it sideways, or it might instead let the femur fall inwards so that our large adductor magnus can help out. We are such clever creatures.

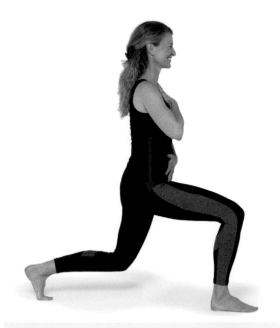

Figure 11.17

Awareness of the trunk and pelvis relationship

Just remember, though, that the hip is a large link in the kinetic chain, and Gmax is a substantial muscle. Any compensations we make increase the stress on other body structures, such as the hamstring, adductor, and knee if they are asked to make up the deficit repetitively.

If the knee is moving inwards, or the pelvis tilting laterally, the body is diverting the movement from the sagittal to the frontal plane. Sometimes the body has the capability to perform the movement differently but needs help to work out how. In the lunge, for example, we could cue from different awareness points.

The first is familiar: the foot. Note whether the pressure has drifted toward the inner border, as this will drag your knee inwards with it. The opposite will apply if your weight settles toward the outside of the foot. (You know what to check: the Listening Foot, so you can ensure there is enough tibiofemoral rotation to achieve a centered foot.)

Next, the pelvis. Remember the car headlight on the front of each side of your pelvis and that, ideally, they shine straight ahead and level. If you notice instead that they are tilted sideways, dipped toward the ground, or have even turned toward the front leg, then it's a sign of the front hip joint "closing" (i.e., the pelvis and femur compressing together). If you shine your pelvic lights straight ahead and open the hip a little to "let it breathe," it sets the hip up in a much easier position for the gluteals to activate.

Finally, the leg itself. If you find that the front knee is wandering inwards or outwards, come back to thinking of the river of water flowing through your leg. Note whether the river is bending to divert the flow, and, if it is, gently adjust yourself to channel the water so that it flows freely in a straight line down your leg.

Instead of a river, some of my clients see a highway between their hip and foot that is lit up by streetlights they can follow; others visualize a stream of colored light. Seeing the path of the movement in our mind's eye directs the intention of the movement for the brain, and engages the whole body to find the solution.

This sense of a shape to the movement direction is just as important as footwork on a Pilates reformer. If we direct the focus from knee bending to hip bending, we channel our intention fully into sagittal plane motion throughout the whole leg. In this case, the straight line of color can be followed in and out of the movement, with the client simply noting changes in its shape and adjusting as necessary.

Adding the springs

By now it should be evident that for the body to be supported adequately on one leg, a variety of factors beyond hip abductor strength are involved. Hunting in the Forest integrated dynamic posture and proprioception of the trunk, as well as the coordination between the joints of the lower limb to make the small vertical motions that help us to contain and use the force of weight bearing between the hip and foot. Our lunges expand the support ability by asking the pelvis to maintain its neuromuscular control pattern at greater hip and knee angles.

With that in place, we can now add the pulsing ability that we trained our powerhouse hip and knee extensors to perform in Chapter 10. This moves us toward developing the shock-absorbent, efficient dynamic leg movement through a single limb that we need in order to hop, skip, and bound.

Movement exploration

Lateral Pulses

Lateral pulses can be practiced in the VHR position, or more deeply in the natural squat.

First, remind your body how to pulse, as you did in Chapter 10 (see Elastic pulses). This wakes up the gluteals and quadriceps, reminding them how to smoothly cycle between eccentric and concentric activity in order to produce the springy movement.

Keeping your shoulders directly positioned over your hips, move that pulse so that your weight is now falling directly through one foot. The other foot is still on the floor, but your weight has moved away from it (see Figs. 11.18 and 11.19).

It is important to remember the "sitting down" intention in the hip when moving the weight laterally. Otherwise, the brain is distracted by the sideways motion, and either tips the shoulders beyond the hip, or pushes the hip beyond the foot (see Fig. 11.20).

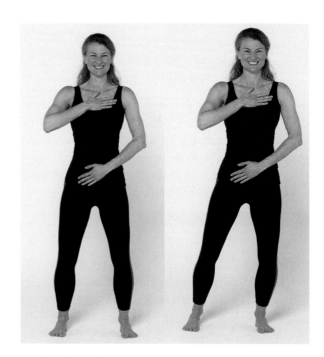

Figures 11.18/11.9

Lateral pulse in the vertical hip release start position

Lateral pulse finish position

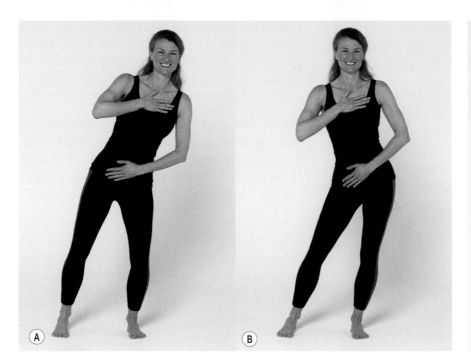

Figure 11.20

When you forget to "sit down" at the hip, your trunk may tip sideways (*A*) or your hips may slide sideways instead (*B*)

Staying aligned over that foot, gradually increase the depth of the movement, pulsing at a few "floors" on the way down and back up again. This challenges the system to maintain the neuromuscular pattern of support through one side of the pelvis while increasing the load at a manageable level.

Pulses are valuable to people of all ages. For the athlete and the dancer, pulses train the neuromuscular timing and coordination in and out of deeper ranges of joint flexion, while teaching the brain to absorb the forces in the large joints of the leg instead of letting them escape upward. Smaller range pulses are just as important for a joint replacement patient to restore the smoothness in their gait; this is achieved by addressing the excessive leg muscle tension that can otherwise develop.

Balance

Balance is not just a case of statuesquely standing utterly still. It is about constant microadjustments, lightning-fast responses constructed from the flow of sensory information coming in from multiple sources.

You are already putting into place many of the factors needed for balance. In Chapter 5, you addressed the position of your head on your neck to optimize the sensory feedback from your upper neck, vestibular system, and eyes. You have established a foot to stand on with your Listening Foot, and you know that if you find yourself weight bearing consistently on either the outside or inside of your foot, you might want to check the Total Body Rotation to make sure that your hips will allow your foot to be placed on the floor.

You have investigated your breathing, learning to spread the breath movement throughout your trunk to minimize excess motion in any one area, and you are aware of releasing held tension so that the joints can absorb the motion caused by the breath.

You have gained proprioceptive awareness of your spine position, and know how to carry your trunk on your pelvis. Now you know support, the ability to integrate these factors in order to stand on a single leg.

Equipped with this wealth of abilities, you can start to further develop balance. For this we can use a simple three-point template to explore it further: maintaining, exploring, and regaining balance.

Maintaining balance

This category involves challenging a posture by altering the conditions around it.

Movement exploration

Stand on a single leg, softening at the hip and knee. Gently pulse into the joints to prevent the fixed leg tension that so often develops as people struggle to keep their balance.

Feel your foot spread over the floor's surface, listening intently. Visualize that helium balloon to establish your CLA.

Balance maintenance 1

Now raise your arms above your head. Staying relaxed, move one arm down to your side and back up again. Repeat with the other arm. You can compare taking the arm down in front of you in the sagittal plane, or out to the side in the frontal plane. This mildly disturbs your center of gravity, asking you to

make small adjustments to maintain your balance (see Fig. 11.21).

Balance maintenance 2

Change the emphasis by keeping your arms relaxed by your sides and slowly move your eyes, gliding them from side to side, up and down, and diagonally without moving your head. Now experiment with turning your head to look around the room, allowing the wobbles to move harmlessly through your body. Eye and head movement influence the feedback coming from your upper neck, eyes, and vestibular system,

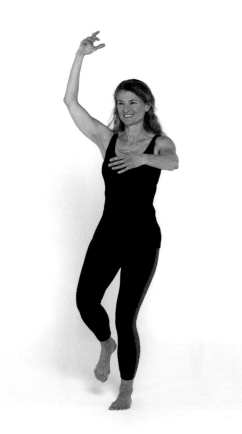

Figure 11.21

Challenging the center of gravity with arm movement

triggering a different set of calculations from the brain (see Fig. 11.22).

Balance maintenance 3

Change the challenge again. Close your eyes, feeling how the body initially reacts with bigger adjustments until you relax and start listening to it. With vision eliminated, the brain will shift from integrating three channels of feedback into the two remaining sources: the sensory feedback from the rest of the body and the vestibular system in the head (see Fig. 11.23).

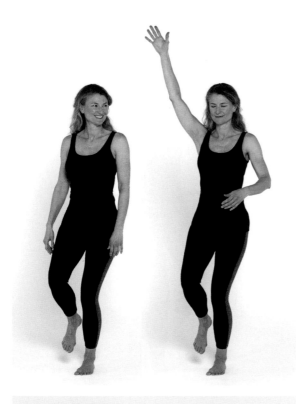

Figures 11.22/11.23

Maintaining balance while smoothly moving the head

Gaining confidence with the eyes closed

Exploring balance

This category invites us to stretch our boundaries by changing our body relationships.

Movement exploration

Balance exploration 1

Taking up your single leg stance with a soft knee and hip, begin by moving your arms in any direction, exploring as many possibilities and combinations as you like. Allow your arms to move your upper body, perhaps turning it, side bending it, curling it inwards or expanding it outwards. Occasionally remind yourself about your soft hip and knee, pulsing a little to reduce your leg tension (see Fig. 11.24).

Balance exploration 2

Extend your exploration now by incorporating the free leg, first imagining it tracing a figure of eight in the air, and then perhaps experimenting with reaching it forward and backward, feeling how this asks for deeper bending at the knee (see Fig. 11.25).

Balance exploration 3

Stretch the free leg right back behind you until your body tilts forward in response, over your stance leg. Again, play with arm movements, head turns, and shoulder turns, acknowledging the tension that can arise, and even attempting the occasional toe touch, as you present more options to the brain (see Fig. 11.26).

Balance exploration 4

The ability to carry ourselves in balance as the whole body moves over the ground is essential to our normal functional movement. This can be explored with Clock Steps.

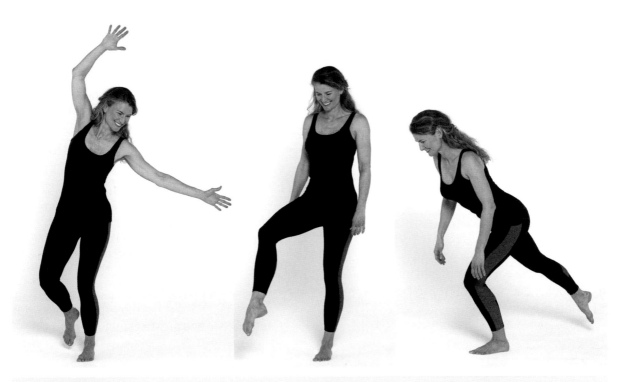

Figures 11.24/11.25/11.26

Exploring balance with the upper body

Exploring the effect of leg movement on balance

Coordinating leg and body angles for balance

Imagine yourself standing in the middle of a large imaginary clock. With your eyes open first, step forward to 12 o'clock, releasing the other leg from the floor. Repeat by stepping backward to 6 o'clock, again keeping the free leg off the floor. Make your way around the clock, between 3 and 9 o'clock, 11 and 5 o'clock, 7 and 1 o'clock, always with one foot off the floor. Once you know that you can organize your trunk as it moves over the ground into each step, repeat the process with eyes closed. It is a very different experience when your vision is excluded: now you really need to sense yourself.

Regaining balance

Sometimes all we need to do to free up our balance is release the idea of controlling it and simply focus on regaining it. This is reflective of our normal lives: we often need the ability to "catch our balance."

Movement exploration

In this practice, the more ungainly the movement is, the better. The aim is to throw yourself off balance, moving your arms, legs, and body in any combination of directions, learning how to coordinate different movements such that you can stay on that single leg without needing to touch the other one down.

This is enormously liberating, and good fun – we relax more when we aren't expecting perfection, and, by removing that pressure, we are willing to take more chances to learn about the size and speed of the movements that push us to the boundaries of our ability to regain our balance.

> There's one key point to understand about balance: the more you try to "keep" it, the more it eludes you.

Power points

- Support, the ability to accept weight through a single leg, involves a large team of muscles not just within the pelvis but also above and below it.

- The sensory feedback from the foot and an awareness of trunk position on the pelvis sets up the gluteals to be able to activate effectively.

- To be functionally relevant, we need to introduce a range of support challenges in different hip angles and body movements.

- Support is one of the key foundations for balance.

- The whole body is involved in balance, not just the three main systems of vision, vestibular, and proprioception. From foot to posture to breathing, you can establish meaningful foundations before even beginning a "balance exercise."

- When aiming to address balance in your programs, consider the three-point template to add greater variety

Methinks that the moment my legs begin to move, my thoughts begin to flow.

Henry David Thoreau

When we see someone running with ease or walking with elegance, their fluent gait catches our eye and arrests our attention. Our brains unconsciously register impressions of vitality, capability, and confidence as we watch them.

As with posture, our gait tells the world something about us.

The effective gait that is our evolutionary heritage is, however, sometimes hard to attain in the modern world. Where once we migrated by necessity, now we exercise in carefully managed doses. Propped up in chairs for hours on end, we forget how to carry ourselves. The steady alternating rhythm that used to simply get us from place to place has been replaced with sitting in a car in order to get to a gym faster to do a time-effective workout.

Yet, we possess all the necessary components to propel ourselves across the ground effectively and even pleasurably if equipped with a few key concepts.

Push, pull, or tip?

The first and easiest place to start is with movement impulse. If you sit on a park bench and watch people walking by, you will see an array of gait interpretations. Despite all that variation, their gaits fall roughly into three categories: pushing, pulling, or tipping.

The pushing gait, even at walking speed, is a beautiful demonstration of our next Functional Force Management strategy, *propulsion*. Propulsion is the creation of momentum, the result of multiple processes integrating to positively move us forward, sideways, or even upward. When you notice someone with a pushing gait, you gain a sense of the entire body being carried forward continuously. In each step, their knee leads the thigh so that it swings like a pendulum under the flexing hip. Their lower leg then swings forward to place the foot on the ground. Their pelvis steadily advances over and then beyond that foot, facilitating the hip extensors to fire. This person uses the ground as a firm resource to push from, using the musculature all the way down the back of the leg from the hip to the foot to propel themselves forward.

The person with a pushing gait consistently carries their body weight in the center of their movement as it progresses over the ground (see Fig. 12.1). Their weight keeps moving forward between the two legs so that their pelvis is placed directly over the foot when they are fully accepting weight through one side. This means that at the moment of mid-stance, the effective walker must already have established "a leg to stand on."

A pulling gait, however, gives a different impression. When the shoulders and pelvis are not stacked over each other, the mechanics change. The person with the compressed look of a sway back or anterior

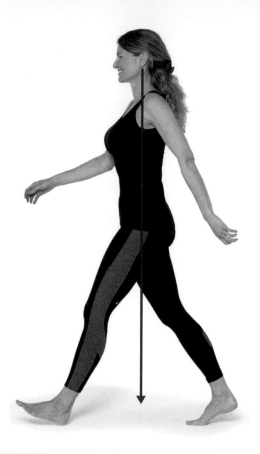

Figure 12.1

Pushing gait: the body is carried directly over the stepping leg

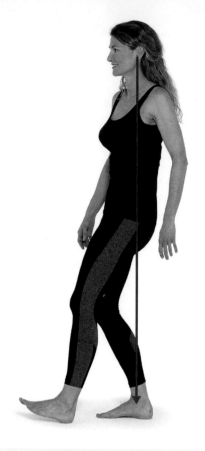

Figure 12.2

Pulling gait: the body trails behind the stepping leg

rib lock posture will carry their upper body slightly behind their pelvis. The line of gravity falls posterior to their hips as they step forward. This person looks as though their body is always following their legs as they walk instead of being carried over them, because the pelvis never truly moves onto and over the foot. The ground is now used as an anchor to pull the body forward, predominantly with the hamstrings. The knee is often pulled into hyperextension, and the gluteals and calves are relatively inactive (see Fig. 12.2).

In terms of hip health, this is a risky strategy to adopt in the long term. In previous chapters, we have described how a healthy, well-moving hip joint needs a secure axis of rotation, which means that the ball (the femoral head) should sit in the middle of the socket (the acetabulum) to create a stable reference point for the movement.

If a person stands with their pelvis slightly in front of their trunk in their normal posture, the hips sit in extension rather than in neutral. This inhibits the gluteals and puts the hip flexors into a lengthened, less effective, and more stressful position.[1] When we step forward, elastic energy storage in the hip flexors and anterior ligaments of the trailing leg should play the dominant role in bringing our femur through, rather than actively pulling it forward with the hip flexors.[2] However, when kept habitually in a lengthened position due to our posture, these structures are unable to store and release energy, and without this low-cost passive assistance, we must compensate with increased muscle activity. This mechanism can make the hip flexors feel tight and irritable as a result of being overworked.

> Many people are stuck in a merry-go-round of stretching and releasing the hip flexors for short-term symptomatic relief. Learning to carry the body in balance, with each segment stacked upon the one below, helps to address the cause of the symptoms and provide a more effective long-term solution.

This is not the only potential problem. As we step forward, we need to extend the hip on the propelling side, but if that hip is already extended due to our posture, we need to find an alternative way to move our pelvis over our foot. We can achieve this by generating a facsimile of hip extension that uses a phenomenon called femoral anterior glide,[3] where the head of the femur translates forward in the socket as the hamstrings pull backward on the femur. In this situation, the deep stabilizing muscles of the hip are not securing the axis of motion of the hip joint as we walk, so the pressures on the structures within and around it are altered.[4,5] This can particularly stress structures like the labrum at the front of the hip, causing discomfort and even pain in response to the compression (see Figs. 12.3 and 12.4).

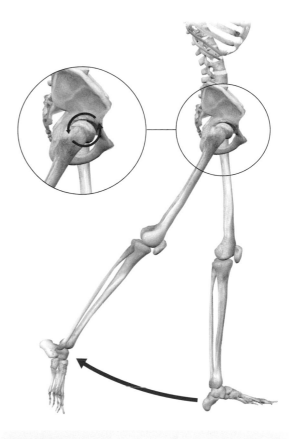

Figure 12.3

Stepping with the intact axis of rotation

With the gluteals in a mechanically disadvantaged position, the hamstrings become the primary hip extensor. However, with their longer line of pull and greater leverage, coupled with insufficient stabilization of the femoral head by the deep hip muscles, they apply greater forces to the unsupported hip. At best, the hamstrings feel overworked, and, at worst, the hip itself can develop pain.

Some people adapt their posture to relieve the pressure at the front of the hip by tipping their trunk forward a little and flexing at the hip and knee.[1] This prevents the hip from extending, which in turn

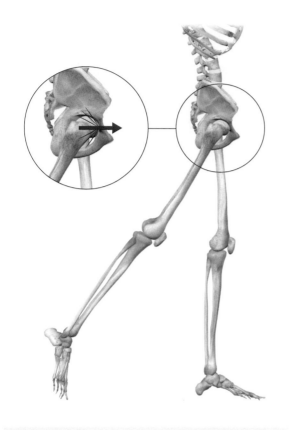

Figure 12.4

Head of femur forced forward, putting pressure on the anterior structures of the hip

Converting a pulling gait into a pushing gait can be relatively simple. First, we need to reconnect the shoulders and pelvis, as balanced self-carriage is the foundation for propulsion.

This begins with awareness of where the weight is borne in the feet. If the body weight falls habitually into the heels, or slides into the toes, the upper and lower body cannot stack themselves over the feet right from the start.

You might offer the balloon cue, or the rabbit ears to decompress the spine (see Chapter 5). Perhaps it will be necessary to open up that anterior rib lock with some imagery, as we did in Chapter 6. Maybe the giant marble is the key to relaxing the overly upright person.

Once you have achieved this, it is important to provide an impulse cue. In a pulling gait, the pelvis or abdomen is drawn forward by an imaginary string, leaving the shoulders to fall behind. To remedy this, imagine your sternum being drawn forward by a tractor beam of light to something far in the distance. If you keep aiming your sternum out to that point, it will encourage the upper trunk to move forward with the pelvis.

reduces the anterior pressure from the femoral head, however, it also reduces the mechanical efficiency of the hip flexors as they cannot store elastic energy. Gluteal weakness is often blamed for this flexed appearance, however, it is a postural solution to a functional problem.

The usual prescription for all of these presentations includes hip flexor and hamstring stretching, in combination with gluteal strengthening. However, these can only have relevance if there is a change in the driving factor: the person's fundamental posture.

The tipping gait

Rather than moving positively forward over the ground, many people sway or tip sideways instead. You will recognize many versions of this, once you know to look for it. From the Hollywood action hero who coolly dips one shoulder on each alternate stride as he saunters toward you on screen, to the knee pain induced lurch of the elderly person who no longer has the muscular control to accept weight fully, the tip is becoming the most predominant gait pattern that you see on the streets.

This gait strategy predominantly uses the frontal plane, yet walking is in fact a rotational phenomenon from the foot right up to the neck. To walk and run beautifully, efficiently, and powerfully, we must get to grips with the transverse plane.

Spiral solutions

One of the myths of gait is that it is a sagittal plane activity, with our arms and legs swinging directly forward and backward. Soldiers marching on parade move like this, but it has little to do with the smooth ease of efficient walking.

Rotation provides the mechanism for us to convert the ground reaction force into a pulse of energy that spirals all the way up through our body to propel us forward. Each body segment turns on the next to open sequential gates for the energy pulse to move through. The timing of this independent motion of one segment upon the next creates a momentary stretch of the tissues between them, storing and then releasing energy as we use ourselves elastically. Rotation is what helps you to flow over the ground.

As soon as the foot strikes the ground, the rotation mechanism is already beginning. As we move into stance, rotation occurs between the small bones within the foot, and then between the foot and the lower leg. At the knee, the tibia and femur rotate relative to each other. Moving up the leg, the hip rotates in its socket. With each stepping foot, one side of the pelvis and then the other is alternately carried forward, subtly turning the pelvis's face from side to side. The spinal segments respond as the thorax rotates on the pelvis and then, finally, there must be rotation at the neck, so that we can keep gazing steadily ahead instead of having our head pulled from side to side by our turning shoulders. That's a whole lot of rotation.

In Chapter 4 we looked at the diagonal elastic strategy, the Functional Force Management mechanism that uses counter-rotation between the pelvis and the upper torso to transfer energy up and down the body. There are in fact multiple myofascial relationships involved in effective dynamic walking, and our ability to access them depends upon the timing and coordination of a number of smaller components.

Swinging it

If your thorax turns a little with each step, an imaginary searchlight on your sternum would sweep from one side of your center line to the other. If your arms stayed in a fixed relationship with your thorax, they would also swing awkwardly across your center line instead of forward and backward. To prevent this, the shoulders must be free to subtly rotate in their sockets. As our chest turns to the left, the right arm must externally rotate a little as it swings forward, and the left arm internally rotates a little as it swings backward to free the arms from the chest. This allows them to sweep through like a pendulum and contribute energy to the walking cycle.

For effective gait, you might remember from Chapter 4 that the counter-rotation between our upper and lower torso stores energy in our posterior oblique myofascial sling. When we allow our shoulder to externally rotate a little as our arm swings forward, we add a little extra stretch to latissimus dorsi, which enhances this effect.

As the pelvis and leg move forward on the opposite side, the diagonal stretch across the back of the body is amplified further, and we gain even greater energy storage as the myofascial tension is engaged beyond the pelvis all the way down the stepping leg and under the foot.[6] From the shoulder to the foot, these adjustments in relative body position help us to "walk our whole body," using and reusing energy to efficiently propel us over the ground.

You might notice that some people walk with the palms of their hands facing backward throughout the entire gait cycle, maintaining their shoulders in constant internal rotation. They do not rotate through their large pelvic and thoracic segments but try to generate momentum by flexing and extending their elbows as they increase their walking speed. This robs them of the entire elastic gait mechanism, and makes walking far less efficient.

Movement exploration

The amount of rotation in the shoulders is subtle, and, for many people, just gaining a sense of relaxation and dissociation between the shoulder and the thorax is enough to make a difference. The Thigh Slide from Chapter 4 is a great opportunity to experience this. You have so far used it to move the rib cage on the pelvis, and to train independence of motion between the neck and the upper back. Now you can notice your shoulders, feeling the sense of opening at the armpit when sliding the hand forward, and feeling it close again as you slide it back along your thigh. To further release the shoulder joint, turn your palm upward as you slide your hand forward to lead your shoulder into external rotation, and turn it downward as you slide it back.

A similar mechanism occurs between the thigh and the pelvis. As we take a step forward, there must be a separation between these two body segments to allow your foot to fall straight in front of you. Otherwise, as the pelvis turns, your foot would follow it, crossing your center line. Instead of imprinting a line of footprints in the sand, you would leave an undulating line more reminiscent of a snake.

Movement exploration

Rock the Boat

To experience the sensation of the hip opening associated with pelvic rotation, we can experiment with a technique called Rock the Boat. Take up a position on your back with your knees bent and feet flat on the floor. If necessary, ease out your upper lock with a folded towel under your head (see Fig. 12.5). Connect with the pressure of your sacrum on the floor, and smoothly move through a few easy sacral rocks to find that reference point where the body can rest on the center of the sacrum. The back of your pelvis is going to be the hull of an imaginary boat.

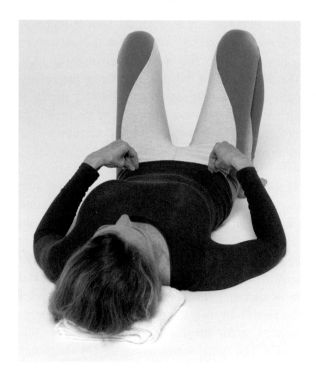

Figure 12.5

Rock the Boat start position with folded towel under the head if necessary to achieve a relaxed neutral head position

Now feel the soles of your feet on the floor. Press one sole into the floor, and then the other, alternating your pressures. Pay attention to whether you are using your whole foot, including the area under your heel. Note where you feel the muscles working: it is likely to be at the back of the leg. You may even find yourself connecting with your glutes on one side and then the other as you alternate.

Now you are going to allow your body to move in response to the foot pressure. As you press down into your right foot, allow the pressure that you generate to move up your leg, past your hip and into the pelvis, causing it to lift a little (see Fig. 12.6). You will feel that your weight has rolled under the left side of your pelvis, and, as the right side has lifted, the pelvis

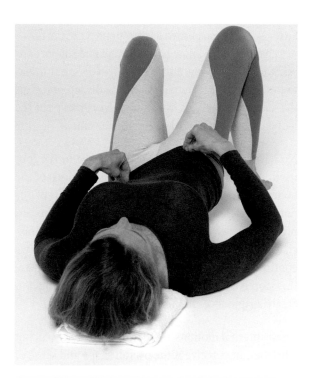

Figure 12.6

Pressing into right foot to lift the right hip and tip pelvis to left

has tipped toward the left. Allow it to return back to the floor, and now press through the left foot, feeling how that pressure can be used to roll your weight into the right side of your pelvis, lifting the left side a little. Explore that connection between the foot and the pelvis, and the sense of the "hull of your boat" rocking from side to side.

Once you have this sensation, notice your knees. They may be swaying from side to side as you move, so now it is time to add the experience of hip opening and closing. As you press through your right foot, aim your knee toward the ceiling, or perhaps think of it as 12 o'clock. It may want to wander off to 10 o'clock or 2 o'clock as your pelvis turns, and if this happens, pause, and see what it might be like to create some space between your upper thigh and your pubic bone. Just experiment with the one side a few times until it becomes easier to allow the front of that hip to open. Then notice that as that hip opens, the other hip closes, with the thigh pressing more closely toward the pubic bone.

As you alternate from side to side, you are establishing new relationships for your brain to utilize for walking. It learns that the pelvis and hip have a relationship to the foot. It learns what pelvic rotation feels like, and it also experiences the hip opening and closing that we need for effective gait.

Now that you can create a separation between your thigh and your pelvis, you can establish the next level of joint rotation. As we step forward in normal gait, the thigh of the leading leg externally rotates, while the trailing thigh internally rotates. As you transfer your weight onto your leg, the motion begins to reverse in preparation for the next step forward. This alternating motion helps us to move forward smoothly through our foot, enabling our pushing gait. If we can't do this because of a block to hip rotation, we skate along on the inner or outer border of our foot, diverting our propulsive energy into a tipping gait.

As we discovered in Chapter 10, some of us have a postural bias into either hip internal or external rotation, and can become more or less stuck there. Our hips forget that they can move through a range of rotation, and although when we are walking it is not a large range, it is an important one. Fortunately, we have already learned the technique of Total Body Rotation, which mobilizes the hips and reminds them of their biomechanical relationship to the feet.

> The obvious sideways tilt of the tipping gait can appear when we divert forces from the blocked rotational plane into the frontal plane. This creates a disturbance to the equilibrium in our trunk, but some people avoid this with a bit of clever compensation. Our brain can opt to perform some biomechanical sleight of hand, absorbing the force by pushing it into the swaggering sideways pelvic tip that we know as the Trendelenberg sign. Hip abductor strengthening can offset some of the effects, but it doesn't address the cause: for this, we need to restore hip rotation.

Between the knee and the foot, multiple joints rotate and counter-rotate through the gait cycle. As we step onto a foot, the femur starts to move into internal rotation as the tibia externally rotates, creating the "screw home" mechanism that tightens the cruciate ligaments inside your knee and transiently locks the joint to support you.[7] This locking mechanism reduces the demand for active muscle activity around the knee to withstand our weight on each step – another beautiful example of our body's drive for efficiency. Then, as your weight passes over your foot, the two bones unlock their relationship to allow your knee to bend and swing through freely.

Working with the Listening Foot from Chapter 5 establishes this critical rotation of the tibia, which will bring the biomechanical benefit at the knee and also at the ankle.

Back to the base

Taking care of the hip and knee mobility components can have a profound effect on our feet. Traditionally, it is considered that the foot mechanics drive what happens in the legs and body, but it is very much a two-way relationship.

So far, we have established a leg to stand on in the previous chapter, so we know how to accept and support our body weight. Having also freed ourselves from a bias toward internal or external rotation of the hip, and done the same with the tibia, we set ourselves up to place the foot on the ground in balance as we step onto it.

Now we can focus on what is happening in the foot itself. As we step onto the foot, small rotations of the bones within it allow it to pronate, which is part of our normal shock-absorbing mechanism. This transient pronation briefly flattens and tensions the strong fascial tissues of our arch, storing elastic energy.[8] As we continue to transition through our step, we release this stored energy to supinate the foot, stiffening it to create a rigid lever to push off from.[9]

These internal motions are too subtle to be sensed, but what we can perceive is the overall shape and sense of the movement that creates a frame for these biomechanics to take place.

This little series integrates our balance, our global body motion, and our awareness of our feet.

Movement exploration

Shoulder swings

Place your fingertips on the points of your shoulders and take one step forward, so that your legs are in a stride stance. Settle your weight onto your front leg, which will lift your back heel. Find the position where you feel the pressure evenly between the front, back, inside, and outside of your foot.

Now imagine the axis passing down through your body. Turn your rib cage rhythmically from side to

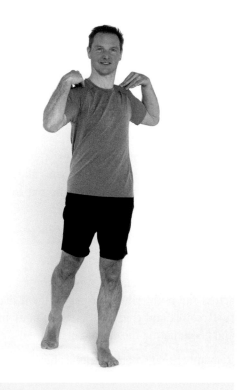

Figure 12.7

Shoulder swings

side using as little muscle as you can around that straight line. Initially, you may find that this pulls you off balance – that is a great discovery, as it allows you to identify unnecessary tension. Relax, perhaps switch your balloon on, and see how effortlessly you can turn your upper body without losing that central connection on your foot (see Fig. 12.7).

Step through

Start with your feet together and your fingertips on the points of your shoulders. Take one step forward, turning your shoulders toward the forward foot. Take a step backward past the start position with that same foot, and turn your shoulders away from it. Now that you have the hang of the movement, you can focus on the leg that is actually doing the supporting. Cast your focus into the sole of this foot. How is the pressure moving through it? Does it feel like a straight line or as if you are going around a corner (see Figs. 12.8 and 12.9)?

In reality there are micro-adjustments going on within your foot so that you are not actually moving straight from heel to toes. However, perceptually if you sense that you are moving straight through your foot, your brain and body can take care of the details.

Perhaps you noticed that your foot turns outwards as you push off it. This is a habit that can contribute to hallux valgus, and eventually to bunions, as the big toe is being pushed outwards at the very moment at which it is bearing the most weight.

Maybe you notice that you are rolling along the outer border of your foot instead. The foot never gets the opportunity to help shock absorb and to store elastic energy for you, so you will need extra muscle activity to compensate. This could be your calves, your hip flexors, even your hamstrings.

It's worth learning to "walk through your feet."

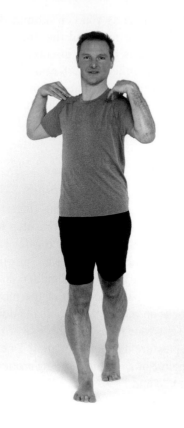 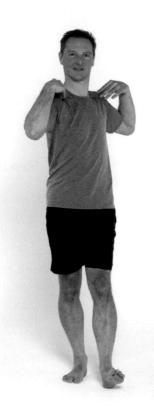

Figures 12.8/12.9

Step through: stepping forward

Step through: stepping back

Punch walking

This is a nice, flowing way to move over the ground, amplifying the sense of rotation in the upper body and feeling it drive the pushing sense from the lower body. Begin with the buoyant sense of self-carriage that can come from the balloon, the long ears, or the puppet master. Do a little exploratory punch – the arm should lead that whole side of the chest forward into rotation, as the other arm counter moves its side back. Test out a few alternating punches, feeling the free turning of the rib cage and noting how the face of the sternum shines from left to right of the center line in response (see Fig. 12.10).

Now, step forward and lead your punch with the opposite arm. Keep alternating as you stride forward,

twisting in the middle with each step. Shift your awareness to your feet: are you gliding straight through them from your heel and out through your toes (see Fig. 12.11)?

Multi-segmental rotation moves forces through and across the body, which disperses them over a large surface area and engages the whole body in creating and perpetuating the motion of gait.

Remember that when rotation is blocked somewhere in the kinetic chain, forces stop moving. When they stop moving and start to accumulate in a specific area, they can cause stress to those structures. Frequently, this is addressed by trying to stabilize

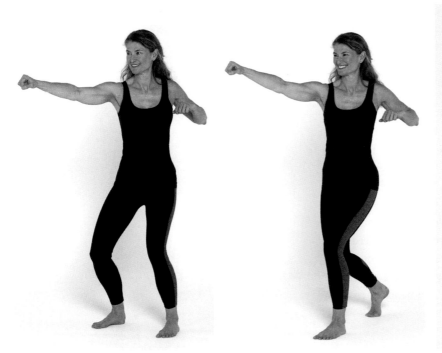

Figures 12.10/12.11

Letting the arm lead the thorax into rotation
Punch walking

the stressed area, because it frequently looks like it is moving excessively. Instead, ask yourself why the movement is amplified in this area, and what is not contributing its fair share.

Simple analysis

The concepts and skills that you have acquired so far put you in a great position to analyze gait. This topic could consume an entire book, and there are many factors that can be considered. However, equipped with these fundamentals, you can appreciate the major factors, and address them simply and relevantly with the techniques provided above.

1. Always begin with the CLA. The CLA will give you the very quickest information about what is happening in the global body. When you look from behind or in front, ask yourself whether the CLA is being carried vertically, or whether the tipping gait is appearing with some sideways motion into the frontal plane, either in the trunk or the pelvis. If you do see some frontal plane movement appearing, it is likely that rotation is missing somewhere in the chain.

    Look at the CLA from the side. Is the upper body stacked over the lower body, with gravity falling vertically through it? Is this a pushing or pulling gait?

2. Next, look at the shoulders. Imagine an unbendable line passing all the way through the person's clavicles from tip to tip. Does this line alternately pivot a little from side to side with each stride? As they come toward you, does the person's sternum turn as they move, or does it stay facing straight ahead? Perhaps it only turns in one direction.

Stay focused on the movement of the shoulder girdle and chest rather than the arm swing: some people are very good at masking a lack of true rotation by increasing the swing from the shoulder joint to make it seem even.

I am often asked, "How much rotation should we see?" This depends upon the speed at which we are moving. The faster we move, the more rotation we use to access our elastic energy mechanism as we walk (see Fig. 12.12). When we run, we increase our rotation as we speed up from a jog to a brisk run. However, if we continue to increase our speed up to sprinting, we need much faster transference of force between our upper and lower bodies. We tighten the coil between our upper and lower body, dramatically reducing the rotation between them.

3. Does the pelvis turn? This is trickier to see. It is easiest to watch only one side at a time, and notice whether the pelvis advances with the foot on that side. If it doesn't, you may see the pelvis tip into the frontal plane with a Trendelenberg sign. Once you have watched one side, then watch the other. Does this side move forward with the foot?

4. Now go all the way down to the feet. As we walk, the specific pressures under the sole of each foot when measured with scanning technology follow a curving trajectory,[10] but our goal in our visual assessment is to determine the general shape of the step, and the direction of movement through the body. We are looking for an overall sense of forward motion through the foot from the back to the front and out through the toes.

Imagine a line from heel through the middle of the foot. Does the person appear to walk straight through the foot on each step? Perhaps you notice that they stay on the outside of their feet from heel strike to toe off, so they cannot adequately

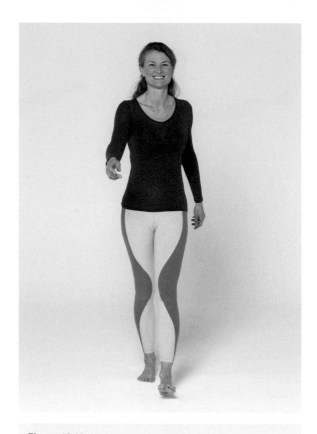

Figure 12.12

Rotation increases with walking speed

shock absorb with transient pronation as they move into the stance phase of their gait.

Or maybe you see that they quickly fall onto the inner border of their foot as they move onto it, blocking the forward trajectory of the pressure as the foot becomes stuck in pronation, and preventing the transition back to supination in preparation for push-off.

Perhaps they pivot off the front of their foot as they push off, dropping their heel inwards and loading that big toe joint that is so often associated with bunions. The line of pressure is turned at an angle as the foot is now pointing outwards instead of forward.

When you see any of these strategies, you will notice a reaction at the knee, as it is either dragged inwards or forced outwards.

For each observation, you know what to do:

- You know how to help someone to find their CLA by releasing their locks and supporting them with a postural cue that is meaningful to them.

- You know how to give them a leg to stand on.

- You know how to help someone to experience rotation in their upper torso with Thigh Slides.

- You know how to help them to find pelvic rotation and hip separation with Rock the Boat.

- You know how to help them to restore rotation at the hip with Total Body Rotation and at the knee with Listening Foot, which will help them to place their foot on the floor.

- You know how to help them to stack themselves over their ankle, with techniques like Stack and Reach if their pronation is prolonged rather than transient in the stance phase.

- You know how to integrate these movements with Shoulder Swings and Punch Walks.

And, of course, you will have a collection of techniques from your own background and training to draw on to enhance and reinforce these basic principles.

For example, when you include a pose or technique that involves hip rotation, you might perhaps take the opportunity for people to explore their walking: do they feel the same parts of their feet before and after? Does their balance feel the same? If your technique has emphasized zone stacking, could you balance it with a rhythmic spinal twist to release the tension and ensure that rotation is available for gait?

When we allow each small component to participate, we get to "walk our whole body," using and reusing energy for maximal efficiency. In doing so, we are working accurately, biomechanically, and neuromuscularly in a way that encourages the flow of motion. We are evolving past "controlling" so that we really do encourage freedom to move.

Power points

- An awareness of whether we push, pull, or tip ourselves over the ground can help our brains to direct our bodies to make different choices.

- Our posture has a profound influence upon our walking. Carrying ourselves with ease sets us up for powerful and flowing gait.

- Effective walking involves rotation at multiple joints throughout the body, from the feet to the neck.

- Sensing the progress and direction of pressure through our feet helps us to propel ourselves effectively with the least stress on our foot structures.

First it is necessary to stand on your own two feet. But the minute a man finds himself in that position, the next thing he should do is reach out his arms.

Kristin Hunter

Supported by our powerful lower body and a balanced erect trunk, our upper limbs have been freed from the incessant weight bearing of our animal ancestors, to develop extraordinary versatility. We have been able not only to reach, climb, hunt, gather, and carry to survive, but to develop creative cultural expression through dance, art, and music. We are capable of using our arms to project force in extraordinary feats of strength, yet pluck the strings of a guitar or remove a stray eyelash from a child's eye with dexterity and exceptional delicacy of touch.

The shoulders and upper limb present a conundrum for this very reason. The extraordinary mobility of the shoulder joint is made possible by compromising on structural stability. Where the hip joint is deep socketed and housed within the substantial bony pelvis, the shoulder joint is formed from the smooth ball of the head of the humerus sitting against a shallow depression on the scapula called the glenoid fossa. It is wrapped loosely in the fibrous sheath of the joint capsule and suspended from the skeleton primarily through muscular and ligamentous attachments. The only point at which the shoulder girdle directly connects with the central skeleton is at the small articulation between the sternum and the clavicle (see Fig. 13.1). Yet, we expect the shoulder to withstand high loads, and indeed it can from a very early age.

This is only possible because the shoulder is well integrated with the rest of the body, and the lower and central zones are able to create and transmit the power that is to be channeled through to the upper limb. It is for this reason that the upper zone comes last in this journey through the body – its functionality and performance depend on the foundations that it sits upon.

Those foundations go deeper than our structure. Before we can consider biomechanics, we need to appreciate some of the drivers for upper-zone posture and function.

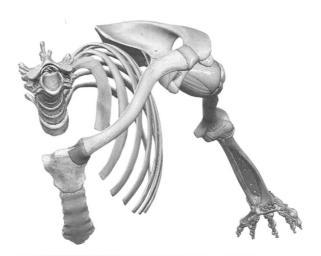

Figure 13.1

The free-floating shoulder girdle, with its sole attachment to the axial skeleton at the sternoclavicular joint, indicated in green

Wearing our emotions

When our three major body zones are feeling connected, we have a sense of occupying our whole selves from our feet to our head. Stress, however, can change that dramatically: many people find themselves predominantly inhabiting their upper zone as they hold themselves together with tension in their neck, shoulders, and arms.

The shoulders are a harbor for emotions in the body. Our language is peppered with references to this phenomenon: we "shoulder the load," and "bear the weight of the world on our shoulders." When startled, we hunch them quickly to protect our neck, and they fold forward to withdraw our heart from potential danger. Some people react in the opposite way, "squaring their shoulders" in resistance to the threat. Whether that threat is physical or emotional, an actual possibility of physical harm or a grinding sense of chronic stress, the physiological and physical response is the same.

The effect is far greater than purely structural: feedback loops within the brain register the body posture and respond with changes in emotion and even in the effectiveness of our cognitive brain processing.[1] Once again, the powerful integration of brain and body reminds us that we are not controlling our matter with our minds but working collaboratively, as minds in and of matter.

Our responses to threat are commonly known as fight, flight, and freeze, and these are features of our autonomic nervous system (ANS). The ANS is a part of our peripheral nervous system and is responsible for regulating the function of our internal organs. Its activity should fluctuate in balance between the *sympathetic* response (which primes our body for action by dampening digestive function and preparing our blood pressure, heart, lungs, muscles and

even eyes, for an intense movement experience) and our *parasympathetic* response (which, when we feel relaxed and safe, promotes sleep, digestion, and repair). When intense or prolonged stress persistently activates the sympathetic branch of the ANS, this balance can be disturbed, affecting multiple aspects of our health.[2,3]

Our sympathetic system also prepares our muscles to actively respond to a survival threat by fighting or fleeing from it. Emotional stress can activate the same physiological responses, and some people instinctively seek to regulate themselves by mirroring the fight/flight strategy with high intensity exercise. This may work as a coping mechanism, but when the stress is ongoing, it can also amplify the demands on the system and lead to exhaustion.

When fight or flight have failed to address the threat, a state of freeze may take over. Arising from a branch of the parasympathetic system, this is a survival strategy for a prey animal when escape is unlikely. The creature effectively "plays dead", becoming temporarily immobile in the hope that their pursuer will become disinterested and leave them alone. Once the danger has passed, their nervous system shifts, and over a few minutes they will shake off the experience and continue on their way. Humans can experience a similar freeze state in traumatic situations and in some cases, become stuck in a functional version of it on a day to day basis. In this state, it can become difficult to sense our bodies, our muscles may feel weaker or less responsive, and movement feels tiring and difficult.

Fight, flight and freeze are all normal defense responses, but they should be transient, and once the threat has passed, our physiology should return to a more relaxed state. When chronically stressed, our defense responses may persist, stiffening our bodies into the flexed protective or the extended resistant posture, and affecting the function of our necks and shoulders. Despite our efforts to show the world that we are coping, our bodies are telling a more honest story.

> You will see this presentation frequently in your clinics and classes as your clients come in with their complaints of neck pain, headaches, and shoulder problems. Instead of just thinking that someone's posture needs to improve, consider the nervous system activity that may be driving it. Conventional body positioning postural cues like scapular or abdominal setting can increase the rigidity. These people need to soften, not stiffen. Use imagery, associations, and awareness to help them to ease out of their contracted state.

The tendency towards immobility or stiffness when the ANS is caught in defense mode affects the whole body. In the upper zone, the upper trapezius, levator scapulae, and pectorals may be persistently tight along with the suboccipital muscles at the base of the skull in the flexed response, or the rhomboids and back muscles may be rigid in the extension response. Neck and shoulder stretches and exercises might offer short-term relief, but to achieve more significant ease in these areas, we need to regulate the ANS to invite the softening that will allow relaxation and mobility.

Messages of calm

Mindful breathing has been shown to be a powerful yet simple strategy for regulating the ANS. In particular, consciously regulating the duration and frequency of each breath cycle has measurable effects upon blood pressure,[7] heart rate variability,[8] anxiety,[9] and hormonal responses to stress.[10] Many teachers will include breath awareness at the end of a class in the cooling down or relaxation section, but the link between breathing, emotional regulation, and function may in fact make it more effective at the beginning, when it can set the body up for better performance.

For very tense upper bodies, unloading the shoulder girdle can support this process. With an individual client, supported sitting with the arms resting on a fitness ball on the thighs invites the neck muscles to relax and the shoulders to drop as they breathe into the ball (see Fig. 13.2). In a class situation, people can unload one another by sitting back to back with their arms resting comfortably on their bent knees.

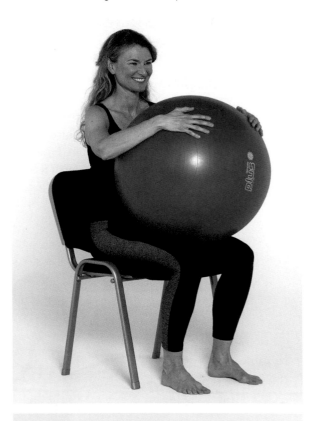

Figure 13.2

Supported relaxation for the shoulders and neck

They can take a moment to sense the breathing of their partner through their backs, and focus on slow counted breaths as they imagine inflating an imaginary ball sitting inside their rib cage (see Fig. 13.3). As their ANS starts to respond, they can become aware of any held tension in the neck and shoulders, and allow it to release.

Once some relaxation has been achieved, integrate it with spinal softening to remind the thoracic spine, neck, and shoulders of their potential mobility. The thoracic spine's mobility is critical for healthy shoulder movement, so it is most helpful to address before shoulder work. An example of this is Sternal Searchlights.

Movement exploration

Sternal Searchlights

Kneel or sit comfortably and place a fist on your sternum. This fist represents a searchlight that you will shine into different parts of the room. First pull it inwards toward your spine, and then push it back out again. Repeat this motion and notice the flexing and extending of your thoracic spine. Now sweep it across to the right, up the wall, across the ceiling, back down the wall, and across the floor. Reverse this motion, and then, for the fun of it, sweep the light in any and every direction, giving your spine an opportunity to iron out any stiff spots. Make the motion as interesting and rich as possible (see Fig. 13.4).

This is also an excellent time to integrate spinal twists, Thigh Slides (see Chapter 4), or the Spinal Elasticizer (see Chapter 7) to mobilize the fixed flexion or extension in the spine.

> High levels of muscle tension are often involved in cases where the ANS is caught in sympathetic overactivation. If the body is forced into motion against its own resistance, it simply induces more tension as it fights itself. Aim to calm and then soften first, as this fosters a sense of ease in motion.

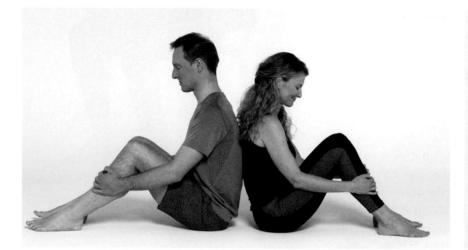

Figure 13.3

Supported breath awareness

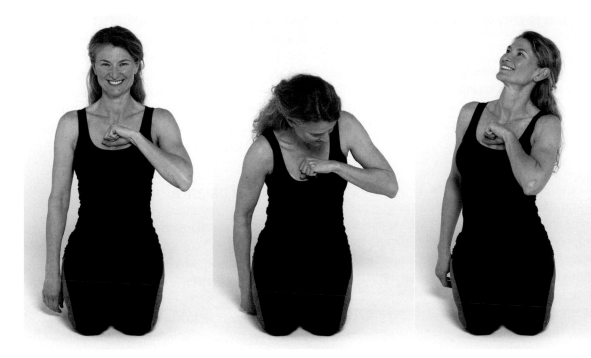

Figure 13.4

Sternal Searchlights

Firm foundations

Having accounted for the way emotions and psychology can obscure a person's true biomechanical potential, we can move on to appreciating the upper zone's physical and functional connections.

Our skeletal structures become progressively more delicate as we move up the body, so our upper zone is effectively the pinnacle of a pyramid of load-bearing and force-production potential. It is balanced upon a supportive central zone, which in turn is carried by a stable and relatively strong lower zone. Robust and well-functioning arms and shoulders are therefore built from the ground up, and their performance involves the coordination of the whole body.

> Movement is built from the functioning level in the body that is closest to the ground. In a wheelchair athlete, therefore, a strong central body is going to be the foundation for powerful arm movement.

For the three zones of the central body to be connected, we need a secure CLA passing through them all. The CLA has a profound effect on shoulder functionality. Relatively small deviations in the sagittal and frontal planes can make a perceptible change in the force output of the upper limb.

The upper lock has a particularly significant effect on shoulder function, and addressing this can have an immediate positive effect on the muscular pattern being used.

It is empowering for someone to discover that their arm performance can change with simple cues, like the "helium balloon" or adjusting the angle of their sternum so that it faces forward instead of up or down.

> In the upper zone, there is a strong temptation to layer on multiple cues before someone begins. Go for the simplest solutions first. Minimal input allows for maximum awareness: make one small change for the CLA and let that register first.

You already know how to establish the CLA from previous chapters. It may be that the person needs to tell a new story with their posture or that a spinal lock needs help to be released. Perhaps they need a foot to stand on, so the Listening Foot and body stacking might come into play.

We have introduced a number of examples of the intimate relationship between the shoulders and the central body over the past few chapters, including:

- Double Arm Raise, which showed us that the control relationship between arms and trunk is achieved with dissociation, or knowing "what to leave behind"

- the Wall Press, which assessed trunk proprioception and control in upper body pushing movements

- the Standing Knee Raise, which identified that the shoulder could be affected by a dependence upon latissimus dorsi to assist with pelvic control.

Everything that you have learned so far in the lower and central zones is relevant to the upper body, as this will determine how you carry and move your neck and shoulders. With a CLA, a stable base, and the ability to move each joint relative to its neighbor, you have established the foundations for optimizing your upper zone potential. Now we can look in more detail at the shoulders themselves.

A complex balance

The delicate cage that surrounds the shoulder joint is made up of two bony projections from the scapula itself: the acromion, which articulates with the clavicle to provide a protective roof over the joint, and the coracoid process, which sits medially to it. Ligaments attach the clavicle to the acromion and coracoid process to complete this lightweight enclosure for the ball and socket joint.

Underneath the bony roof of the acromion sits a small fluid sac, the subacromial bursa. This acts as a cushioning and antifriction device to protect the supraspinatus tendon, which folds over the head of the humerus to insert on the outer surface of the greater tubercle (see Fig. 13.5).

The shallowness of the glenoid fossa (the socket of the shoulder joint) allows maximum movement of the arm. However, to make the shoulder a little more stable without compromising this mobility, a ring of fibrocartilage called the labrum runs around the rim of the fossa, deepening it slightly and creating a seal with the head of the humerus.

The scapula itself is extraordinarily mobile. Depending upon the arm movement, it is able to glide in all directions over the rib cage, demonstrating elevation and depression, protraction and retraction, upward and downward rotation, and combinations of these movements. It can do this because it is not constrained by a

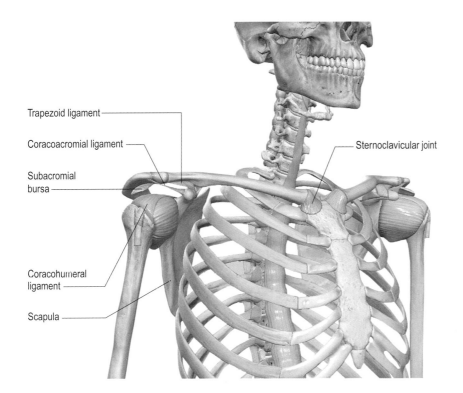

Trapezoid ligament

Coracoacromial ligament

Subacromial bursa

Sternoclavicular joint

Coracohumeral ligament

Scapula

Figure 13.5

A protective arch of bone and ligament is created over the head of the humerus

bony joint; instead it is attached to the central skeleton solely by soft tissues that can move it through large ranges of motion.

The scapula is this mobile for a reason: it must dynamically position the shallow cup of the shoulder socket to maintain its relationship with the head of the humerus as the arm moves. If you imagine the extravagant and varied arm movements of a dancer, you can appreciate the speed, accuracy, and coordination of the scapular movement needed to achieve this. If you then consider a tennis player, whose arm also moves through large ranges of motion but must also absorb force and deliver power, you are confronted with the dilemma of stability versus mobility. How can we be so mobile yet stable at the same time?

This conundrum has led to practices built on mis-understandings about the normal movement of the

shoulder. The cues of scapular setting and drawing the shoulder blade down and back, for example, are ubiquitous in almost every training environment, although they can actually contribute to shoulder problems, rather than alleviating them.

Consider the process of arm elevation. Normal bio-mechanics of the scapula dictate that as the arm is lifted overhead, the scapula rotates upward, which moves the bony "roof" out of the way in order for the shaft of the arm to freely lift without compressing the sensitive structures occupying the space between them (see Fig. 13.6). If this normal motion does not occur, the supraspinatus tendon is squeezed between the humerus and the acromion, which in turn can lead to impingement pain on lifting the arm.

Now think about the client in front of you. Perhaps they initiate their arm lifting with scapular elevation

scapula must be mobile in order to support normal arm function. Imagine how unnatural it would be just to reach into the back of your kitchen cupboard while keeping your shoulders fixed back and down. Try winding up into a golf backswing without allowing one scapula to slide forward around your rib cage, and the other to slide back toward the spine. Feel how restrictive it is to reach upward while keeping your scapula fixed back and down. It feels awkward for a reason, and that reason is that it interferes with your biomechanics. It quite simply is not normal movement.

It is routine for the "draw back and down" cue to be given to people to prepare them for lifting their arms overhead, whether in sitting, standing, or lying down. However, as this interferes with the scapula's free upward rotation in response to arm movement, it increases the possibility of tendon compression. This is why it is not surprising that we see many people with shoulder impingement pain that has developed as an unfortunate consequence of their attempts to improve their posture and function.

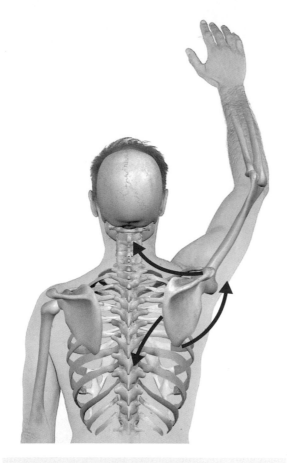

Figure 13.6

Upward rotation of the scapula creates space for the supraspinatus tendon and bursa as the arm lifts

(i.e., their shoulder hikes upward with their arm). Alternatively, they might glide the scapulae away from the spine into protraction, putting them into a forward shoulder position. In either of these cases, cueing for the shoulder blades to be drawn back and down might seem quite logical. And yet, actively holding the scapulae in this position, even "gently," can have some undesirable effects.

This type of anti-movement cue actively places the scapulae in a fixed position. As we know, the

The bilateral nature of the cue is also associated with diminished trunk rotation and arm swing. Normal, efficient gait requires alternating rotation of the upper torso against the lower torso. This centrally generated rotation initiates natural, connected arm swing, which in turn relies on freely moving scapulae. When the scapulae are actively drawn back and down, rotation is blocked, altering the mechanics of walking and running. (Incidentally, when this happens, people can begin to over-push with their calves to compensate for the loss of efficiency, so a cue at the top of the body can create issues at the other end of the chain.)

If this is the case, how do we avoid creating a problem while trying to solve another?

We often start on the right track, cueing to softly lengthen the spine through the top of the head, and then sense the balance point where the weight feels as though it falls through the center of the feet. For those who cannot let their shoulders drop, you may find that you first need to address the upper lock with the Head Slide in order to tell the brain that it can release the upper trapezius. Remember that these people may be caught in a stress response and are therefore often in need of breath regulation.

This often goes a long way toward placing the upper body in a more supported position. In such a case, resist the urge to layer on additional positional cues for the shoulders, because that can instantly transform a dynamic posture into a static one. Instead, direct your client's attention to the upper body and have them move between their normal posture and a more buoyant, light, and expansive posture, using comparison to increase their awareness of position, shape, and motion in their chest, sternum, upper back, and scapulae. With this connection made, you can enhance the experience with awareness cues rather than positional holding.

> Think of the clavicles as two long arrows extending out beyond your body. When you round your shoulders, the arrows point forward, and as you pull your shoulders back, the arrows point backward. Can you the expand the arrows straight out to the sides?

> Just as you did with the trunk, can you gain a sense of the shape and length across the front of your upper body compared with the back? Does one side curve inwards as the other curves outwards? Can you ease them into a similar length and shape?

> When we use awareness and imagery, we retain the ability to move freely.

This is all very well standing still, but what happens when we want to move the arm? In the upper limb, it is not a case of being stable *or* mobile: we cannot in fact be stable without being mobile. To maintain the integrity of the ball and socket joint, the scapula must be able to move in all directions, not just to position the socket but also to allow the scapula to absorb and transmit force to and from the rest of the body. If a scapula has been habitually stuck in a certain postural position, locking it into an alternative position simply replaces one dysfunction with another. Instead, we need to discover our other options.

Movement exploration

Scapula exploration

Reach under one arm and find the bottom of your scapula on that side. Feel around it and notice its shape. Now feel how it moves up and down as you raise and lower your shoulder. Notice how your scapula slides away from your spine as you reach around as if giving yourself a hug, and then how it glides back toward your spine as you reverse the motion, taking your arm out wide to open your chest. Trace the shape of a rainbow in front of you with your hand, and feel the scapula in continuous motion across your rib cage as your arm sweeps across from one side to the other. How about just reaching upward? The scapula rotates upward, so its bottom point moves away from the spine. Compare this to the hug motion again: can you feel the difference, as the whole scapula moves away from the spine? (see Fig. 13.7)

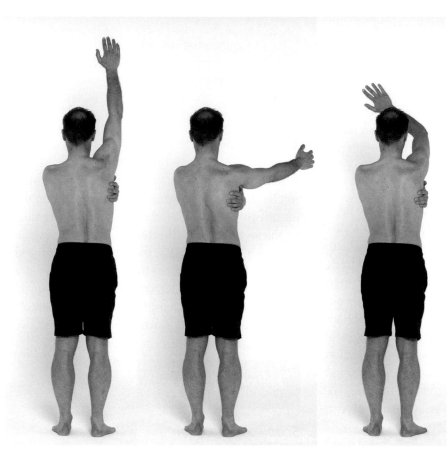

Figure 13.7

Feel how the scapula moves in response to your arm motion

Once the scapula is free to move in all directions, you open new cueing possibilities for the arm movement.

For people who hunch their shoulder upward when lifting an arm, the point of focus needs to be shifted along the arm. The arm is a long lever acting on the shoulder, and most people will feel the weight of it in their upper arm and shoulder when they lift normally. Invite them to choose an arm to investigate and then rest their opposite hand on the top of that shoulder to note whether their shoulder becomes tense and rises during the movement. Cue them to float the hand of the lifting arm upward as if they have a balloon on their thumb. By making the hand the perceived point of initiation, the shoulder relaxes and the scapula

tends to drop and upwardly rotate naturally, making the entire motion feel simpler and easier. The sense of engagement is spread through the entire arm at a low level, reducing the experience of load at the shoulder.

You can also use the imagery of lifting the arm from its underside, as if it is supported in a sling. This has the effect of balancing the front to back muscle activity, similar to what we saw with the hip in Chapter 8. We shift the brain's attention from the front of the shoulder and upper side of the arm, which can tend to trigger the neck muscles, to the back of the arm, which creates a sense of connection to the posterior shoulder and shoulder blade. The muscles that primarily move the arm are, of course, on the front of the shoulder, but casting our awareness to the back can bring the stabilizing partnership into play.

The same principle works in the four-point position. If you cue someone who is on their hands and knees to lift an arm, they frequently elevate the scapula. However, when you cue them to float the arm, the movement changes, and, in most people, the scapula will upwardly rotate, making the movement feel longer, easier, and more comfortable.

Extra credit: If you look at someone raising their arms into bilateral abduction, you might notice that one of their scapulae races away from the spine much more quickly than the other, giving the appearance of lack of control. Rather than diving straight into stability work, consider the possibility that the muscles that link the scapula and the humerus – muscles that include teres major and minor and the long head of triceps – may be contributing to the problem. If these muscles are restricted, as soon as the arm starts to lift, the scapula will be dragged with it. To restore a more normal rhythm between the two bones, the shoulder will benefit from these muscles being released and lengthened.

Once again, it seems that to be stable in the shoulder, we must also be mobile.

Suspending the arms

Whether the arms are working in open or closed chain, forces are being transferred between the arm and the body. As we saw in Chapter 3, using the arms with elevated shoulders disconnects the upper zone from the substantial support of the central zone, leaving us with the finer, strap-like muscles around the neck to provide the anchor for force transfer. This is called "working above your power zone," and fails the principle of force sharing by primarily using small structures to bear the load of the arms. To reconnect, there are several possibilities.

First, allow the upper zone to "land" on your central body. The sense of landing on yourself lets the upper zone dock into the rest of the body. Rather than being directed upward toward the neck, awareness drops downward, increasing the connection with our legs and feet on the ground. This initiates a positive feedback loop. For example, if we allow our upper zone to float down and land on our central body during a warrior pose, our sense of the hips and pelvis carrying our body increases, and this support in turn allows the shoulders to settle further into relaxed connection. The pose becomes stronger and more stable.

Build the image of a force field (or power zone) that encircles the mid-chest – an energy source from which the arms can move in any direction, including overhead, with both strength and ease. This is a much broader sensory experience than scapular setting: it is the more diffuse awareness of fully supported arm movement projecting from a substantial region of the body. There is no sense of isolated muscles working, because in reality to have a stable shoulder, multiple muscles are acting cooperatively (see Fig. 13.8).

An alternative cue that works on the same principle is that of the front and back circle.

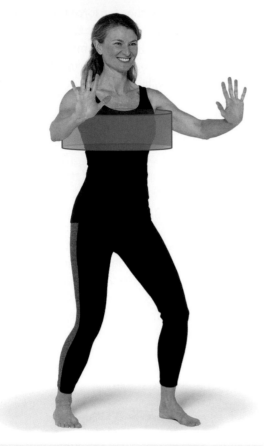

Now rub the back of one hand, and continue up the back of the arm all the way to your shoulder blade, and then swapping hands continue from the shoulder blade on the other side down the back of your arms to your hand. This is your back circle. Again, hold your arms in front of you at shoulder height in a loose arc, and picture them suspended from your back circle. Let your arms bob up and down a little, and see if you notice how secure they feel. Now see if you can change your intention and move between using your front circle and back circle. Can you notice that there is a subtle difference in where you feel the support, and the comparative sense of stability? Most people will identify that the back circle automatically broadens and activates the upper back and makes the shoulders feel more secure (see Fig. 13.9).

The back circle can be used in any position, whether supporting the open chain movements of the ballet dancer or the powerful pushing of a bench press. It is a simple way of accessing a large muscular surface

Figure 13.8

Working in the power zone circle around chest

Movement exploration

Rub your palms together and then trace a line from one hand along the inside of your arm, across your chest and then, swapping hands, continue along the inside of the other arm to the hand. This line represents your front circle. Hold your arms in front of you at shoulder height in a loose arc, and picture them suspended from your front circle. Let the arms bob gently up and down a few times.

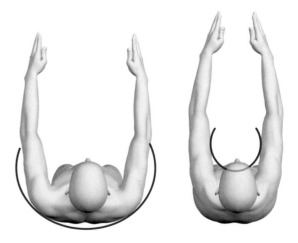

Figure 13.9

You can change your arm support pattern by focusing on the front or back circles area for force transfer while opening and decompressing the front of the shoulders.

Now that we can carry our shoulders with greater ease, we have a powerful foundation for the activation of our shoulder girdle muscles.

Power points

- The shoulder and neck posture that you see may be the visible representation of a person's emotional status, so calming the system may be the most effective start point.

- A supportive lower zone and secure CLA are essential foundations for upper body performance, and if there are functional difficulties in the trunk and pelvis, they can emerge as shoulder issues. When this is the case, shoulders will have only limited potential for improvement until the global foundations are addressed.

- Setting the shoulders and scapulae into place to address postural issues creates robotic, stiff motion that does not promote normal function.

- To have a stable shoulder, we need a mobile but dynamically controlled scapula.

Winning our wings 14

She walked with the Universe on her shoulders and made it look like a pair of wings.

Ariana Dancu

We are constantly transferring forces between the central body and the upper limb as we use it. It doesn't matter whether you are moving a computer mouse, cleaning your teeth, or swinging from a crossbar, the arm is dependent upon its proximal connections. It performs most effectively when these connections provide support over a substantial surface area of the central body. As with the trunk and the lower zone, we have many potential neuromuscular strategies for this force transfer, but we frequently limit our choice to a habitual strategy that we use as our all-purpose solution.

When considering movement control in the upper zone, ask yourself this question: "where are the forces going?"

Force management in the upper zone

Ideally, we can transfer our forces not only to the substantial mid back area but also around the anterolateral wall of the rib cage, creating a wrap-around effect that enables further fascial connections down into the trunk itself. Serratus anterior plus the lower and middle fibers of trapezius have a predominant role in achieving this large area for force transfer between the shoulder girdle and the central body, which we will refer to as the *support pattern* (see Fig. 14.1).

Nevertheless, some of us habitually use an *anterior pattern* instead, where the pectorals, biceps, and anterior deltoid are dominant. In this case, the brain

has a stronger connection to the muscles on the front of the body and directs our upper-limb forces to the anterior chest wall. We forfeit the neuromuscular connection to the back of our body, so the wrap-around effect of the support pattern is lost. The available surface area for force transfer is therefore diminished, affecting our potential for safe and efficient strength output.

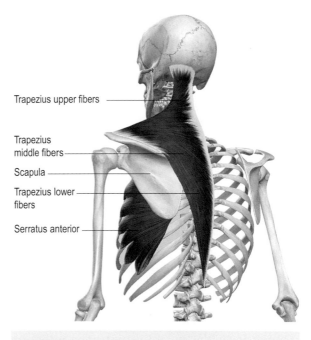

Trapezius upper fibers

Trapezius middle fibers

Scapula

Trapezius lower fibers

Serratus anterior

Figure 14.1

The support partnership of scapular stabilizers, providing a large surface area for skeletal attachment

229

When the forces are not being shared, the balance of muscle work must shift. If someone habitually uses the anterior pattern, the scapulae will not be adequately connected at the back of the rib cage in functional movements, even if the posterior shoulder and upper back muscles have the appearance of being well developed. Isolated strengthening exercises can develop muscles without necessarily initiating a scapular control pattern.

Lacking the wider muscular support network, the anterior shoulder and chest muscles become tight and tense. Pectoralis minor attempts to help through its attachments onto the upper front ribs, but this can tip the scapula forward, making it appear winged. Being a stabilizer of the glenohumeral joint[1] means that the biceps tendon can be put under more pressure, and grumbly tendons are common. Our priority, before we can successfully load the system, is to help the brain find its posterior surface again.

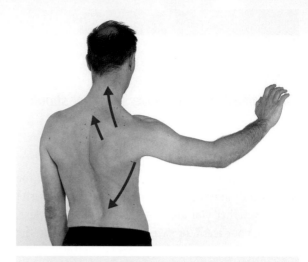

Figure 14.2

The muscle partnership that contributes to the downwardly rotated scapula

Practically, connecting with a sense of the back circle will help to rebalance this pattern. It will be especially important to reconnect the triceps, which tend to disengage in the anterior pattern – we will explore this presently in the Stalking Cat.

Some of us may draw the scapula down into a depression pattern, or may even drag it into downward rotation. Habitual downward rotation of the scapula can contribute to shoulder impingement because the bony arch of the acromioclavicular joint doesn't lift out of the way quickly enough to prevent compression of the supraspinatus tendon as the arm lifts. The muscles that tend to be involved include latissimus dorsi, levator scapulae, and the rhomboids (see Fig. 14.2).

You might already have noticed this pattern when you looked at the Standing Knee Raise test in Chapter 11. This is because it frequently shows up in combination with pelvic stability issues on the opposite side via the posterior oblique myofascial sling. It will appear as the arm being pulled down a little as the person stands on the opposite leg (see Fig. 14.3).

To help reset the global body pattern, Heaven and Earth (see Chapter 11) coaxes the scapula to upwardly rotate and the body to lengthen through the reaching side while encouraging pelvic activation on the opposite standing side. In doing so, it not only encourages the brain to reduce its reliance on latissimus dorsi for trunk and pelvic stability, it liberates the shoulder.

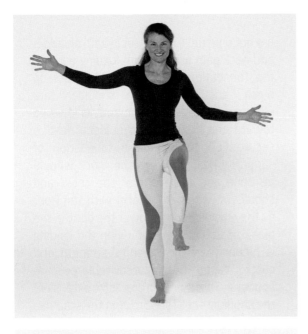

Figure 14.3

When shoulder pain is present, check the Standing Knee Raise for latissimus dorsi dependence

As we discussed earlier, many people use the elevation pattern, tightening the muscles connecting the shoulder girdle to the neck and forcing these smaller structures to bear the majority of the load. Addressing the foundation posture, working from the power zone rather than above it, and connecting with the back circle cue are all relevant possibilities here.

Another common pattern is that of *retraction*: a learned habit of narrowing the back by drawing the shoulder blades together with the rhomboids. The rhomboids connect the scapula to the thoracic spine between C7 and T5 but don't attach it to the rib cage, so this strategy doesn't offer an optimal surface area for force transfer and support. It is a tricky strategy to unpick, as this person is particularly vigilant about avoiding a forward shoulder posture and often feels inadequately supported unless they can sense a strong rhomboid contraction.

> To have an independent shoulder, you need a leg to stand on.

In loaded tasks like a bicep curl, for example, you may observe that the upper arm squeezes in toward the body, or that the elbow pulls downward. Both are signs that latissimus dorsi is being engaged as a primary stabilizer, and you may also notice the scapula has turned in a downward direction.

> The image of a marshmallow in your armpit, which you don't want to squash, can release the arm and allow the scapula to float back to a level position again without any increase in effort.

> Ask your client whether they would prefer a narrow, pinched upper back or a broad, balanced, strong back. Then ask them to notice whether the front and back of their upper body feel as though they are of a similar length. Can they experiment with making them more equal?

> As an alternative, the clavicle arrows (Chapter 13) may deliver a positive directional cue for their shoulders. Finally, when these people raise their arms, ask them to think of the bottom points of the shoulder blades creating a smile across their back, spreading away from each other as the arms move upward.

Last, we have the *collapse* pattern. Imagine for a moment that you have a closed system between your hand and your scapula, which is sitting securely on your rib cage. For optimal upper limb performance, you would contain any forces acting through your upper limb within this closed system. What we see in the collapse pattern is the scapula disengaging from the rib cage, effectively "springing a leak" at the back. Load moves up the arm and out past the scapula, which appears to lift from the posterior rib wall into a winged position (see Fig. 14.4).

To unlock any of these presentations, the brain needs the opportunity to explore different strategies. Remember, if the loading on the body is high, the brain sticks with what it knows to minimize risk. To promote change, we need to reduce the load and make the cerebellum sit up and take notice by altering the conditions.

It's not unusual to see people with shoulder and neck pain arising from loading without the foundations to support it. "Press-up pinch" and "Chaturanga shoulder" are common examples. As the body is lowered toward the floor, the shoulders need a secure CLA to provide a foundation of support. The back of the neck should be open and the front of the chest and shoulders wide and parallel with the floor as the elbows bend to lower the body in the plank position. However, when the loading is higher than the person's strength and control capabilities, a predictable posture appears. The spine drops into extension, the shoulders roll forward, and the scapulae pinch together, sometimes accompanied by shortening and compression of the back of the neck, and sometimes with the head dropping (see Fig. 14.5). No amount of cueing will sort this problem out until the load is reduced to allow for change.

Remember the concept of the lever from Chapter 4? Simply dropping the knees to the floor will decrease the load that the body must manage by shortening the lever. With less load, expanding through the spine and across the chest becomes possible. Once this is learned and secure, the person can be progressed to the full position again.

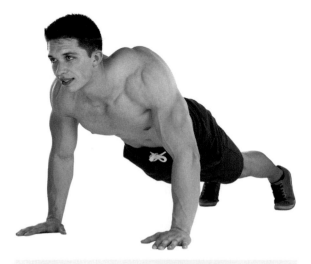

Figure 14.4

The collapse pattern

Wandering shoulders

As with any joint, for optimal strength, there needs to be a stable point to pull from. It therefore follows that if you are performing a bicep curl, for example, you ideally want the shoulder to remain in place in order for that muscle to exert an efficient concentric pulling action upon the forearm to bend the elbow (see Fig. 14.6).

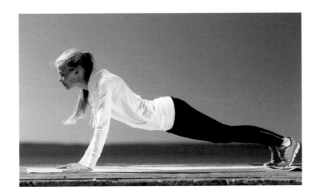

Figure 14.5

When the lever is long, the load may be too high to permit an effective upper body pattern

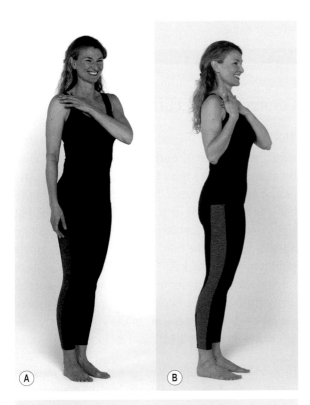

Ⓐ   Ⓑ

Figure 14.6

A. Start position. B. Shoulder stays securely in place as the elbow bends

However, you will frequently see a different pattern altogether. Instead of the forearm moving toward the shoulder using the elbow as a simple hinge, the shoulder is drawn forward toward the forearm. The elbow still bends, but it is a less effective movement without a stable point to pull from. The same thing occurs with the triceps: instead of supporting a clean and simple elbow-straightening action, the shoulder rolls forward, and sometimes even pops upward. This is the wandering shoulder.

Although weakness of the scapular muscles is frequently blamed, the wiring of the movement pattern is an equally crucial element in this presentation. It is tempting to default to the old "back and down" cue again to prevent the problem by immobilizing the scapula, but this provokes contrived, robotic movement that doesn't foster dynamic stability. To wire in a new program for the movement, we need to activate our old friend "awareness."

Taming a wandering shoulder can be done as an awareness exercise in a class without any weight in the hand. By keeping the motion unloaded, we can eliminate weakness as the primary problem and focus on the brain/body wiring.

Movement exploration

In standing, place the fingertips of one hand on the front of the other shoulder. Find your self-carriage posture with whichever cue has been most effective for you (balloon, puppet, rabbit ears, stacking, etc.) and see if the shoulder remains in place as you bend your elbow.

If it slides forward or pops upward (see Fig. 14.7), there is no need to fight with it. Calmly start again, but this time decide to leave your shoulder resting in place. If it wants to dive forward, pause to interrupt

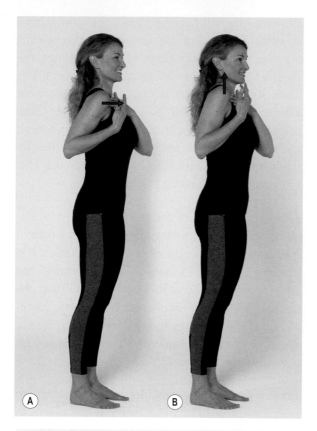

Figure 14.7

A. Shoulder drifts forward as elbow bends. *B.* Shoulder draws upward as elbow bends

> It is important not to try too hard. An intention to allow something new to emerge activates a different pathway compared to trying to make it happen.

The same technique can be used for any shoulder or elbow movement. You can play with active elbow straightening, and even shoulder rotation, turning your straight arm inwards and then outwards while maintaining the head of the humerus in place. There is no need for the shoulder to dive forward, shunt upward, or slide back and forth unless the loading is too high. To sort out the wandering shoulder, take the time to address the wiring before focusing on strengthening.

Connecting the cuff

The rotator cuff, comprising supraspinatus, infraspinatus, subscapularis, and teres minor, is so called because it wraps supportively around the humeral head. Each muscle has a dual function: they act individually to move the arm in a specific direction, but when working as part of the collective, they exert an inward draw on the humeral head to keep it snugly stabilized in the socket. This is a key component in solving the stability/mobility conundrum: by stabilizing the ball in the socket, the rotator cuff creates a secure axis for movement, in the same way that we saw earlier in the hip joint (see Fig. 14.8).

the overexcited muscles from playing out the old habitual pattern and let it fall back into its start position. Begin again, and investigate what it is like to allow the shoulder to be still, without forcing it into a consciously fixed position. Different muscles will become active around the shoulder girdle as it stays in place, but, importantly, you won't detect any specific direction of movement for the scapula. You have told the brain what you want to happen and have allowed it to coordinate the solution, which involves both the scapular stabilizers and the rotator cuff muscles in a more sophisticated balance than you could achieve consciously.

How do we train this? If you have tamed the wandering shoulder, you have already begun: maintaining the head of humerus in a consistent position while performing the arm movements described in the last exploration requires your rotator cuff to activate its muscular partnership.

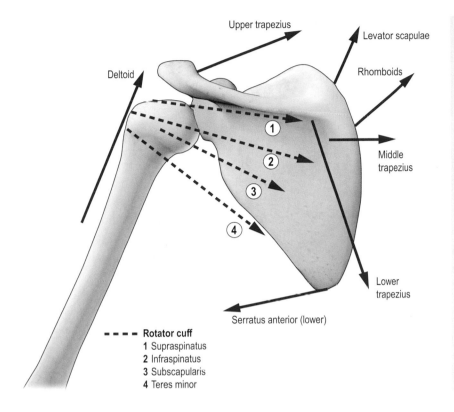

Upper trapezius

Levator scapulae

Rhomboids

Deltoid

Middle
trapezius

1

2

3

4

Lower
trapezius

Serratus anterior (lower)

- - - - Rotator cuff
1 Supraspinatus
2 Infraspinatus
3 Subscapularis
4 Teres minor

Figure 14.8

Force vectors of the
shoulder. Notice the inward
direction of force applied
by the rotator cuff muscles
as they stabilize the head
of the humerus against the
pulling forces of arm motion

From this point, there are two different cueing approaches, depending on whether you are working with open or closed chain movements.

Open chain

Whether your arm is freely moving or you are picking up a load, open chain movements of the arm will exert a pulling force on the shoulder joint. By reversing this action, we can activate the stabilizing role of the rotator cuff. To experience this, bend forward with your trunk and let your arms hang straight to the floor. Keeping the arms loosely hanging straight, imagine sucking them upward as if plugging the shoulders into their sockets. Release and repeat, this time becoming aware that as you plug the shoulders in, the muscles around the scapula also firm up, securing the entire shoulder girdle on the rib cage.

This is a strong and protective position from the shoulder. If you were to pick up a barbell, the broad connection across the upper back would also engage farther down through your posterior chain, and you might be able to sense this all the way to your pelvis. The shoulder becomes supported by the whole body.

If this is difficult to feel, it is sometimes helpful to hold a small weight in your hands to increase the sensory feedback of the action.

The "plugging in" happens around the shoulder joint, but if you initially try too hard, you might jump over your shoulder and retract your scapulae instead. This action calls in the rhomboids but misses the wider scapular connections. Having jumped over the shoulder joint, you are less likely to have activated the rotator cuff collective in its stabilizing role.

Scapular retraction is often used because it is an easy movement to cue, whereas plugging in requires more patience and skill to instruct. We need to be clear, however, that retraction moves the scapula, whereas plugging in secures the ball in the socket of the shoulder while stabilizing the scapula.

Real life study

In my own practice, I have encountered many young, athletic individuals who have had to give up their sport due to recurrent shoulder dislocations. They have frequently been strong, well conditioned, and accustomed to lifting weights in the gym. Without exception, they used the retraction pattern to set their scapulae, unaware that this compromised their shoulder stability. They had strengthened their rotator cuff in the individual movement roles for each muscle, so they had trained shoulder abduction and both internal and external shoulder rotation, but they had no experience of the collective action of these muscles in securing the humeral head. This was the root of the problem: without the inward draw of the rotator cuff muscles working together on the head of the humerus, it can slide across the glenoid fossa when put under the pressure of loaded arm movement, compromising the stability of the joint. All of these clients improved quickly once they established a relaxed neutral CLA, tamed their wandering shoulder, and learned to plug in.

We can also work with the rotator cuff in its dual role of stabilizing and mobilizing the humerus while integrating the scapular stabilizers.

First, we need to address a misunderstanding based on passive anatomy. The lower fibers of trapezius, which contribute to the stability of the scapula on the rib cage, have a medial and inferior orientation.

This makes it possible for the scapula to be drawn down and in toward the origin of the muscle on the spine, working concentrically toward the inner range of the muscle fibers. This is the root of the "back and down" cue for the lower trapezius, and, indeed, this action does activate these fibers.

However, as we raise our arms, the varying fiber angles of the three sections of the trapezius along with serratus anterior promote a rotational action of the scapula (see Fig. 14.9), while upper trapezius enables further motion of the entire shoulder girdle by acting upon the clavicle. The lower fibers of trapezius are ideally orientated to prevent serratus anterior from pulling the scapula too far laterally, and they also oppose the levator scapulae from pulling it upward into elevation. By controlling these actions, the lower fibers of trapezius contribute to stabilizing the scapula as it upwardly rotates. However, the scapula is turning up and away from the spine, not drawing down and in towards it. Imagine, for example, a violin player, whose arms must be beautifully supported yet fluently mobile. Setting their scapulae back and down will compromise their arm movement. They cannot function with their lower fibers of trapezius fixed in inner range. When considering upward rotation of the scapula, it makes sense to train in a more relevant position, as we will now explore with Diamonds.

Movement exploration

Diamonds

Take up a position lying on your front with your forehead resting on the floor. Make a diamond shape with your arms on the floor, connecting the fingertips of both hands at a point several inches beyond your head. If necessary, place a folded blanket under your hips to relieve any pressure on the spine (see Fig. 14.10A).

pivot points. Pause for a moment, and replace them on the floor. If your neck has remained relaxed, you will have accessed the scapular stabilizers of your mid back. If your hands and wrists have remained relaxed with your palms facing down as your forearm lifts and your upper arm turns, you will have activated your rotator cuff. As you repeat the motion, become aware of the area of the mid back that is giving you support. This is your upper zone (see Fig. 14.10B).

The closed circuit

In the closed chain situation, gravity is now pushing the ball into the socket. We have a new challenge now, which is to carry ourselves lightly and dynamically

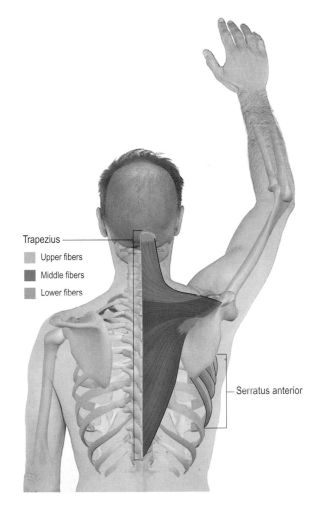

Figure 14.9

The muscle partnerships for upward rotation of the scapula

You may find that your shoulders are a little hunched – if so, gently create a little more space between your ears and your shoulders. There is no need to pull down hard: just ease out your neck muscles.

Imagine inflating a ball of air under the front of each shoulder: this will help them to plug in.

Now, keeping the hands and wrists relaxed, rotate your forearms off the floor, using your elbows as

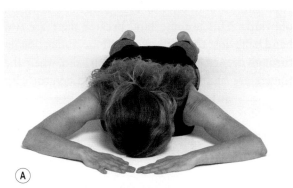

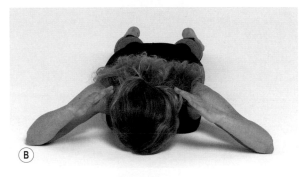

Figure 14.10

A. Diamond start position. *B.* Diamond finish position

over our arm, rather than switching off and loading our joints by leaning passively on them. Fortunately, we have reflex activity in the arm that is much like the positive support response in the leg. This enabled us to crawl successfully as babies: the stimulus through our palms triggered responses throughout the arm so that we could alternately accept our weight as we made our way across the floor.

As adults, we can benefit from this underlying response by using closed chain positions, because our rotator cuff still responds to the compression stimulus.

To fire up the reflex responses, first we need a responsive hand. Start in a hands and knees position. Imagine elastic bands crossing your palms between your fingers and thumbs and gently stretch them outwards. This is important, because there are two hand behaviors that will switch off the connection up through the arm. The first is the tight palm, where the fingers are slightly curled and the skin contact with the floor is lost. The second is the switched off, passive hand, which is often associated with the elbows facing forward in a locked position and the body hanging between the shoulders (see Fig. 14.11). Both of these presentations cause high compression in the wrist, leading to discomfort in weight-bearing positions. When you use elastic band hands, they become active and ready to talk to the rest of the body.

Position your shoulders, elbows, and wrists in a vertical stack, with your elbows softened just a little so that they are not locked out. This is the active support position for the arms. As you open and connect your palms to the floor, imagine a circular doorway forming in the center of each one. These doorways lead to pipelines that pass all the way up each arm. Think of energy from the ground surging up through these tubes, filling them right up through your shoulders and into the breadth of your upper back. This is a closed pressure circuit between your hands and your upper body, and it is going to form the basis for the closed chain work for the rotator cuff and scapula.

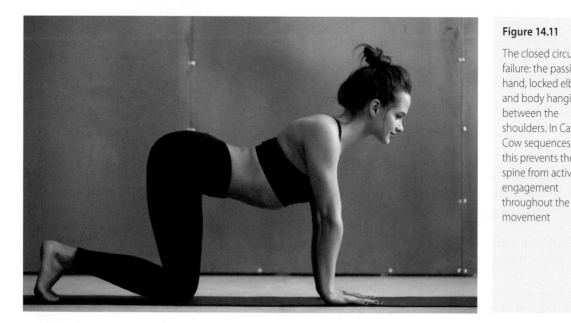

Figure 14.11

The closed circuit failure: the passive hand, locked elbows and body hanging between the shoulders. In Cat/Cow sequences, this prevents the spine from active engagement throughout the movement

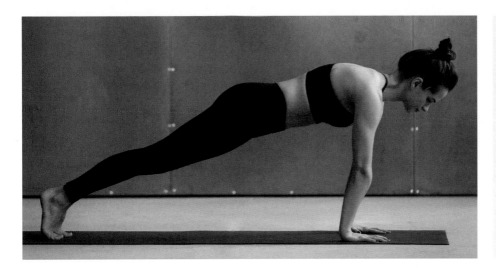

Figure 14.12

Thoracic flexion masquerading as scapular stability. Loss of vertical arm stacking: passively locked, non-dynamic arms, hyperextended elbows, increased wrist extension

You might wonder why I haven't simply asked you to press the floor away. For some people this works, but others rush straight past the scapula and into the mid back, causing thoracic flexion instead of achieving stable shoulders (see Fig. 14.12).

The next little-known element for closed chain shoulder stability is the controlled and coordinated mobility in the wrist and elbow. Almost without exception, when someone has poor shoulder control, they lock out their elbow or keep it in a fixed angle of bending whenever they can. Imagine for a moment pushing open a heavy door. The wrist and elbow must make small dynamic adjustments to modulate how much pressure is pushed up the arm to the scapula and how much is contained and pushed outwards to the door. If the joints stiffen too much, the full force is transmitted up the arm, and the scapula must manage all of it. This often causes the appearance of winging, where part of the scapula lifts off the rib cage. We have leaked force "out the back door" instead of using it to project outwards, so our push is weakened.

In the hands and knees position, stretch your hands and fill the imaginary tube in your arms with that upward surging earth energy. Test the springs in your elbows, feeling that the scapula is securely settled on the rib cage while the elbows bend, and maintaining the closed circuit of pressure. Whenever you are doing closed chain or pushing work, whether it is on the reformer, the yoga mat, or the gym floor, focus on the surface contact through your hands to allow the elbows to bend smoothly, and then to squeeze into straightening without locking out. To share forces through the upper limb and maintain a stable scapula, keep the arms dynamically engaged.

Now you are ready for some crawling.

Movement exploration

Stalking Cat Crawls

Crawling has become quite commonplace now in the training arena, but the emphasis on stability often compromises the movement quality that translates into true dynamic control. For this, we need to channel the quietly stalking cat, understanding that the placement of its paws determines the response that happens above it.

Begin with elastic band hands, but pulse and relax the stretch through the fingers to soften the hand and increase its responsiveness. Stack your shoulder, elbow, and wrist to establish stable support through your arms. Now peel one hand from the floor, beginning at the heel of the hand and ending in the fingertips. Replace it a short distance ahead, fluidly pressing it onto the floor from the heel to the palm (see Fig. 14.13). The more graceful you make this

movement, the more effective you will be in your arm and shoulder. Graceful is not weak: it is the controlled motion of the panther.

Connect the palm with the floor and transition your weight onto the hand, absorbing it with a gentle spring in your elbow as your opposite knee allows your body weight to progress forward. It will be tempting to lock the elbow, which creates a passive arm that shunts all of the weight straight up to the scapula, making it appear unstable. This is force management in action: if the weight-bearing load on the

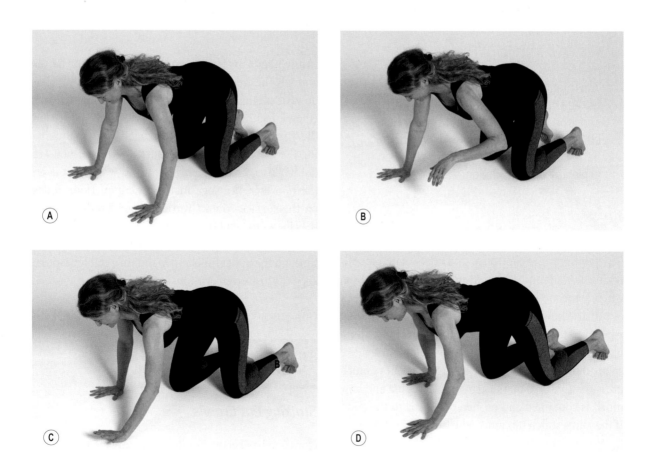

Figure 14.13

Stalking cat (*A–D*): shoulder stability begins with the coordination of hand and elbow

arm is not modulated by an accommodating elbow and responsive triceps, it races to the next most easily moveable area, which is generally the scapula.

As your body moves forward to place the other hand, the weight-bearing elbow should compress and decompress a little to store and release the energy that assists the movement. In a dynamically controlled arm, the elbow does not stay in a fixed position.

It is not unusual for people with seemingly well-developed triceps but persistent shoulder problems to feel fatigue after only a few of these movements, despite being able to press heavy loads in the gym. Locking and lifting doesn't train the finely tuned coordination that we use in normal functional movement.

This multijoint coordination throughout the upper limb also applies in open chain movement. What you may not have expected, however, is that to throw a ball, swing a baseball bat, hit a tennis serve, or drive a golf ball, we need to know how to crack the whip.

Cracking the whip

Picture for a moment the long traditional bullwhip used by a cowboy. The cowboy's body initiates the pulse of potential force and delivers it through the whip handle; the whip then becomes an extension of his arm. The energy visibly ripples away from his central body to culminate in the stinging crack at the end of the whip. The entire movement is dependent on a continuous flow of energy between body segments, beginning with the part of the body closest to the ground and surging up and out to the hand.

Now visualize your arm as the whip. Your hand is the tip of the whip. You create power in your lower body, and then transmit it upward through your body until it funnels out through your arm, finally releasing it from your hand, perhaps to throw or hit a ball.

Think of the arms as delivering the force created in the body.

Tension in the arms, particularly in the wrists and elbows, blocks this force delivery. The tennis player who grips the racquet too hard will find that they need to use more arm strength to hit the ball powerfully when compared to the relaxed player who uses the whip action. Too much hand tension robs the violinist of finger dexterity and precision, and wrist tension will diminish the fluency in her bowing arm, demanding more from the elbow and shoulder instead. From a force-sharing perspective, if you block a joint in the kinetic chain, you will push more pressure into those that remain. If the wrist and elbow are tense, the shoulder must pick up the slack.

For more power and less load on our body structures, we need highly coordinated, quick multijoint movement throughout the entire kinetic chain.

Seaweed Arms

This might feel a little strange at first, but there is serious purpose behind the technique. It is about discovering and resolving arm tension, and coordinating the shoulder, elbow, and wrist.

In relaxed standing, create a circle with your arms in front of you (see Fig. 14.14A). Open out from the backs of the upper arms, and then allow the elbows to open, and finally your wrists, so that the arms unfold all the way out to the fingertips (see Fig. 14.14B). Just as your fingers straighten, start to draw in from the wrists, following with the arms as if scooping the air in front of you into your chest (see Fig. 14.14C). As your fingertips meet, start the outward movement

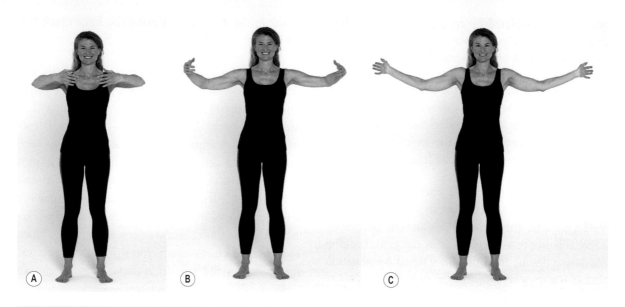

Figure 14.14

A. Seaweed Arms start position. *B.* Opening from the elbows. *C.* Returning from the wrists

again from the upper arms. Let the motion continue as a ripple, in and out, like seaweed in the water.

Those with relaxed arms find this easy, but those trapping their forces in their hands, wrists, and elbows will initially find the motion jerky and unnatural. These are the people who most need this technique, to relieve uncomfortable, and sometimes painful, tension and to enable their movement intention to be freely transmitted through their arms.

Encourage an open but relaxed hand and wrist when teaching exercises. "Tin soldier hands" increase peripheral tension, which robs the upper limb of fluency. The nervous system learns rigidity rather than control.

Coordinated mobility like this allows us to use our magic myofascial system to store and release energy.

Myofascial mates

We have a good idea of the shoulder's relationship with the back of the body, but its connections with the front of the body are just as critical.

The central body provides a great deal of support for the shoulder, but in open chain tasks, it needs to do this elastically. At this point in the book, you are well aware of the progressive lengthening through the trunk that accompanies overhead arm movements. Consider how the sides of the ribs open a little and the thoracic spine extends as the arm raises: the trunk muscles must be active yet allow for this expansion. Traditional core work and abdominal setting don't permit this because they set the trunk muscles at a fixed length. If the body is prevented from responding, the shoulder becomes functionally disconnected past a certain point in range. We therefore need to think of the trunk muscles less as static anchors and more like the rope of a rock climber being let out under control as they abseil down the side of a cliff.

> To support the shoulder, the trunk muscles must be able to change in length. Bracing or setting the abdominals opposes this.

Remember the Greyhound Hand Slide exercise from Chapter 6? We used it to promote the CLA and balance the central body, but it is also the first step in promoting the elastic connection between the trunk and the arms. You might remember that there was no conscious setting of the abdominals involved, yet you were able to securely rest on your mid sacrum with your spine relaxed. The abdomen was allowed to respond reflexively to the arm moving overhead, active enough to dynamically support the arm but not restricted in any way. We are going to use the same principle in Drawing the Sword.

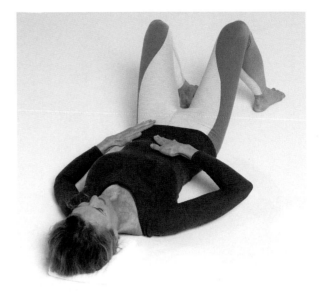

Figure 14.15

Waking up the support muscles of the abdomen

Movement exploration

Drawing the Sword

Take up the Greyhound starting position, lying on your back with knees bent and feet flat on the floor. You may need the folded towel under your head to ease the neck into a neutral position and to breathe away any other spinal locks. Finally, do a little sacral rock to find the place where you can just settle onto the floor without effort. This mid-sacrum position will remain consistent throughout the movement.

Now place your left hand on the left side of your lower abdomen (see Fig. 14.15). Rub diagonally from this point up and across to your right rib cage, letting the brain know where the connections are, and then return the hand to its place on the left side of the lower abdomen (see Fig. 14.16). Let it be heavy, because this is the scabbard for your sword.

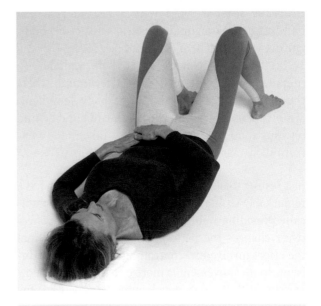

Figure 14.16

Drawing the Sword start position

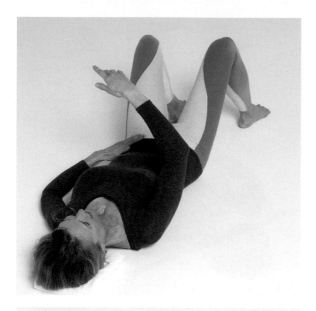

Figure 14.17

Drawing the Sword movement trajectory

With your right hand, draw the imaginary sword from the scabbard and with a relaxed arm and hand, sweep it diagonally up and across your body, ending with your arm overhead (see Figs. 14.17 and 14.18). There is no need to tense the abdomen in preparation. This is just like a Greyhound, where the spine stays relaxed and the body lengthens. Simply focus on leaving your scabbard hand behind on your abdomen, and taking your other hand away from it.

Just resting that scabbard hand on the abdomen has a remarkably strong effect on the brain: it is not physically providing stability, but the sensory input effectively changes the pattern. People usually find that the effort involved in controlling their trunk diminishes, so the movement is more efficient. You are now working with the myofascial connections between the trunk and the shoulder.

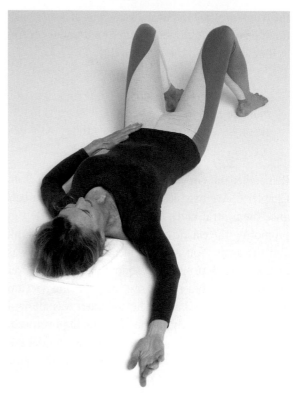

Figure 14.18

Drawing the Sword finish

The conventional approach to a technique like this is to attempt to stabilize one area against the resistance of another. This sets up the impression of fighting for control. Draw the Sword instead applies two of our previous movement intention cues: "leaving something behind" and "taking one part away from the other." These facilitate movement ease, and there are many opportunities in Pilates, yoga, and general movement training to apply this type of cueing.

Movement integration

We started this upper limb journey in the emotional nervous system, and then explored the postural foundations and connections between the three zones. We have discovered that to be stable, we must also be mobile in our upper limb, and now we will investigate coordinating that movement through the whole body.

Let's focus on the upper half of the body moving over a relaxed but grounded lower body.

Movement exploration

Reach and pull

Stand comfortably with your weight centered in your feet and soften your hips and knees. Bend your elbows so that your forearms are parallel to the floor.

Notice that your sternum is pointing straight ahead (see Fig. 14.19).

You are going to lead your upper body into rotation with your left hand by moving it away from your body until the arm is straight in front of you. If you keep moving it away from you, you might notice that you can let your scapula slide away from your spine to follow it, and – if you allow still more motion – that you can let it tug on that side of your rib cage, which turns your sternum to the right (see Fig. 14.20).

Grasp an imaginary rope with your hand and draw it back toward you, allowing your elbow to brush past your side, gently pushing the scapula back toward the spine and inviting the ribs to follow so that your sternum is now facing left. Let your right arm stretch

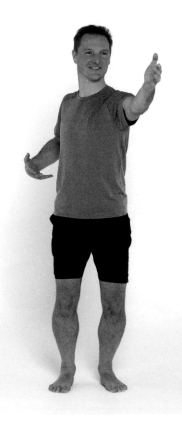
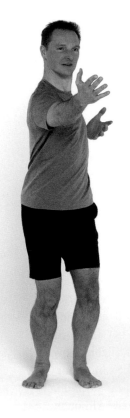

Figures 14.19/14.20

Reach and pull: feel how the arm draws the rib cage into rotation as you reach

Feel the rib cage and scapula respond as you draw your arm back forward into the reach as your left hand pulls back, and feel how much easier the turn is when both sides participate.

Slowly repeat the movement and explore the link between the hand, arm, scapula, and trunk, and the richness that emerges when your left and right sides seamlessly coordinate with each other.

These links are critically important for the biomechanics of upper limb power and efficiency, yet so many people's brains have lost the connections. This is hardly surprising, given how many people spend many hours with their arms in a fixed position on a computer keyboard. As a movement teacher, you have the opportunity to reintegrate these movements by being aware of the natural synergy between the arm, scapula, and rib cage.

Beginner students in yoga and Pilates can be helped enormously by discovering their shoulder blades in twisting poses, for example. Often the focus is on ensuring that the turn is being correctly driven from the waist and not by the arms, but, if overdone, we lose the natural chain of movement connection that would integrate this single element into actual functional movement. We absolutely need to help people to find the ability to rotate the trunk on the pelvis, but a blocked scapula can put the handbrake on the global movement.

You can feel this for yourself. Sit with your spine in its buoyant position, on the floor with crossed legs or legs outstretched, or even on a chair. Bring your arms into the back circle position as if encircling a large tree. Turn your rib cage to the left and then the right, feeling how much motion is available. Now repeat the process using the same position but stabilizing the scapulae in the "back and down" position. Can you still rotate as easily? It is unlikely. Although

you have told your body to twist at the waist instead of using the arms, just as you did before, the mobility has become restricted.

> Replacing scapular setting with either the back circle or "landing on the upper zone" (see Chapter 13) avoids creating rotational restriction.

In Thread the Needle, for example, many people become stuck at the shoulder on their reaching side, compressing the front of the joint and struggling to access the upper body twist that the pose has to offer. Let them understand that the arm, shoulder blade, and rib cage "hold hands" in a chain, so as the arm reaches away, the scapula follows it by sliding away from the spine and then brings the rib cage with it. The link is made between the arm, shoulder blade, and rib cage, enabling a richer turn (see Fig. 14.21).

In twisting poses, those people whose leading shoulder seems jammed forward are encouraged to "open

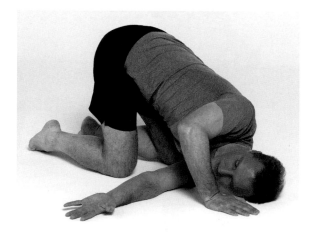

Figure 14.21

The arm talks to the scapula, which in turn leads the rib cage into rotation

the shoulder," but sometimes they aren't sure how to achieve this. If, for example, in a high lunge twist you cue the arm to sweep up to the ceiling as the chest turns, it is easy for the beginner's shoulder to be caught forward, restricting their turn. If you cue the turn from the elbow first to open the chest, the scapula naturally moves out of the way by gliding back toward the spine (see Fig. 14.22). Because it "holds hands" with the rib cage, it encourages an easier turn of the thoracic spine. Each time you encourage someone to open at the front of the shoulder, remember that you are also cueing the scapula to slide back.

In the Pilates Bow and Arrow, as one arm "holds the bow" the other draws the imaginary bowstring back, rotating the rib cage as it follows the elbow (see Fig. 14.23). To find the richness in the pose, be aware of the scapulae: the drawing arm should gently slide the scapula back toward the spine, which then naturally turns the ribs. At the same time, the other scapula reaches forward to support the bow arm, taking the ribs with it. In this way, the left and right sides work in partnership to create the turn, preserving the elasticity of the motion.

In the gym, whether you are rowing on a machine or punching a bag, performing pulley pushes and pulls, or even monkey crawling, your scapula should be sliding across your power zone as you reach or rotate. You need this in order to maintain an open channel

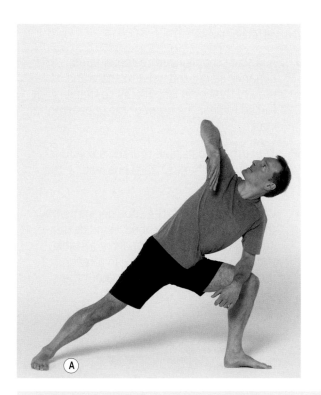
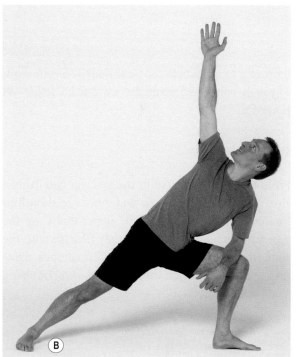

Figure 14.22

Leading from the elbow can often assist the trunk into rotation (*A* and *B*)

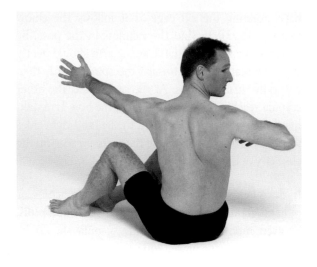

Figure 14.23

Allowing the scapula to move enables the ribs to turn more easily

for forces to move between your body and your arms. Through connected mobility, we can be stable yet powerful.

Winning our wings

From the highly forceful to the graceful and expressive, the arms rely on their wider body relationships for optimal performance. The upper limbs are the social butterflies of the body: they flourish with the support of the rest of the body and need open channels of communication throughout the kinetic chain,

all the way from the foot to the hand. Although they need to be stable, they require mobility to achieve that dynamic control. They seem to be capricious and contradictory, yet once we embrace these apparent paradoxes, they are fascinating to explore and work with.

Power points

- We have a number of different possibilities for force transfer between the arm and the central body. Some are more suited to load bearing than others.

- The rotator cuff muscles have dual functions. Working their individual movement actions and persuading them to engage in their cooperative stabilizing role are two different concepts for the brain and require different tasks.

- A stable scapula needs a coordinated, dynamic elbow and wrist to share and modify the upper limb forces so that it is not forced to bear the brunt of the upper limb load.

- The arm, scapula, and thoracic spine functionally "hold hands," each one leading the next into motion.

- When working with the shoulder, remember the importance of the hand. Hand dexterity depends upon the support of a stable shoulder, but hand tension can affect the fluency and control throughout the entire arm.

Before embarking on our discussion about moving the body, we began with moving the brain. Now that we have explored different aspects of functionality, we can come full circle and focus on speaking the brain's language as we teach.

If you are expanding people's movement vocabulary, working on the quality and efficiency of their movement, and improving technique, then it is fundamental to your practice to instruct in a way that facilitates learning. From our discussion so far, it will have become evident that using our senses is essential for motor learning, and understanding more about our senses equips us with more possibilities.

The senses can broadly be divided into three categories: those that tell us about the world outside our bodies, those that help us to locate and recognize our relative body parts and body position as we interact with the world, and those that tell us about the world inside our bodies (i.e., the experience of the "lived body"). These sources interact to provide a comprehensive real-time conceptualization of ourselves.

The feeling of warm sun on your face, the wind lifting your hair, and the smell of hot coffee are all features of *exteroception*[G]. Exteroceptive feedback is that which originates outside the body. It provides inputs such as vision, sound, smell, and touch to help us construct our perception of the world around us.

To inform us about the moving or positional relationships between our body parts, proprioceptive feedback is drawn from sensors in our soft tissues, such as our skin, muscles, ligaments, and even fascia. Through proprioception[G], we sense effort, force, and the sense of heaviness in our limbs.[1] When you hold your arm out to the side with your eyes closed, the proprioceptive quality of joint position sense allows you to know where your arm is. If you move it in a sweeping loop in front of you, you can sense the motion as a result of the proprioceptive quality of kinesthesia.

We understand how our body is orientated in the external world with the help of the sensors within our vestibular system – our inner ear – which provides us with finely tuned information about the angle and positioning of our head. Strongly integrated with our senses of vision, touch, and body-generated proprioception, the vestibular system is central in adjusting the balance between our sensory systems as our physical relationship with the external environment changes.[2] As such, it is involved in the perception we have of our body relative to our external environment.[3]

The critical element to the construction of our experience as a lived body is *interoception*[G]. Right at this moment, your brain is receiving a torrent of information arising from the processes taking place in your body. Even as you sit still, your entire system is in motion – your lungs are expanding and emptying as your diaphragm descends and rises, your heart is rhythmically sending blood on its voyage through your arteries, your gut is busily digesting and moving food matter through itself, lymph fluid is moving through its own separate circulatory system, and your organs are sliding across one another to make room for these adjustments, like passengers on a crowded bus. Some of these things you will not be consciously able to detect, but other messages from within will be familiar: you might be aware of feeling uncomfortably warm, for example, or perhaps hungry or thirsty.

Interoceptive awareness is linked to how you experience yourself, and how you respond emotionally to these sensations. As research scientist Bud Craig describes it, "Interoceptive integration generates the feeling of being alive."[4] Our language is peppered with references to this phenomenon. We speak of our "gut feeling," and "feeling something in our hearts," so it is no surprise that recent research uses the ability to detect one's own heartbeat as a measure of interoceptive perception.[5,6]

The study of interoception has heralded a leap forward in understanding the fully integrated body and mind, because the way in which we construct emotions is mediated by these sensations coming from the body. Previous theories postulated that what we thought (our cognitive processes) created the emotions and sensations that we felt, a "top-down" mechanism. However, it seems instead that it is the signals arising from our bodies that bias our emotions and thus influence our decisions and behaviors.

As the brain is creating simulations in advance of our actions, it pulls from past experiences to create a context for the interoceptive sensations that you experience, and according to Seth,[7] this shapes the emotion that you feel. Sensing a rapid heartbeat might fill you with satisfaction and motivation if you relish hard physical training, and you associate it with rewards like greater performance, fitness, or weight loss. Your perception may even be further positively biased by the environment you are in, stimulated by exteroceptive information like the sights, smells, and sounds of your exercise environment. The feeling of a rapid heartbeat is therefore experienced as positive, even pleasant.

However, if you are about to make a presentation to an audience, waiting for a medical diagnosis to be delivered, or checking your bank balance to suddenly find that it is well below your monthly expenses, the same interoceptive sensation of increased heartbeat might be associated with anxiety instead. The sensation in this case is not a pleasant experience, but it is the context rather than the actual sensation that differentiates the emotional response.

Interoception is being investigated in an array of health presentations, and discussions have arisen around both positive and negative implications of high interoceptive awareness. People with anxiety, for example, have been found to pay close attention to interoceptive signals, although they seem to be selective in the ones to which they choose to attend. They also tend to overestimate the implications of harmless somatic cues. Anxious people, therefore, do not necessarily have better interoception: they can be very sensitive to their body signals, but not accurate in their interpretation of them.[8]

This means that you as a professional must be both a careful listener and an astute questioner in order to help these people to be able to more calmly and accurately understand and articulate what they are feeling. You can then decide whether there is an actual physical need to modify the exercise due to its position, loading, or excessive motor skill requirement, or whether the issue is the interface between the person's perception of sensation and their interpretation of its meaning.

If the latter is the case, your action will be to continue with the task at hand while providing reassurance. You may need to reframe the meaning they are attributing to their sensory experience and direct their attention to other sensory possibilities, such as comparative pressure, light touch, and motion.

Combined, the qualities of proprioception (where I am) and interoception (how I am) are thought to be key to the experience of embodiment. This is thought to be essential for the experience of self-awareness and self-connection; truly, modern research is dissolving the distinction between mind and body.

The associative brain

Each movement that you make is the creation of a whole "family" of contributing associations, and this involves multiple areas of the brain. Without you realizing, a simple movement carries with it your pre-existing assumptions and beliefs about it: the feelings that it provokes and imagery that it carries; the sensory associations such as smell, temperature, sound, and touch; and the emotional state associated with movement or exercise. It is all happening with lightning speed from moment to moment without you even being aware of it.

What is even more fascinating is that the family of associations, which arises from a network of neuronal connections, can change radically from moment to moment, task to task. Multiple interactions from all over the brain are involved, and the networks of neuronal connections are highly dynamic, with neurons constantly working in different relationships.

> To achieve change, we need to address the "family dynamic" at the beginning of the process, rather than simply correcting the movement output at the end. We need some family members to sit this one out, and invite others to join the party.

How do we do this?

The most interesting moment in a movement is the one *just prior* to its beginning. This is where the brain sets up the action, transforming your movement intention into a movement impulse that fires up the supportive foundation muscles, prepares your center of gravity, and takes the handbrake off by releasing tension in opposing muscle groups.

It is often the moment that we miss as practitioners, as our eyes catch up somewhere in the middle of the movement when the biomechanical outcome of this preparation becomes most obvious, and we then set about correcting this. In other words, we actually treat the reaction rather than the root of the movement strategy. The real issue happened well before this.

You might observe it as an involuntary in-breath. Perhaps it is an expression that flits across the person's face, telling you that the association for their preparatory movement is anxiety. Maybe their face speaks of a determination to "try hard" that is destined to become excessive effort. It could be that the expression in their eyes tells of past efforts that have defeated them, or that their minds are handcuffed by a head full of instructions. What you are observing are visible indicators of the neuronal network family involved with the movement task.

This magic moment, a split second before the movement commences, is where the change must be made, so don't rush past it – pause, investigate, and reframe the person's mindset before proceeding.

You can make your intervention before the movement begins by creating the opportunity to choose different neuronal network family members. The thought or attitude that you have before you start a movement engages the family members associated with it. To change some of these members in the neuronal network for that movement task, you therefore need to begin by adjusting the attitude that precedes it.

Set a different objective: perhaps frame the task as one of exploration rather than achievement, removing performance pressure and replacing it with a process of collaborative inquiry. Using "What do you notice?" questions redirects the focus from results to process. Reach into the brain's rich resources to trigger different associations by asking, for example, "What can you imagine filling your legs with, to allow them to reach smoothly away from your body?"

The imagery is totally individual but allows the person to activate different brain relationships and thus alter the association family for that movement. One of my young adolescent patients chose to fill his legs with rich hot chocolate as he ran, which immediately reduced his muscle tension, increased his joint mobility, and created a rhythm and fluency that had not been there moments before. When he opened a window for change in his nervous system by activating new associations, he was rewarded with a powerfully comprehensive shift in his neuromuscular relationships.

Other clients have filled their pelvic bowls with flowers, their arms with music, sunk their feet into grass, melted candle wax down their necks, and sent movement through themselves like ocean waves. Whatever they choose, they hold the keys to their own neuroplasticity by drawing on their sensory memory bank.

Making connections

As we can see, the systems do not work independently but through multisystem integration. This is exceptionally useful for us as teachers of movement, because once again we can choose from a variety of tools to help people to make connections.

Have you ever asked somebody what they feel as they perform a movement, and they answer, "I don't know?" You think to yourself that if all the wiring is available, and you can see the muscles working and the joints moving, how is it possible that they can't feel anything?

It is perfectly possible. Sometimes you have to teach someone how to feel. Research has identified that at rest, our brain's "sense of self" centers tick away, integrating a broad spectrum of proprioceptive and interoceptive information.[9,10] However, in people who have been traumatized, anxious, or are depressed, the part of the brain that processes the meaning of sensation no longer functions normally.[11-13] When they tell you that they can't feel anything, they are not kidding.

For other people, the problem is an inability to filter out a specific sensation amidst the large amount of feedback coming into the brain. They may be highly attentive to pain sensation, for example, but don't know how to identify and refine other sensations. For these people, the experience of learning how to feel is much like a social drinker attending a wine appreciation course – they already have the structures and neurological systems in place to receive the sensory information but need some coaching to develop their palate.

Here are just a few methods for helping someone to feel:

1. **Provide a filter** to decrease the amount of sensory noise that the person must decipher. It's important to understand that people are not always very confident about answering a question on what they feel, because they don't know what kind of information you are asking for. They don't want to feel foolish: they are new to this, and they don't want to get it wrong. Avoid flabby questions like, "What do you feel?" if you don't want to hear the reply, "I don't know."

   Narrow the focus of your question so that it becomes much more precise, for example: "What is different about what you feel here, compared to here?," or "What does it feel like in this body part when you perform the movement this way compared to that way?" If you give people specific options to choose between, they can come forward with an answer, because they clearly understand what you want to know. This gives them the confidence to simply tell you what their felt experience is right now, and there is no right or wrong about that.

2. **Use contrast as an aid.** Sometimes it is not easy to feel something until it changes.

Example: I am working with a professional footballer with chronic groin and hamstring problems, and he is performing a leg press using the reformer. I ask whether he can feel any muscles working.

"Dunno," he replies.

This is not unusual. I encounter many athletes who can sense strong muscle activation associated with high load but can't otherwise connect with themselves. A seemingly innocuous situation like this can pose a threat to their confidence. Struggling as he is to understand how and what to feel, I must catch him before he shuts down and withdraws completely. I ask whether he can tell that there is a movement happening. He says yes. I comment that as there is movement occurring, there will be some muscles working somewhere, so we just need to investigate a little further.

To help him to identify and understand a sensation, we begin with learning to detect change. I invite him to place his hand on his thigh, which I can see is working as he moves, so I know it will be easy to feel and learn from. As he presses out, I ask whether he notices anything moving or changing under his hand. He tells me that he is able to identify a change, and when I tell him this is great, he is a little surprised at his success. As it didn't seem too difficult, he is open to the next suggestion. I explain that the change is actually the muscle contracting.

As he performs a few more repetitions, I ask him whether he can notice the difference between when it contracts and when it relaxes. This associates meaning with the sense of change.

Having mastered feeling something under his hand, he is ready to investigate the sensation arising from the muscle itself. I ask him if he can describe the feeling of the muscle contracting under his hand. By this time he is gaining confidence, and buoyed by his success and the understanding that there is no wrong response, he is more willing to articulate his experience.

Finally, we see if he can identify the sensation without the additional feedback from the hand. I ask whether, if he takes his hand away, he can still feel the muscle working as he presses out. By this time, he trusts me and is quite comfortable with the process, so he spontaneously volunteers that he can now also feel other muscles working in his leg.

The simplicity of detecting change is a way in for a person like this, enabling him to perceive, interpret, and articulate his experience. This is a transferable skill – he is not just learning to sense a specific muscle, but to sense muscles in general. If I invest time here, meeting him where he truly is, he will progress quickly and learn more easily.

3. **Use your assets.** If someone has had an injury, the sensory feedback in that area can be compromised. It may be necessary to boost confidence by first practicing in an easier, less emotionally charged area for a few repetitions. This will help them to understand how to listen to their sensations and learn the sense of the movement's quality. For example, a person with a chronically painful knee may find it easier to press out with their leg having first experienced the rhythm, timing, and sensation of a pushing movement with the arm.

4. **Clarify expectations.** Sometimes, the person tells you that they feel nothing because they are expecting something bigger or in some way different to what they are experiencing.

Example: I was working with a woman who had been struggling to regain normal function following major hip surgery. On this occasion we were performing a leg press into a fitness ball, aiming to take advantage of the sensory feedback that it provided. Despite clearly creating a force into that ball, she could not feel anything. We had tried a few techniques to see if we could elicit some sense of the leg, but nothing was working. So, we moved into the realm of associations. She had previously been a keen skier, so drawing on that, the relevant question was, "Can you sense different snow qualities through your boots or your skis? Hard icy snow, or powdery fragile snow, for example?" She replied that, yes, that was easy.

"Can you tap into the sensory memory of that right now, and how your legs would adapt to each different condition?" She answered again that this was clear and easy.

"Guess what? That is feeling!" I said. She was astonished.

We returned to the leg pressing task, with that idea in mind. Instead of frantically trying to find something without knowing what she was looking for, she began investigating the feel of the gently resistant ball against the sole of her foot and how she used her leg muscles to respond to its pressure. Using her existing associations switched on a light bulb – she learned how to sense her leg.

5. **Find yourself from outside in.** The sensory systems work collaboratively to enhance one another's performance, and this is powerful in helping people to sense themselves.

Tactile input, the interface between the outside world and your body's surface, can help to support proprioceptive and interoceptive processes. Research on balance demonstrated that just touching a single fingertip on a stable surface, without pressure, was enough to improve single leg balance.[14] Even more interestingly, lightly grasping a walking stick improved not just single leg balance while touching the cane but the next repetition when not touching it.[15] This demonstrates the usefulness of tactile input in enhancing proprioception. The input was tiny, yet the performance gain for the whole body was significant.

Tactile input also helps a body part to tell the brain, "Here I am!" Martial artists have long known the benefits of tactile muscle stimulation, slapping and sometimes pounding their muscles rhythmically with their hands as part of their warm up. Rubbing, tapping, and slapping an area prior to asking it to actively work can make connecting with it markedly easier. It is a simple, achievable way to tap into our ability to integrate our senses.

Visual input is also a source of intriguing effects. A study on interoception found that when people gazed quietly at themselves in a mirror, they became more aware of interoceptive signals arising from their bodies.[16] They connected what they saw reflected in the mirror with their sense of self: their interoceptive perception was improved by exteroceptive feedback.

Mirrors are frequently used purely to see visual markers. Although it can initially be helpful simply to observe that shoulders are raised, backs are arched, or knees are falling inwards, this isn't where the power lies. Take it further so that when somebody notes a particular visual marker, you ask them about the feeling of the movement when they perform it this way (e.g., where do they note the most pressure or work). Modify the movement and ask the same question. When the movement looks like this, does it feel the same or different? For some people, making the connection between what they see and what they feel is the transformative moment.

> When we learn to dance with the sensory systems, we are teaching mindful movement.

These applications can be applied to any form of movement training, and at any level. Some can be smoothly integrated into classes, whereas others lend themselves to more detailed individual work.

Respecting the sensory system and understanding its integration with the associative brain and how it links memory, imagery, and emotion, can bring a richness and subtlety to your work, and a deeper sense of ownership and involvement for your client.

Which part of the brain are you talking to?

Educating our clients and patients plays an incredibly important role in helping them to make positive choices, better understand their perceptions and beliefs, and boost their confidence through ownership of new knowledge.

Sometimes, however, our earnest and well-meaning stream of information appears to fall upon fallow ground, which can be frustrating! A student of mine once declared in a course, "Sometimes, I just want to tell the person to go away and only come back

when they are ready to listen!" This is not an unusual feeling, I am sure, but it is possible that in the case of some people, they are listening, but their brains cannot hear you.

When a person is experiencing stress, trauma, or fear, the amygdala (a part of the limbic system in the brain associated with survival-related emotional response) experiences a shift in its activity and behavior,[17] which, if sustained, can lead to feelings of helplessness and anxiety. When in this state, sensory information can be blocked from reaching memory and associative circuits. Learning then becomes exceptionally difficult, because we depend upon those associative circuits to make sense of the information that we are hearing.

Furthermore, when the limbic system is highly active under conditions of emotional stress or fear, activity can become suppressed in the prefrontal cortex,[18] which is the part of the brain involved in logical reasoning, decision making, planning, focus and attention, working memory, and a range of other features that come under the heading of executive function.[19]

This state contributes to what is called affective filter, a term coined by linguistics expert Stephen Krashen[20] to describe an emotional state of stress during which people are not responsive either to learning or to storing new information. Krashen used this term to describe barriers to learning a new language, which in many ways parallels the experience of a client stepping into the realms of training or rehabilitation for the first time.

How does this information help us?

First, in our interaction with a client, we might ask ourselves which part of their brain we are talking to. If providing technical information – on anatomy or muscle function, for example – we are speaking to the "executive brain," the prefrontal cortex. However, if the person is highly stressed, exhausted, nervous, and struggling with confidence, then from a brain perspective, this rational, thinking part of the brain might not be available. No matter how interesting and valuable your information is, the person just can't get it. Their thinking and reasoning brain is offline, while their emotional switchboard – the limbic system – is flashing colored lights of activity (see Fig. 15.1).

> A calm receptive state is fundamental for learning.

If you understand that someone's emotional circuitry needs to settle in order for them to be able to engage that executive brain, you need to set up your session accordingly.

It is helpful to begin with sensory connection tasks. Easy things, like slapping and vigorously rubbing the legs, arms, and abdomen are simple yet so powerful at bringing people into their bodies and lighting up parts of the brain affected by stress. Make it a ritual at the start of a session as a precursor to the warm-up, regardless of whether you are going to begin vigorously or peacefully.

Framing is helpful here. If your client is the type who prefers to burn off those fight and flight hormones with a "go hard or go home" session, give them the message that sensation input helps to prime neuromuscular performance, that connecting with the surface of the feet will boost the reflexes that drive leg muscle performance, and that taking a few moments on breathing awareness can make the biggest part of the lungs available for oxygen transfer. You are speaking to them in the language of performance and action, which bypasses their mental barriers, so that despite themselves, they start to connect and focus.

In terms of the environment, a person needs to feel safely able to experiment and explore, and to know that "mistakes" are simply learning opportunities.

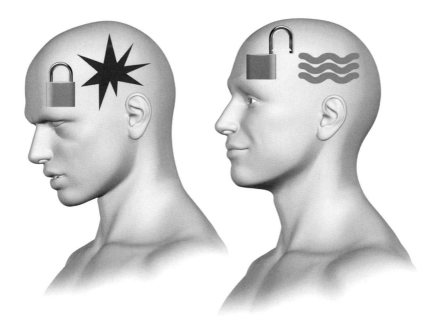

Figure 15.1

Calming the emotional brain unlocks the thinking brain

Often people are given a rule, are trained to practice based on that rule, and are judged on how well they adhere to it. These are people who don't dare to practice on their own in case they "get it wrong," and feel apprehension when introduced to something new. This amplifies the affective filter. We can overcome this by teaching in a way that encourages a person to articulate what they notice about themselves when performing a movement or task. To improve that performance, offer cues that allow them to compare and contrast their sensory experience. An example might be: "Where do you notice the pressure under your foot right now? And when your pressure is there, what do you notice about your knee? I wonder what would happen if you moved the pressure toward the center/front/outside/inside of your foot – where does your knee go now? Ah, so it seems that your foot and your knee talk to each other – what conversation would you like them to have?"

Teaching this way not only establishes a collaborative relationship with your clients, it boosts self-confidence by stimulating a very personal level of knowledge – one that is developed through their own senses.

Power points

- We are able to effectively navigate our lives in real time because our brains are constantly making predictions based on our huge database of previous experiences and associations, assets that we can use in our movement teaching.

- To improve movement, traditional approaches talk to the thinking brain. Neuroscience guides us to talk to the "feeling brain," accessing wider networks through our sensory experience.

- By integrating mind, emotion, and body, we truly work holistically.

I can't go back to yesterday because I was a different person then.

Alice, *Alice's Adventures in Wonderland*, Lewis Carroll

And so, we reach the end of what is really just a beginning.

There is no way to capture in a single book the magnitude and scope of what it is to work with movement. I have always been predisposed to a sense of wonder, but as this journey has unfolded, I have found myself even more awestruck, beguiled, and humbled by the vastness and promise of what is yet to be learned.

There are so many valuable approaches, techniques, and philosophies to draw from as we develop our movement kaleidoscope. Personally, I roll and crawl, jump and hop, swing and curl, lift some weights, dance a bit when I can, work in some yoga, and generally mix up my physical explorations regularly. It all has value when done mindfully, with curiosity and the intention to respectfully yet persistently expand capability and capacity based on the principles of normal movement.

Normal healthy movement, as it turns out, is variable, adaptable, responsive, and individual. It resists rigid rules, and explores possibilities. As we have tracked it through these pages together, we have discovered that physics is a friend to us, and that the ease with which we manage forces sets our movement free. We have learned that control is a dance, not a fight, and that stability does not arise from the strength of our resistance but from the breadth of our choices. Above all, we can appreciate that the interplay between our sensory selves, our emotions, our memories, beliefs, and

perceptions has more power to change our movement than any magic exercise.

For the movement professional, there is an assurance that you don't have to choose between being science based or heart centered, and that to work holistically is not a choice but an imperative if we are to help people to overcome their barriers and learn to own and love their movement.

The field of movement research is perhaps at its most fluid and dynamic ever. Anatomy, which until relatively recently we thought we had pretty much mastered, has turned out major advances in the past few years with the help of new technology. Our understanding of our mechanics and how we use ourselves is a continuously evolving field, and many long-held assumptions about how our bodies work have been overturned. That's even before we consider the advances in brain science – a subject that gives us a wonderland of new insights to explore. It means that some things that we thought were facts are actually no more than widely perpetuated beliefs. That can sting, and sometimes we resist what is unfamiliar.

Just remember, though, that when you feel that disturbing sense that your footing is unstable, you may simply be standing on an escalator. Let it carry you to a higher level. If you maintain a sense of wonder, it dissolves the discomfort of uncertainty, transforming it instead into a space for your curiosity to roam. Have the courage to evolve your practice to truly reflect the interface between the emerging science and your own personal experiences and observations, without fear of censure from those who prefer to stay safely in their boxes. The kaleidoscope of our interrelated systems is a limitless playground for this process of independent inquiry and exploration.

And, finally, we finish where we began: in our pursuit of the power and the grace. Power is the ability to access your potential and unleash it to manifest your will. Grace is the deployment of that power under the conditions of choice and freedom. I hope that through these pages, you will discover them both for yourself.

GLOSSARY

Anti-movement: a stabilizing strategy that limits global body motion for the purpose of resisting force.

ASIS: anterior superior iliac spine. The most easily palpable bony points on the front of the pelvic bones.

Body segment: the link between two joints.

Catastrophizing: a common cognitive distortion, causing a tendency to imagine the worst possible outcome in response to an event, experience, or sensation.

Co-contraction: the simultaneous contraction of muscles with opposing actions about a joint to enhance joint stability.

Concentric: as the muscle contracts, it shortens (e.g., the biceps in a bicep curl).

Dissociation: the ability to move a body part smoothly and independently of other parts.

Distal: the part of a body structure that is farthest from your body's center (e.g., your foot is more distal to the hip than your knee).

Eccentric: as the muscle contracts, it lengthens (e.g., the quadriceps as you move into a deep squat).

Exteroception: the perception and processing of stimuli originating outside the body (e.g., heat, light).

Fascia: the continuity of connective tissue lying beneath the skin that encloses, supports, and provides attachments for body structures such as muscles and the internal organs. Also involved in proprioception and energy transfer during movement.

Flexibility: the range of motion allowed by the joints and soft tissues; this available range of motion is a pre-requisite for *functional mobility*.

Force: an interaction that can induce motion of an object and involves both magnitude and direction.

Functional Force Management®: the array of strategies that enable the body to create, control, and withstand the forces associated with movement.

Functional mobility: the ability to move freely and with control through the full range of motion required.

Functional stability: the ability to meet the load and control demands of the required movement task.

Grey matter: consisting of nerve cell bodies and nerve fibers, this is a major component of the central nervous system, from which the central core of the spinal cord and the cerebral cortex is composed.

Ground reaction force (GRF): the force exerted by the ground on a body in contact with it.

Held tension: an unconscious tendency to maintain muscles in a persistently heightened level of contraction.

Inner range: the muscle is acting when it is shortest (e.g., bend your elbow all the way and then try to squeeze it towards your shoulder a little further).

Interoception: the sense of one's own internal body and its workings (e.g., hunger, heartbeat).

Isometric: the muscle does not change length as it contracts.

JEMS®: Joanne Elphinston Movement Systems

Kinetic chain: the interaction between linked body segments involved in a specific motion.

Mid-range: the point between the most shortened and most lengthened position of the muscle, where the contraction is strongest.

Movement impulse: the sense of intended movement direction and quality.

Neuromuscular responses: automatic, unconscious patterns of muscle activity that prepare for, or react to expected or unexpected forces.

Neuroplasticity: the nervous system's constant reorganization of its structure, function, and connections in response to the stimuli that it encounters.

Outer range: the muscle is contracting at its longest (e.g., in a pull-up, starting with your elbows straight would be starting in outer range as the biceps are at their longest).

Pandiculation: a behavior that regulates tension in the nervous system via the active, self-resisted lengthening of muscles across multiple body segments.

Point of preparation: the area of the body that first responds to the impulse to move.

Priming: the use of a specific stimulus, cue, or experience to influence the response to a subsequent stimulus.

Proprioception: awareness of joint position or joint motion generated from sensory feedback from the body.

Proximal: the part of a body structure that is closest to your body's center (e.g., your elbow is more proximal than your hand).

Self-efficacy: an individual's intrinsic belief in their capability to achieve a goal.

Stability: the ability to maintain a state of postural equilibrium and joint integrity in the body.

Strength: the ability to exert sufficient force to overcome resistance.

Tensegrity: the balance of tension and compression acting on a skeletal structure to preserve its integral stability.

Vestibular system: the sensory system housed within our inner ear that plays a major role in balance, orientation of the body, and control of eye movements with respect to head position.

REFERENCES

Chapter 1

1. Campbell A, Kemp-Smith K, O'Sullivan P, Straker L. Abdominal bracing increases ground reaction forces and reduces knee and hip flexion during landing. J Orthop Sports Phys Ther. 2016;46(4):286–92.

2. Hodges PW, Richardson CA. Feedforward contraction of transversus abdominis is influenced by the direction of arm movement. Exp Brain Res. 1997;114(2):362–70.

3. Hodges PW. Changes in motor planning of feedforward postural responses of the trunk muscles in low back pain. Exp Brain Res. 2001;141(2):261–6.

4. Mannion AF, Caporaso F, Pulkovski N and Sprott H. Spine stabilisation exercises in the treatment of chronic low back pain: a good clinician outcome is not associated with improved abdominal function. Eur Spine J. 2012;21(7):1301–10.

5. Beales D, Smith A, O'Sullivan P, Hunter M, Straker L. Back pain beliefs are related to the impact of low back pain in baby boomers in the Busselton Healthy Aging Study. Phys Ther. 2015;95(2): 180–9.

6. O'Sullivan PB, Caneiro JP, O'Keeffe M, Smith A, Dankaerts W, Fersum K, O'Sullivan K. Cognitive functional therapy: an integrated behavioral approach for the targeted management of disabling low back pain. Phys Ther. 2018;98(5):408–23.

7. Saragiotto BT, Maher CG, Yamato TP, Costa LO, Menezes Costa LC, Ostelo RW, Macedo LG. Motor control exercise for chronic non-specific low-back pain. Cochrane Database Syst Rev. 2016 Jan 8; (1):CD012004.

8. Miyamoto GC, Costa LO, Cabral CM. Efficacy of the Pilates method for pain and disability in patients with chronic nonspecific low back pain: a systematic review with meta-analysis. Braz J Phys Ther. 2013;17(6):517–32.

9. Grenier SG, McGill SM. Quantification of lumbar stability by using 2 different abdominal activation strategies. Arch Phys Med Rehabil. 2007;88(1):54–62.

10. Tsao H, Hodges PW. Immediate changes in feedforward postural adjustments following voluntary motor training. Exp Brain Res. 2007;181(4):537–46.

11. Meisingset I, Woodhouse A, Stensdotter AK, Stavdahl Ø, Lorås H, Gismervik S, Andresen H, Austreim K, Vasseljen O. Evidence for a general stiffening motor control pattern in neck pain: a cross sectional study. BMC Musculoskelet Disord. 2015 Dec;16(1):56.

12. Tsai LC, McLean S, Colletti PM, Powers CM. Greater muscle co-contraction results in increased tibiofemoral compressive forces in females who have undergone anterior cruciate ligament reconstruction. J Orthop Res. 2012;30(12):2007–14.

13. Hodges PW, Coppieters MW, MacDonald D, Cholewicki J. New insight into motor adaptation to pain revealed by a combination of modelling and empirical approaches. Eur J Pain. 2013;17(8):1138–46.

14. Mok NW, Brauer SG, Hodges PW. Changes in lumbar movement in people with low back pain are related to compromised balance. Spine. 2011;36(1):E45–52.

15. Cholewicki J1, Silfies SP, Shah RA, Greene HS, Reeves NP, Alvi K, Goldberg B. Delayed trunk muscle reflex responses increase the risk of low back injuries. Spine 2005;30(23): 2614–20.

16. Hodges P, van den Hoorn W, Dawson A, Cholewicki J. Changes in the mechanical properties of the trunk in low back pain may be associated with recurrence. J Biomech. 2009;5:42(1):61–6.

17. Granacher U, Gollhofer A, Hortobágyi T, Kressig RW, Muehlbauer T. The importance of trunk muscle strength for balance, functional performance, and fall prevention in seniors: a systematic review. Sports Med. 2013;43(7): 627–41.

18. Martinez AF, Lessi GC, Carvalho C, Serrao FV. Association of hip and trunk strength with three-dimensional trunk, hip, and knee kinematics during a single-leg drop vertical jump. J Strength Cond Res. 2018;32(7):1902–8.

19. Willy RW, Davis IS. The effect of a hip-strengthening program on mechanics during running and during a single-leg squat. J Orthop Sports Phys Ther. 2011;41(9):625–32.

20. Willson JD, Kernozek TW, Arndt RL, Reznichek DA, Scott Straker J. Gluteal muscle activation during running in females with and without patellofemoral pain syndrome. Clin Biomech. 2011;26(7):735–40.

21. Noehren B, Scholz J, Davis I. The effect of real-time gait retraining on hip kinematics, pain and function in subjects with patellofemoral pain syndrome. Br J Sports Med. 2011;45(9):691–6.

22. Willy RW, Scholz JP, Davis IS. Mirror gait retraining for the treatment of patellofemoral pain in female runners. Clin Biomech (Bristol, Avon). 2012;27(10):1045–51.

23. Barendrecht M, Lezeman HC, Duysens J, Smits-Engelsman BC. Neuromuscular training improves knee kinematics, in particular in valgus aligned adolescent team handball players of both sexes. J Strength Cond Res. 2011;25(3): 575–84.

24. Online Etymology Dictionary. [accessed 15 May 2019] Available at: www.etymonline.com/word/kaleidoscope#etymonline_v_1769

Chapter 2

1. Kleim JA, Jones TA. Principles of experience-dependent neural plasticity: implications for rehabilitation after brain damage. J Speech Lang Hear Res. 2008;51(1):S225–39

2. Tsao H, Danneels LA, Hodges PW. ISSLS prize winner: smudging the motor brain in young adults with recurrent low back pain. Spine (Phila Pa 1976). 2011 Oct 1; 36(21):1721–7.

3. Makin TR, Filippini N, Duff EP, Henderson Slater D, Tracey I, Johansen-Berg H. Network-level reorganisation of functional connectivity following arm amputation. Neuroimage. 2015;114:217–25.

4. Schwenkreis P, El Tom S, Ragert P, Pleger B, Tegenthoff M, Dinse HR. Assessment of sensorimotor cortical representation asymmetries and motor skills in violin players. Eur J Neurosci. 2007;26(11):3291–302.

5. Last N, Tufts E, Auger LE. The effects of meditation on grey matter atrophy and neurodegeneration: a systematic review. J Alzheimers Dis. 2017;56(1):275–86.

6. Woollett K, Maguire EA. Acquiring 'the Knowledge' of London's layout drives structural brain changes. Curr Biol. 2011;21(24):2109–14.

7. Müller P, Rehfeld K, Schmicker M, Hökelmann A, Dordevic M, Lessmann V, Brigadski T, Kaufmann J, Müller NG. Evolution of neuroplasticity in response to physical activity in old age: the case for dancing. Front Aging Neurosci. 2017;9:56.

8. Mah L, Szabuniewicz C, Fiocco AJ. Can anxiety damage the brain? Curr Opin Psychiatry. 2016;29(1):56–63.

9. McEwen BS. Glucocorticoids, depression, and mood disorders: structural remodeling in the brain. Metabolism. 2005;54(5 Suppl 1):20–3.

10. McEwen BS. In pursuit of resilience: stress, epigenetics, and brain plasticity. Ann NY Acad Sci. 2016;1373(1):56–64.

11. Braden BB, Pipe TB, Smith R, Glaspy TK, Deatherage BR, Baxter LC. Brain and behavior changes associated with an abbreviated 4-week mindfulness-based stress reduction course in back pain patients. Brain Behav. 2016;16;6(3):e00443.

12 Bullmore E, Sporns O. The economy of brain network organization. Nat Rev Neurosci. 2012;13:336–49.

13. Voogd J, Barmack NH. Oculomotor cerebellum. Prog Brain Res. 2006;151: 231–68.

14. Sens PM, Almeida CI, Souza MM, Gonçalves JB, Carmo LC. The role of the cerebellum in auditory processing using the SSI test. Braz J Otorhinolaryngol. 2011;77(5):584–8.

15. Parsons LM, Petacchi A, Schmahmann JD, Bower JM. Pitch discrimination in cerebellar patients: evidence for a sensory deficit. Brain Res. 2009;15;1303:84–96.

16. Narayanan S, Thirumalai V. Contributions of the cerebellum for predictive and instructional control of movement. Curr Opin Physiol. 2019;8:146–51.

17. Moberget T, Ivry RB. Cerebellar contributions to motor control and language comprehension: searching for common computational principles. Ann N Y Acad Sci. 2016;1369(1):154–71.

18. Adamaszek M, D'Agata F, Ferrucci R, Habas C, Keulen S, Kirkby KC, Leggio M, Mariën P, Molinari M, Moulton E, Orsi L, Van Overwalle F, Papadelis C, Priori A, Sacchetti B, Schutter DJ, Styliadis C, Verhoeven J. Consensus Paper: Cerebellum and emotion. Cerebellum. 2017;16(2):552–76.

19. Manto, M and Bastian, AJ. Cerebellum and the deciphering of motor coding. The Cerebellum. 2007;6(1):3–6.

20. Strick PL, Dum RP, Fiez JA.Cerebellum and nonmotor function. Annu Rev Neurosci. 2009;32:413–34.

21. Kipping JA, Grodd W, Kumar V, Taubert M, Villringer A, Margulies DS. Overlapping and parallel cerebello-cerebral networks contributing to sensorimotor control: an intrinsic functional connectivity study. Neuroimage. 2013;83:837–48.

22. Sokolov AA, Miall RC, Ivry RB. The Cerebellum: Adaptive prediction for movement and cognition trends in cognitive sciences, 2017;21(5):313–32.

23. Aridan N, Mukamel R. Activity in primary motor cortex during action observation covaries with subsequent behavioral changes in execution. Brain Behav. 2016;6(11):e00550.

24. Helm F, Marinovic W, Krüger B Munzert J, Riek S. Corticospinal excitability during imagined and observed dynamic force production tasks: effortfulness matters. Neuroscience. 2015;290:398–405.

25. Eaves DL, Haythornthwaite L, Vogt S. Motor imagery during action observation modulates automatic imitation effects in rhythmical actions. Front Hum Neurosci. 2014;8:28.

26. Dimberg U, Thunberg M, Elmehed K. Unconscious facial reactions to emotional facial expressions. Psychol Sci. 2000;11(1):86–9.

27. Hennenlotter A, Dresel C, Castrop F, Ceballos-Baumann AO, Wohlschläger AM, Haslinger B. The link between facial feedback and neural activity within

central circuitries of emotion—new insights from botulinum toxin-induced denervation of frown muscles. Cereb Cortex. 2009;19(3):537–42.

28. Strack F, Martin LL, Stepper S. Inhibiting and facilitating conditions of the human smile: a nonobtrusive test of the facial feedback hypothesis. J Pers Soc Psychol. 1988;54(5):768–77.

29. Mori K, Mori H. Another test of the passive facial feedback hypothesis: when your face smiles, you feel happy. Percept Mot Skills. 2009;109(1):76–8.

30. Larsen RJ, Kasimatis M, Frey K. Facilitating the furrowed brow: an unobtrusive test of the facial feedback hypothesis applied to unpleasant affect. Cogn Emot. 1992;6(5):321–38.

31. Grossi JA, Maitra KK, Rice MS. Semantic priming of motor task performance in young adults: implications for occupational therapy. Am J Occup Ther. 2007;61(3):311–20.

32. Wulf G, Chiviacowsky S, Lewthwaite R. Altering mindset can enhance motor learning in older adults. Psychol Aging. 2012;27(1):14–21.

33. Tomasino B, Weiss PH, Fink GR. To move or not to move: imperatives modulate action-related verb processing in the motor system. Neuroscience. 2010;169(1):246–58.

34. Bar M. The proactive brain: using analogies and associations to generate predictions. Trends Cogn Sci. 2007;(7):280–9.

Chapter 3

1. Zhao R, Zhang M, Zhang Q. The effectiveness of combined exercise interventions for preventing postmenopausal bone loss: a systematic review and meta-analysis. J Orthop Sports Phys Ther. 2017;47(4):241–51.

2. Ma D, Wu L, He Z. Effects of walking on the preservation of bone mineral density in perimenopausal and postmenopausal women: a systematic review and meta-analysis. Menopause. 2013;20(11):1216–26.

3. Zhao R, Zhao M, Xu Z. The effects of differing resistance training modes on the preservation of bone mineral density in postmenopausal women: a meta-analysis. Osteoporos Int. 2015;26(5):1605–18.

4. Zhao R, Zhao M, Zhang L. Efficiency of jumping exercise in improving bone mineral density among premenopausal women: a meta-analysis. Sports Med. 2014;44(10):1393–402.

5. Xu J, Lombardi G, Jiao W, Banfi G. Effects of exercise on bone status in female subjects, from young girls to postmenopausal women: an overview of systematic reviews and meta-analyses. Sports Med. 2016;46(8):1165–82.

6. Belavý DL, Quittner MJ, Ridgers N, Ling Y, Connell D, Rantalainen T. Running exercise strengthens the intervertebral disc. Sci Rep. 7: 45975. PMCID: PMC5396190 Published online 2017 Apr 19. doi: 10.1038/srep45975.

7. Stanley LE, Lucero A, Mauntel TC, Kennedy M, Walker N, Marshall SW, Padua DA, Berkoff DJ. Achilles tendon adaptation in cross-country runners across a competitive season. Scand J Med Sci Sports. 2017 Apr 28. doi: 10.1111/sms.12903. [Epub ahead of print]

8. Narici MV, Maganaris CN. Adaptability of elderly human muscles and tendons to increased loading J Anat. 2008;208(4):433–43.

9. Hodges PW and Richardson CA. Feedforward contraction of transversus abdominis is influenced by the direction of arm movement. Exp Brain Res. 1997;114(2):362–70.

Chapter 4

1. Wilke J, Schleip R, Yucesoy CA, Banzer W. Not merely a protective packing organ? A review of fascia and its force transmission capacity. J Appl Physiol (1985). 2018;124(1):234–44.

2. Schleip R, Muller DG. Training principles for fascial connective tissues: scientific foundation and suggested practical applications. J Bodyw Mov Ther. 2013;17:103–15.

3. Findley T, Chaudhry H, Dhar S. Transmission of muscle force to fascia during exercise. J Bodywork & Movement Therapies 2015;19, 119–123.

4. Maas H, Sandercock TG. Force transmission between synergistic skeletal muscles through connective tissue linkages. J Biomed Biotechnol. 2010;2010:575672. Accessed 17 May 2019. doi: 10.1155/2010/575672. PubMed Central ID: PMC2853902.

5. Wager JC, Challis JH. Elastic energy within the human plantar aponeurosis contributes to arch shortening during the push-off phase of running. J Biomech. 2016;49(5):704–9.

6. Eng CM, Arnold AS, Lieberman DE, Biewener AA. The capacity of the human iliotibial band to store elastic energy during running. J Biomech. 2015;48(12):3341–8.

7. Elphinston J. Stability, sport and performance movement. Chichester, UK: Lotus; 2013.

8. Myers T. Anatomy trains. London: Churchill Livingstone; 2001.

9. Mooney V, Pozos R, Vleeming A, Gulick J, Swenski D. Exercise treatment for sacroiliac pain. Orthopedics. 2001;24: 29–32.

10. Willard FH, Vleeming A, Schuenke MD, Danneels L, Schleip R. The thoracolumbar fascia: anatomy, function and clinical considerations. J Anat. 2012;221(6):507–36.

11. Bertolucci LF. Pandiculation: nature's way of maintaining the functional integrity of the myofascial system? J Bodyw Mov Ther. 2011;15(3):268–80.

12. Myers T. Foam rolling and self-myofascial release. 2015. [Accessed August 20, 2019] Available: www.anatomytrains.com/blog/2015/04/27/foam-rolling-and-self-myofascial-release.

Chapter 5

1. Rosário JL, Diógenes MS, Mattei R, Leite JR. J Bodyw Mov Ther. Angry posture. 2016;20(3):457–60.

2. Cuddy, A. Presence: Bringing your boldest self to your biggest challenges. Orion-London. 2016; pp 156–157.

3. Canales JZ, Fiquer JT, Campos RN, Soeiro-de-Souza MG, Moreno RA. Investigation of associations between recurrence of major depressive disorder and spinal posture alignment: a quantitative cross-sectional study. Gait Posture. 2017;52:258–64.

4. Michalak J, Mischnat J, Teismann T. Sitting posture makes a difference-embodiment effects on depressive memory bias. Clin Psychol Psychother. 2014;21(6):519–24.

5. Nair S, Sagar M, Sollers J 3rd, Consedine N, Broadbent E. Do slumped and upright postures affect stress responses? A randomized trial. Health Psychol. 2015;34(6):632–41.

6. Wilkes C, Kydd R, Sagar M, Broadbent E. Upright posture improves affect and

fatigue in people with depressive symptoms. J Behav Ther Exp Psychiatry. 2017;54:143–9.

7. Carney DR, Cuddy AJ, Yap AJ. Power posing: brief nonverbal displays affect neuroendocrine levels and risk tolerance. Psychol Sci. 2010;21(10):1363–8.

8. Laird JD. Self-attribution of emotion: the effects of expressive behavior on the quality of emotional experience. J Pers Soc Psychol. 1974;29(4):475–86.

9. Söderkvist S, Ohlén K, Dimberg U. How the experience of emotion is modulated by facial feedback. J Nonverbal Behav. 2018;42(1):129–51.

10. Strack F, Martin LL, Stepper S. Inhibiting and facilitating conditions of the human smile: a nonobtrusive test of the facial feedback hypothesis. J Pers Soc Psychol. 1988;54(5):768–77.

11. Hodges PW, Gurfinkel VS, Brumagne S, Smith TC, Cordo P. Coexistence of stability and mobility in postural control: evidence from postural compensation for respiration. Exp Brain Res. 2002;144(3):293–302.

12. Grimstone SK, Hodges PW. Impaired postural compensation for respiration in people with recurrent low back pain. Exp Brain Res. 2003;151(2):218–24.

13. Kiers H, van Dieën JH, Brumagne S, Vanhees L. Postural sway and integration of proprioceptive signals in subjects with LBP. Hum Mov Sci. 2015;39:109–20.

14. Fujitani R, Jiromaru T, Kida N, Nomura T. Effect of standing postural deviations on trunk and hip muscle activity. J Phys Ther Sci. 2017;29(7):1212–15.

15. Reeve A, Dilley A. Effects of posture on the thickness of transversus abdominis in pain-free subjects. Man Ther. 2009;14(6):679–84.

16. Beer A, Treleaven J, Jull G. Can a functional postural exercise improve performance in the cranio-cervical flexion test? – a preliminary study. Man Ther. 2012 Jun;17(3):219–24.

17. Dichgans J, Diener HC. The contribution of vestibulo-spinal mechanisms to the maintenance of human upright posture. Acta Otolaryngol. 1989;107(5–6):338–45.

18. Kulkarni V, Chandy MJ, Babu KS. Quantitative study of muscle spindles in suboccipital muscles of human foetuses. Neurol India. 2001;49(4):355–9.

19. Kogler A, Lindfors J, Odkvist LM, Ledin T. Postural stability using different neck positions in normal subjects and patients with neck trauma. Acta Otolaryngol. 2000;120(2):151–5.

20. Johnson MB, Van Emmerik R EA. Effect of head orientation on postural control during upright stance and forward lean. Motor Control. 2012;16(1):81–93.

21. Treleaven J. Dizziness, unsteadiness, visual disturbances, and sensorimotor control in traumatic neck pain. J Orthop Sports Phys Ther. 2017;47(7):492–502.

22. Johnson MB, Van Emmerik RE. Is head-on-trunk extension a proprioceptive mediator of postural control and sit-to-stand movement characteristics? J Mot Behav. 2011;43(6):491–8.

23. Roll R, Kavounoudias A, Roll JP. Cutaneous afferents from human plantar sole contribute to body posture awareness. Neuroreport. 2002;13(15):1957–61.

24. Masi AT, Nair K, Evans T, Ghandour Y. Clinical, biomechanical, and physiological translational interpretations of human resting myofascial tone or tension. Int J Ther Massage Bodywork. 2010;3(4):16–28.

25. Stecco C, Gagey O, Belloni A, Pozzuoli A, Porzionato A, Macchi V, Aldegheri R, De Caro R, Delmas V. Anatomy of the deep fascia of the upper limb. Second part: study of innervation. Morphologie. 2007;91(292):38–43.

26. Gogola A, Saulicz E, Kuszewski M, Matyja M, Myśliwiec A. Development of low postural tone compensatory patterns – predicted dysfunction patterns in upper part of the body. Dev Period Med. 2014;18(3):380–5.

27. Gogola A, Saulicz E, Kuszewski M, Matyja M, Myśliwiec A. Development of low postural tone compensatory patterns in children – theoretical basis. Dev Period Med. 2014;18(3):374–9.

28. Alghadir A, Zafar H, Whitney SL, Iqbal Z. Effect of chewing on postural stability during quiet standing in healthy young males. Somatosens Mot Res. 2015;32(2):72–6.

29. Alghadir AH, Zafar H, Iqbal ZA. Effect of tongue position on postural stability during quiet standing in healthy young males. Somatosens Mot Res. 2015;32(3):183–6.

30. Gurfinkel V, Cacciatore TW, Cordo P, Horak F, Nutt J, Skoss R. Postural muscle tone in the body axis of healthy humans. J Neurophysiol. 2006;96(5):2678–87.

Chapter 6

1. Hodges PW, Coppieters MW, MacDonald D, Cholewicki J. New insight into motor adaptation to pain revealed by a combination of modelling and empirical approaches. Eur J Pain. 2013;17(8):1138–46.

2. Tsao H, Galea MP, Hodges PW. How fast are feedforward postural adjustments of the abdominal muscles? Behav Neurosci. 2009;123(3):687–93.

3. Lee LJ, Coppieters MW, Hodges PW. Anticipatory postural adjustments to arm movement reveal complex control of paraspinal muscles in the thorax. J Electromyogr Kinesiol. 2009;19(1):46–54.

4. Müller R, Häufle DF, Blickhan R. Preparing the leg for ground contact in running: the contribution of feed-forward and visual feedback. J Exp Biol. 2015;218(Pt 3):451–7.

5. Cholewicki J, Silfies SP, Shah RA, Greene HS, Reeves NP, Alvi K, Goldberg B. Delayed trunk muscle reflex responses increase the risk of low back injuries. Spine. 2005;30(23):2614–20.

6. Vleeming A, Schuenke MD, Danneels L, Willard FH. The functional coupling of the deep abdominal and paraspinal muscles: the effects of simulated paraspinal muscle contraction on force transfer to the middle and posterior layer of the thoracolumbar fascia. J Anat. 2014;225(4):447–62.

7. Ward SR, Kim CW, Eng CM, Gottschalk LJ 4th, Tomiya A, Garfin SR, Lieber RL. Architectural analysis and intraoperative measurements demonstrate the unique design of the multifidus muscle for lumbar spine stability. J Bone Joint Surg Am. 2009;91(1):176–85.

8. Regev GJ, Kim CW, Tomiya A, Lee YP, Ghofrani H, Garfin SR, Lieber RL, Ward SR. Psoas muscle architectural design, in vivo sarcomere length range, and passive tensile properties support its role as a lumbar spine stabilizer. Spine. 2011;15;36(26):E1666–74.

9. Laird RA, Keating JL, Ussing K, Li P, Kent P. Does movement matter in people with back pain? Investigating "atypical" lumbo-pelvic kinematics in people with and without back pain using wireless movement sensors. BMC Musculoskelet Disord. 2019;20(1):28.

10. Bordoni B and Marelli F. Failed back surgery syndrome: review and new hypotheses. J Pain Res. 2016;9:17–22.

11. Bordoni B and Zanier E. Anatomic connections of the diaphragm: influence of respiration on the body system. J Multidiscip Healthc. 2013;6:281–91.

12. Liao D, Lottrup C, Fynne L, McMahon BP, Krogh K, Drewes AM, Zhao J, Gregersen H. Axial movements and length changes of the human lower esophageal sphincter during respiration and distension-induced secondary peristalsis using functional luminal imaging probe. 2018;24(2):255–67.

13. Li C, Chang Q, Zhang J, Chai W. Effects of slow breathing rate on heart rate variability and arterial baroreflex sensitivity in essential hypertension. Medicine (Baltimore). 2018;97(18):e0639.

14. Eherer AJ, Netolitzky F, Högenauer C, Puschnig G, Hinterleitner TA, Scheidl S, Kraxner W, Krejs GJ, Hoffmann KM. Positive effect of abdominal breathing exercise on gastroesophageal reflux disease: a randomized, controlled study. Am J Gastroenterol. 2012;107(3):372–8.

15. Skandalakis PN, Zoras O, Skandalakis JE, Mirilas P. Transversalis, endoabdominal, endothoracic fascia: who's who? Am Surg. 2006;72(1):16–18.

16. Abu-Hijleh MF, Habbal OA, Moqattash ST. The role of the diaphragm in lymphatic absorption from the peritoneal cavity. J Anat. 1995;186(Pt 3):453–67.

17. Talasz H, Kremser C, Kofler M, Kalchschmid E, Lechleitner M, Rudisch A. Phase-locked parallel movement of diaphragm and pelvic floor during breathing and coughing—a dynamic MRI investigation in healthy females. Int Urogynecol J. 2011;22(1):61–8.

18. Hodges PW, Eriksson AE, Shirley D, Gandevia SC. Intra-abdominal pressure increases stiffness of the lumbar spine. J Biomech. 2005;38:1873–80.

19. Bordoni B and Morabito B. Symptomatology correlations between the diaphragm and irritable bowel syndrome Cureus. 2018;10(7):e3036.

20. Hagman C, Janson C, Emtner M. Breathing retraining – a five-year follow-up of patients with dysfunctional breathing. Respir Med. 2011;105(8):1153–9.

21. Jerath R, Crawford MW. How does the body affect the mind? Role of cardiorespiratory coherence in the spectrum of emotions. Adv Mind Body Med. 2015;29(4):4–16.

22. Herschorn S. Female pelvic floor anatomy: the pelvic floor, supporting structures, and pelvic organs. Rev Urol. 2004; 6(Suppl 5):S2–S10.

23. Tuttle LJ, Nguyen OT, Cook MS, Alperin M, Shah SB, Ward SR, Lieber RL. Architectural design of the pelvic floor is consistent with muscle functional subspecialization. Int Urogynecol J. 2014;25(2):205–12.

24. Rejano-Campo M, Desvergée A, Pizzoferrato AC. Relationship between perineal characteristics and symptoms and pelvic girdle pain: a literature review. Prog Urol. 2018;28(4):193–208

25. Hetrick DC, Ciol MA, Rothman I, Turner JA, Frest M, Berger RE. Musculoskeletal dysfunction in men with chronic pelvic pain syndrome type III: a case-control study. J Urol. 2003;170: 828–31.

26. Faubion S, Shuster L, Bharucha A. Recognition and management of nonrelaxing pelvic floor dysfunction. Mayo Clin Proc. 2012;87(2):187–93.

27. Gilpin SA, Gosling JA, Smith ARB, Warrell DW. The pathogenesis of genitourinary prolapse and stress incontinence of urine. A histological and histochemical study. Br J Obstet Gynaecol. 1989;96:15–23.

28. Strasser H, Steinlechner M, Bartsch G. Morphometric analysis of the rhabdosphincter of the male urethra. J Urol. 1997;157(Suppl 4):177–80.

29. Aydın Sayılan A, Özbaş A. The effect of pelvic floor muscle training on incontinence problems after radical prostatectomy Am J Mens Health. 1997;12(4):1007–15.

30. Van Kampen M, De Weerdt W, Claes H, et al.. Treatment of erectile dysfunction by perineal exercise, electromyographic biofeedback, and electrical stimulation. Phys Ther. 2003;83:536–43.

31. Rosenbaum TY. Pelvic floor involvement in male and female sexual dysfunction and the role of pelvic floor rehabilitation in treatment: a literature review. J Sex Med. 2007;4:4–13.

32. Teixeira RV, Colla C, Sbruzzi G, Mallmann A, Paiva LL. Prevalence of urinary incontinence in female athletes: a systematic review with meta-analysis. Int Urogynecol J. 2018;29(12):1717–25.

33. Hodges PW, Gandevia SC. Activation of the human diaphragm during a repetitive postural task. J Physiol. 2000;522 Pt 1: 165–75.

34. Gandevia SC, Butler JE, Hodges PW, Taylor JL. Balancing acts: respiratory sensations, motor control and human posture. Clin Exp Pharmacol Physiol. 2002;29(1-2):118–21.

35. Nygaard IE, Glowacki C, Saltzman CL. Relationship between foot flexibility and urinary incontinence in nulliparous varsity athletes. Obstet Gynecol. 1996;87(6):1049–51.

Chapter 7

1. Patwardhan AG, Havey RM, Meade KP, Lee B, Dunlap B. A follower load increases the load-carrying capacity of the lumbar spine in compression. Spine. 1999;24(10):1003–9.

2. Patwardhan AG, Meade KP, Lee B. A frontal plane model of the lumbar spine subjected to a follower load: implications for the role of muscles. J Biomech Eng. 2001;123(3):212–17.

3. Christiansen BA, Bouxsein ML. Biomechanics of vertebral fractures and the vertebral fracture cascade. Curr Osteoporos Rep. 2010;8(4):198–204.

4. Noguchi M, Gooyers CE, Karakolis T, Noguchi K, Callaghan JP. Is intervertebral disc pressure linked to herniation?: An in-vitro study using a porcine model. J Biomech. 2016;49(9):1824–30.

5. Barrett JM, Gooyers CE, Karakolis T, Callaghan JP. The impact of posture on the mechanical properties of a functional spinal unit during cyclic compressive loading J Biomech Eng. 2016;138(8). Paper No: BIO-15-1516.

6. Parkinson RJ, Callaghan JP. The role of dynamic flexion in spine injury is altered by increasing dynamic load magnitude. Clin Biomech. 2009;24(2):148–54.

7. Kim SH, Kwon OY, Yi CH, Cynn HS, Ha SM, Park KN. Lumbopelvic motion during seated hip flexion in subjects with low-back pain accompanying limited hip flexion. Eur Spine J. 2014;23(1):142–8.

8. Sjolie AN. Low-back pain in adolescents is associated with poor hip mobility and high body mass index. Scand J Med Sci Sports. 2004;14(3):168–75.

9. Hasebe K, Sairyo K, Hada Y, Dezawa A, Okubo Y, Kaneoka K, Nakamura Y. Spino-pelvic-rhythm with forward trunk bending in normal subjects without low

back pain. Eur J Orthop Surg Traumatol. 2014;24 Suppl 1:S193–9.

10. Prather H, Cheng A, Steger-May K, Maheshwari V, Van Dillen L. Hip and lumbar spine physical examination findings in people presenting with low back pain, with or without lower extremity pain. J Orthop Sports Phys Ther. 2017;47(3):163–72.

11. Harris-Hayes M, Sahrmann SA, Van Dillen LR. Relationship between the hip and low back pain in athletes who participate in rotation-related sports. J Sport Rehabil. 2009;18(1):60–75.

12. Burnett A, O'Sullivan P, Ankarberg L, Gooding M, Nelis R, Offermann F, Persson J. Lower lumbar spine axial rotation is reduced in end-range sagittal postures when compared to a neutral spine posture. Man Ther. 2008;3(4): 300–6.

13. Added M, de Freitas DG, Kasawara KT, Martin RL, Fukuda TY. Strengthening the gluteus maximus in subjects with sacroiliac dysfunction. Int J Sports Phys Ther. 2018;13(1):114–20.

14. Cibulka MT, Sinacore DR, Cromer GS, Delitto A. Unilateral hip rotation range of motion asymmetry in patients with sacroiliac joint regional pain. Spine (Phila Pa 1976). 1998;23(9): 1009–15.

15. Bussey MD, Bell ML, Milosavljevic S. The influence of hip abduction and external rotation on sacroiliac motion. Man Ther. 2009;14(5):520–5.

Chapter 8

1. Abt JP, Smoliga JM, Brick MJ, Jolly JT, Lephart SM, Fu FH. Relationship between cycling mechanics and core stability. J Strength Cond Res. 2007;21(4):1300–4.

2. Sheeran L, Sparkes V, Caterson B, Busse-Morris M, van Deursen R. Spinal position sense and trunk muscle activity during sitting and standing in nonspecific chronic low back pain: classification analysis. Spine. 2012;37(8):E486–95.

3. Tong MH, Mousavi SJ, Kiers H, Ferreira P, Refshauge K, van Dieën J. Is there a relationship between lumbar proprioception and low back pain? A systematic review with meta-analysis. Arch Phys Med Rehabil. 2017;98(1): 120–36.

4. Kane K, Barden J. Frequency of anticipatory trunk muscle onsets in children with and without developmental coordination disorder. Phys Occup Ther Pediatr. 2014;34(1):75–89.

5. Johnston LM, Burns YR, Brauer SG, Richardson CA. Differences in postural control and movement performance during goal directed reaching in children with developmental coordination disorder. Hum Mov Sci. 2002;21(5-6): 583–601.

6. Zazulak BT, Hewett TE, Reeves NP, Goldberg B, Cholewicki J. Deficits in neuromuscular control of the trunk predict knee injury risk: a prospective biomechanical-epidemiologic study. Am J Sports Med. 2007;35(7):1123–30.

7. Zazulak BT, Hewett TE, Reeves NP, Goldberg B, Cholewicki J. The effects of core proprioception on knee injury: a prospective biomechanical-epidemiological study. Am J Sports Med. 2007;35(3):368–73.

Chapter 9

1. Lieberman D, Raichlen D, Pontzer H, Bramble D, Cutright-Smith E. The human gluteus maximus and its role in running. Journal of Experimental Biology. 2006;209:2143–155.

2. Dix. J, Marsh S, Dingenen B, Malliaras P. The relationship between hip muscle strength and dynamic knee valgus in asymptomatic females: a systematic review. Phys Ther Sport. 2018;37: 197–209. doi: 10.1016.

3. Al-Hayani A. The functional anatomy of hip abductors. Folia Morphol. 2009;68(2): 98–103.

4. Nelson-Wong E, Gregory DE, Winter DA, Callaghan JP. Gluteus medius muscle activation patterns as a predictor of low back pain during standing. Clin Biomech (Bristol, Avon). 2008;23(5):545–53.

5. Winter DA. Gait & posture. Human balance and posture control during standing and walking. 1995;3:193 214.

6. Winter DA, Prince F, Frank JS, Powell C, Zabjek KF. Unified theory regarding A/P and M/L balance in quiet stance. J Neurophysiol. 1996;75(6):2334–43.

7. Nelson-Wong E, Callaghan JP. Is muscle co-activation a predisposing factor for low back pain development during standing? A multifactorial approach for early identification of at-risk individuals. J Electromyogr Kinesiol. 2010;20(2): 256–63.

8. Prior S, Mitchell T, Whiteley R, O'Sullivan P, Williams BK, Racinais S, Farooq A. The influence of changes in trunk and pelvic posture during single leg standing on hip and thigh muscle activation in a pain free population. BMC Sports Sci Med Rehabil. 2014;6(1):13.

9. Franklyn-Miller A, Richter C, King E, Gore S, Moran K, Strike S, Falvey EC. Athletic groin pain (part 2): a prospective cohort study on the biomechanical evaluation of change of direction identifies three clusters of movement patterns. Br J Sports Med. 2017;51(5): 460–8.

10. Kim TW, Kim YW. Effects of abdominal drawing-in during prone

hip extension on the muscle activities of the hamstring, gluteus maximus, and lumbar erector spinae in subjects with lumbar hyperlordosis. J Phys Ther Sci. 2015;27(2):383–6.

11. Walters J, Solomons M, Davies J. Gluteus minimus: observations on its insertion. Journal of Anatomy. 2001;198: 239–42.

Chapter 10

1. Elphinston J. Stability, sport and performance movement: practical biomechanics and systematic training for movement efficacy and injury prevention. Chichester: Lotus; 2013.

2. Seroyer S, Nho S, Bach B, Bush-Joseph C, Nicholson G, and Romeo A. The kinetic chain in overhand pitching: its potential role for performance enhancement and injury prevention. Sports Health. 2010;2(2):135–46.

3. Chu SK, Jayabalan P, Kibler WB, Press J. The kinetic chain revisited: new concepts on throwing mechanics and injury. PM R. 2016;8(3 Suppl):S69–77.

4. Martin C, Bideau B, Bideau N, Nicolas G, Delamarche P, Kulpa R. Energy flow analysis during the tennis serve: comparison between injured and noninjured tennis players. Am J Sports Med. 2014;42(11):2751–60.

5. McGinty G, Irrgang J, Pezzullo D. Biomechanical considerations for rehabilitation of the knee. Clinical Biomech (Bristol, Avon). 2000;15:160–6.

Chapter 11

1. Bullock-Saxton JE, Janda V, Bullock MI. Reflex activation of gluteal muscles in walking. An approach to restoration of

muscle function for patients with low-back pain. Spine. 1993;18(6):704–8.

2. Bullock-Saxton JE, Janda V, Bullock MI. The influence of ankle sprain injury on muscle activation during hip extension. Int J Sports Med. 1994;15(6):330–4.

3. Kelly LA, Kuitunen S, Racinais S, Cresswell AG. Recruitment of the plantar intrinsic foot muscles with increasing postural demand. Clin Biomech. 2012;27(1):46–51.

4. Prior S, Mitchell T, Whiteley R, O'Sullivan P, Williams BK, Racinais S, Farooq A. The influence of changes in trunk and pelvic posture during single leg standing on hip and thigh muscle activation in a pain free population. BMC Sports Sci Med Rehabil. 2014;6(1):13.

5. Grimaldi A, Mellor R, Hodges P, Bennell K, Wajswelner H, Vicenzino B. Gluteal tendinopathy: a review of mechanisms, assessment and management. Sports Med. 2015;45(8):1107–19.

Chapter 12

1. Lewis CL, Sahrmann SA. Effect of posture on hip angles and moments during gait. Man Ther. 2015;20(1):176–82.

2. Simonsen EB. Contributions to the understanding of gait control. Dan Med J. 2014;61(4):B4823.

3. Sahrmann S. Diagnosis and treatment of movement impairment syndromes. St Louis: Mosby; 2002, p. 144.

4. Lewis CL, Sahrmann S, Moran DW. Effect of hip angle on anterior hip joint force during gait. Gait Posture. 2010;32(4):603–7.

5. Lewis CL, Khuu A, Marinko LN. Postural correction reduces hip pain in adult with acetabular dysplasia: a case report. Man Ther. 2015;20(3):508–12.

6. Myers T. Anatomy trains: myofascial meridians for manual and movement therapists. Edinburgh: Churchill Livingstone; 2001.

7. Ha Yong Kim, Kap Jung Kim, Dae Suk Yang, Sang Wook Jeung, Han Gyeol Choi, Won Sik Choy. Screw-home movement of the tibiofemoral joint during normal gait: three-dimensional analysis. Clin Orthop Surg. 2015;7(3):303–9.

8. Kelly LA, Cresswell AG, Farris DJ. The energetic behaviour of the human foot across a range of running speeds. Sci Rep. 2018;12;8(1):10576.

9. Wager JC., Challis JH. Elastic energy within the human plantar aponeurosis contributes to arch shortening during the push-off phase of running. Journal of Biomechanics. 2016;49(5):704–9.

10. Lugade V, Kaufman K. Center of pressure trajectory during gait: a comparison of four foot positions. Gait Posture. 2014;40(1):252–4.

Chapter 13

1. Martina WL, Murraya PS, Batesa PR, Leea PSY. Fear-potentiated startle: a review from an aviation perspective. The International Journal of Aviation Psychology. 2015;25(2):97–107.

2. Lampert R, Tuit K, Hong K, Donovan T, Lee F, Sinha R. Cumulative stress and autonomic dysregulation in a community sample. Stress. 2016;19(3):269–79.

3. Payne P, Levine P, Crane-Godreau MA. Somatic experiencing: using interoception and proprioception as core elements of trauma therapy. Front. Psychol. 4 February 2015 | https://doi.org/10.3389/fpsyg.2015.00093.

4. Levine P, Frederick A. Waking the tiger: healing trauma. Berkeley, CA: North Atlantic Books; 1997.

5. Van der Kolk. The body keeps the score. London: Penguin; 2014, p. 54.

6. Roelofs K, Hagenaars MA, Stins J. Facing freeze: social threat induces bodily freeze in humans. Psychol Sci. 2010;21(11):1575–81.

7. Howorka K, Pumprla J, Tamm J, Schabmann A, Klomfar S, Kostineak E, Howorka N, Sovova E. Effects of guided breathing on blood pressure and heart rate variability in hypertensive diabetic patients. Auton Neurosci. 2013;179(1–2): 131–7.

8. Zaccaro A, Piarulli A, Laurino M, Garbella E, Menicucci D, Neri B, Gemignani A. How breath-control can change your life: a systematic review on psycho-physiological correlates of slow breathing. Front Hum Neurosci. 2018;12:353.

9. Jerath R, Crawford MW, Barnes VA, Harden K. Self-regulation of breathing as a primary treatment for anxiety. Appl Psychophysiol Biofeedback. 2015;40(2):107–15.

10. Xiao Ma, Zi-Qi Yue, Zhu-Qing Gong, Hong Zhang, Nai-Yue Duan,Yu-Tong Shi, Gao-Xia Wei, You-Fa L. The effect of diaphragmatic breathing on attention, negative affect and stress in healthy adults. Front Psychol. 2017;8: 874.

Chapter 14

1. Chalmers PN, Cip J, Trombley R, Cole BJ, Wimmer MA, Romeo AA, Verma NN. Glenohumeral function of the long head of the biceps muscle: an electromyographic analysis. Orthop J Sports Med. 2014 Feb 26;2(2):2325967114523902. doi: 10.1177/2325967114523902.

Chapter 15

1. Proske U, Gandevia S. The proprioceptive senses: their roles in signaling body shape, body position and movement, and muscle force. Physiological Reviews. 2012;92(4):1651–97.

2. Ferrè ER, Bottini G, Iannetti GD, Haggard P. The balance of feelings: vestibular modulation of bodily sensations. Cortex. 2013;49(3):748–58.

3. Ferrè ER, Haggard P. Vestibular-somatosensory interactions: a mechanism in search of a function? Multisens Res. 2015;28(5-6):559–79.

4. Craig AD (Bud). How do you feel? An interoceptive moment with your neurobiological self. New Jersey: Princeton University Press; 2015, p. 182.

5. Christensen JF, Gaigg SB, Calvo-Merino B. I can feel my heartbeat: dancers have increased interoceptive accuracy. Psychophysiology. 2018;55(4):e13008.

6. Stern ER, Grimaldi SJ, Muratore A, Murrough J, Leibu E, Fleysher L2, Goodman WK, Burdick KE1. Neural correlates of interoception: effects of interoceptive focus and relationship to dimensional measures of body awareness. Hum Brain Mapp. 2017;38(12):6068–82.

7. Seth AK. Interoceptive inference, emotion, and the embodied self. Trends Cogn Sci. 2013;17(11):565–73.

8. Krautwurst S, Gerlach AL, Gomille LHiller W, Witthöft M. Health anxiety—an indicator of higher interoceptive sensitivity? J Behav Ther Exp Psychiatry. 2014;45(2):303–9.

9. Craig AD. How do you feel—now? The anterior insula and human awareness. Nat Rev Neurosci. 2009;10(1):59–70.

10. Van der Kolk. The body keeps the score. London: Penguin; 2014, pp. 90–3.

11. Connolly CG, Wu J, Ho TC, Hoeft F, Wolkowitz O, Eisendrath S, Frank G, Hendren R, Max JE, Paulus MP, Tapert SF, Banerjee D, Simmons AN, Yang TT. Resting-state functional connectivity of subgenual anterior cingulate cortex in depressed adolescents. Biol Psychiatry. 2013;74(12):898–907.

12. Paulus MP, Stein MB. Interoception in anxiety and depression. Brain Struct Funct. 2010;214(5–6):451–63.

13. Avery JA, Drevets WC, Moseman SE, Bodurka J, Barcalow JC, Simmons WK. Major depressive disorder is associated with abnormal interoceptive activity and functional connectivity in the insula. Biol Psychiatry. 2014;76(3):258–66.

14. Baldan AM, Alouche SR, Araujo IM, Freitas SM. Effect of light touch on postural sway in individuals with balance problems: a systematic review. Gait Posture. 2014;40(1):1–10.

15. Oshita K, Yano S. Effect and immediate after-effect of lightly gripping the cane on postural sway. J Physiol Anthropol. 2016;35(1):14.

16. Ainley V, Maister L, Brokfeld J, Farmer H, Tsakiris M. More of myself: manipulating interoceptive awareness by heightened attention to bodily and narrative aspects of the self. Conscious Cogn. 2013;22(4):1231–8.

17. Sah, P. Fear, anxiety and the amygdala. Neuron. 2017;96(1):1–2.

18. Van der Kolk. The body keeps the score. London: Penguin; 2014, pp. 62–4.

19. Siddiqui SV, Chatterjee U, Kumar D, Siddiqui A, Goyal N. Neuropsychology of prefrontal cortex. Indian J Psychiatry. 2008;50(3):202–8.

20. Krashen, SD. Principles and practice in second language acquisition. Pergamon Press Inc. 1982. [Accessed August 20, 2019] Available: http://www.sdkrashen. com/content/books/principles_and_ practice.pdf.

INDEX